Applied Artificial Intelligence

This book explores the advancements and future challenges in biomedical application developments using breakthrough technologies like Artificial Intelligence (AI), Internet of Things (IoT), and Signal Processing. It will also contribute to biosensors and secure systems, and related research. *Applied Artificial Intelligence: A Biomedical Perspective* begins by detailing recent trends and challenges of applied artificial intelligence in biomedical systems.

Part I of the book presents the technological background of the book in terms of applied artificial intelligence in the biomedical domain. Part II demonstrates the recent advancements in automated medical image analysis that have opened ample research opportunities in the applications of deep learning to different diseases. Part III focuses on the use of cyberphysical systems that facilitates computing anywhere by using medical IoT and biosensors and the numerous applications of this technology in the healthcare domain. Part IV describes the different signal processing applications in the healthcare domain. It also includes the prediction of some human diseases based on the inputs in signal format. Part V highlights the scope and applications of biosensors and security aspects of biomedical images.

The book will be beneficial to the researchers, industry persons, faculty, and students working in biomedical applications of computer science and electronics engineering. It will also be a useful resource for teaching courses like AI/ML, medical IoT, signal processing, biomedical engineering, and medical image analysis.

Biomedical and Robotics Healthcare

Series Editors:
Utku Kose, Jude Hemanth, Omer Deperlioglu

Applied Artificial Intelligence
A Biomedical Perspective

Edited by
Dr. Swati V. Shinde, Dr. Varsha S. Bendre, Dr. Jude Hemanth, and Dr. M. A. Balafar

CRC Press
Taylor & Francis Group
Boca Raton London New York

CRC Press is an imprint of the
Taylor & Francis Group, an **informa** business

Cover image: © Shutterstock

First edition published 2024
by CRC Press
2385 NW Executive Center Drive, Suite 320, Boca Raton FL 33431

and by CRC Press
4 Park Square, Milton Park, Abingdon, Oxon, OX14 4RN

CRC Press is an imprint of Taylor & Francis Group, LLC

ISBN: 978-1-032-34914-5 (hbk)
ISBN: 978-1-032-34915-2 (pbk)
ISBN: 978-1-003-32443-0 (ebk)

DOI: 10.1201/9781003324430

Typeset in Times
by KnowledgeWorks Global Ltd.

Contents

PART I Applied Artificial Intelligence for Biomedical Applications

PART II Medical Image Processing Using Deep Learning Algorithms

PART III   Medical IOT and Recent Trends

PART IV Biomedical Signal Processing

PART V Recent Trends in Biomedical Applications

List of Figures and Tables

Part I

*Applied Artificial Intelligence
for Biomedical Applications*

1 Healthcare Fees-Centric to Value-Centric Transformation through Data, Analytics, and Artificial Intelligence

Sanjeev Manchanda and Mahesh Kshirsagar
Tata Consultancy Services, Mumbai, Maharashtra, India

CONTENTS

1.1 INTRODUCTION

The United Nations (**UN**) Sustainability Development Goals (**SDG**) agenda **#3** is "**Good Health and Well-Being**." The UN has set the target year 2030 to achieve these goals.

One of the key dimensions of "Good Health and Well-Being" is linked to healthcare, and in the context of healthcare it essentially translates into following: everyone on the planet, irrespective of the individual being rich or poor, living in an urban or

DOI: 10.1201/9781003324430-2

rural area, literate or illiterate, male or female, child or aged individual or youth or adult individual, resident of a developed nation or a developing nation, should get affordable and quality healthcare services.

To make affordable and quality healthcare services available to everyone, it is important to understand the overall healthcare ecosystem, and the kind of transformation it needs to achieve this goal.

Today we are living in the world dominated by technology, and with this technology a humongous amount of data are getting generated every day. These data definitely have the capability to contribute to driving the required transformation in healthcare services.

1.2 HEALTHCARE ECOSYSTEM

1.2.1 KEY TREND

The **healthcare ecosystem** predominantly consists of:

Patients
Providers (which include hospitals, doctors, therapists, laboratories, etc.)
Payers (health insurers)
Suppliers (which include pharmaceutical and medtech companies, pharmacies, etc.) **government, regulators, and policy makers**

Among the many emerging trends in healthcare, one of the key trends is its moving from a **fees-centric** model to a **patient-centric model**. In the patient-centric model, patients expect a **retail-like personalized experience**.

To be patient-centric, **holistic patient care management** becomes very critical, and to be patient-centric, the **healthcare ecosystem** necessarily must become **data-centric**.

1.2.2 DATA CENTRICITY

While the core healthcare-related data (such as *patient information, patient history, patient services, patient encounter, provider operations, caregiver acts, facility operations, medical material and devices, health insurance plan, billing, and order management*) are continuously generated in the ecosystem, a huge amount of data related to healthcare, known as *complementary data* (such as *data from the Internet and social media*) is also getting generated. These data come in all forms and shapes, and cut across structured, semistructured, and unstructured data.

Analysis of these data and deriving intelligent and actionable insights from that data are about using the power of the data to drive the vision of value-based healthcare through descriptive, causal, predictive, and prescriptive analytics.

Leveraging the power of the data by having data core to all the operations in the healthcare ecosystem, and continuously enhancing the usage of the data, is about treading on the path of **data centricity**.

1.2.2.1 Impact on the Healthcare Ecosystem

Data centricity, which has analytics and artificial intelligence (AI) solutions as its core pillars, will lead the following game-changing elements in the healthcare ecosystem:

Patient centricity
Revolutionized providers
Payers' agility and adaptiveness
Higher distributors' efficacy
Ecosystem cognizant
Compliant by design

Representative examples of how data centricity, analytics, and artificial intelligence would bring about this change are covered in this chapter.

1.2.2.2 Expected Outcome

Treading on the path of data centricity will lead to following **4-A(s)**:

Affordability in medical treatment (MT)
Accuracy in MT
Accelerated outcome in MT
Augmenting the **healthcare professionals** for **higher-efficacy** MT through **artificial intelligence**

These expected outcomes are definitely aligned with **UN SDG #3**, "**Good Health and Well-Being**."

1.3 HEALTHCARE INDUSTRY TRANSFORMATION

The healthcare industry, which is witnessing value-based care, is enabling the rise of health and wellness, which is characterized by being:

I. Personalized and value-based
II. Integrated and frictionless
III. Affordable and equitable
IV. Trustworthy and secure

The transformation is already on for all the entities in the healthcare ecosystem, and with data centricity it will become further enhanced and accelerated.

1.3.1 DATA MODERNIZATION

The most fundamental prerequisite to tread on the path of data centricity is **data modernization**. Like any other industry, the healthcare industry has a typical information technology (IT) solutions landscape comprising of online transaction processing (OLTP) systems (such as enterprise resource planning [ERP] and supply chain management [SCM], whether commercial or homegrown), supportive business applications (such as human capital management [HCM] and governance, risk management, and compliance [GRC]), data warehouse, business intelligence applications, enterprise content management (ECM), and collaboration suites. While this constitutes enterprise data, supporting and complementary data are often sourced from healthcare ecosystem partners, and the healthcare industry then also sources additional data (huge but with lot of noise) from the worldwide web (the Internet and social media). The majority (85+%) of these data are unstructured, while the remaining data are structured.

Data fluidity is a well-known term in the healthcare industry that describes the ability to consume data at any point of exposure within an organization in the form desired. This necessitates all kinds of data:

Core data linked to healthcare operations (such as patient history)
Complementary data to healthcare operations (such as patient behavior from wearables/medical Internet of Things [M-IoT])
Orthogonal data (such as weather conditions at the patient's residence)

Such data related to the healthcare ecosystem emitting from various sources should be collected, sanitized, integrated, contextualized, and enriched to get into the consumable form to enable a single version of the truth.

Data fluidity also requires catering to following critical aspects:

I. Managing **semantics** (focused on **unstructured data**) in addition to **metadata** (focused on **structured data**)
II. Managing integration-based **ontology** (focused on **unstructured data**) in addition to **master data** and **reference data** (focused on **structured data**)
III. **Data quality** focused to be **adaptive** when managing **unstructured data**
IV. Ability to manage **streaming real-time data** in addition to offline, near-real-time data
   a. Here it is also required to process on the edge (such as wearables) for timely decision making
V. Representation of the data in form of a **knowledge graph** for better understanding
   a. Here also the ability to **query** that data using **natural language** is required
VI. Focus on **DecisionOps,** which is a combination of **EnggOps, DataOps, and AIOps**

And last but not the least, all the data should be **migrated** and available on the **cloud,** where it remains available all the time **without compromising data privacy and data sovereignty**.

While migration of data to the cloud creates a good foundation for data fluidity, the real power of data can only be realized when these data can get **contextually exchanged** between the key entities (such as payers, providers, and distributors) of the healthcare ecosystem. To enable this data exchange, a **data marketplace** solution that connects providers and consumers of data is needed.

However, it is just not about data exchange, it is also about **data interoperability**, and thus **data interoperability standards** (such as Fast Healthcare Interoperability Resource [**FIHR**]) are required to provide a default data marketplace type of solution.

The data centricity enabled by data fluidity plays the major role in enabling the transformation in the healthcare industry amounting to patient centricity, revolutionized providers, payers' agility and adaptiveness, higher efficacy for distributors, ecosystem cognizance, and compliance by design.

1.3.2 PATIENT CENTRICITY

The healthcare industry is witnessing transformation where individuals are expecting personalized retail-like experience. While that is true, the true patient centricity will be achieved when an individual, irrespective of being rich or poor, living in urban or rural area, literate or illiterate, male or female, child or aged, youth or adult, resident of developed nation or developing nation, will get timely, accurate, affordable, and quality healthcare services.

The healthcare solution powered by data, analytics, and AI has the capability to bring this radical transformation as it helps in creation of patient persona.

I. **Preventive healthcare**

The very first aspect here is preventive healthcare, that is, to avoid any medical treatment in first place. The preventive healthcare enabled by data can be managed in an aggregated manner.

Patients should get data-driven insights about their health and also their surroundings so that they can take better care of themselves, which would include recommendations about diet, physical activities, and mental stress management. These data will be about patients' demographics and medical history and include orthogonal data such as weather conditions. The surroundings include the patient's family, residence area, locality, and village or city.

The next level of aggregation is for the family of the patient, by providing data-driven insights into taking better care of the family.

As the aggregation moves up, data-driven insights would lead to the entire society being advised to take better care of their health.

II. **Healthcare insurance**

One size does not fit all. How precise an insurance benefit policy can be worked out for an individual is the key here. The more precise it is, in terms of being personalized, the better it would be both in terms of its price and its tenure. Typically, the coverage for chronic and serious illness is high and thus availed by limited people, but with data centricity, that too can get managed at lower price points, and thus coverage can become more inclusive.

III. **Healthcare advice**

A unified healthcare data ecosystem would lead to the foundation of personalized advice, where it would be omnichannel (email, phone calls, video chats, social media, website, and in-person meeting) and multimodal (written, voice, gestures) interactions, where a patient would have a consistent experience by getting contextually connected with the right healthcare professionals based on the patient's current state, which would include at minimum their demographic details, current health status, and location.

A primary care physician would be better empowered to advise patients on what treatment would fit best for them and how they should pursue it.

IV. **Treatment**

Data centricity can bring in complete game-changing experience, as complete diagnosis and therapy would be driven by the data, historic as well as current. It would effectively distinguish among healthy, acute, chronic, and terminal states.

Here technology advancement would even capture the data linked to emotions of the patient, if the patient is not able to express them in oral or written form.

This would be applicable for both the outpatient department (OPD) cases as well as hospitalization cases, where the patient would have to undergo only required minimal, but accurate, tests and treatments.

V. **Services**

a. **Pharmacy**

With a connected data ecosystem and AI-based algorithms, the pharmacy can both recommend best possible and cost-effective medicines to the patients and ensure that they serve the patients in a timely fashion.

b. **Ambulance**

The connected data ecosystem can provide in-time availability ambulance service at competitive price points.

c. **Caregivers**

Matching the demand-supply equation, taking into account needs and preferences of an individual and also skills and preferences of the caregiver, would be much more effective with data.

VI. **Hospitalization on-boarding**

With data centricity and a connected healthcare ecosystem, the patient should experience very smooth customer on-boarding. If patient has been advised to get admitted in a particular hospital, then by the time patient arrives at that hospital, they should be directly taken to the ward/bed allocated to them, with required healthcare professionals being there to take care of the patients. The patient should not experience any waiting time and procedural delays that are counterproductive to patient treatment.

VII. **Hospitalization discharge**

This should be as smooth as on-boarding; that is, once the patient is ready for discharge, they should just walk out the hospital, as with data centricity, advanced analytics, and AI algorithms, the entire claims processing would observe straight though processing (STP). As the patient will be undergoing only required minimal tests and treatments, the medical expenses would also be minimal.

VIII. **Posthospitalization care**

This would be on similar lines as preventive care, with the only difference being that patients would have to follow discharge guidelines until they fully recover.

With more and more nonhealthcare providers such as retail, e-commerce, and banks who too are offering healthcare services, the aforementioned focus on patient centricity is becoming more and more critical.

1.3.3 REVOLUTIONIZED PROVIDERS

The providers' benefits would be wide-ranging and lead to a revolutionized stage.

I. **Patient engagement**

From patient registration, eligibility verification, benefit validation, and patient liability estimation to appointment scheduling, data-driven solutions will result in a personalized and frictionless experience for the patient.

II. **Medical treatment** and **collaborative intelligence**

The providers' space is dominated by healthcare professionals (HCP), and typically there is a wide gap between the demand for quality HCP and their availability. The data centricity, analytics, and especially AI are leading to the era of collaborative intelligence, wherein HCP are assisting the machines, and the machines are assisting HCP.

Using the healthcare data, the HCP professional trains the machines to do the job similar to what they do, and then when the machine gets trained, it helps the HCP to do the job they are trained for at a much higher scale, speed, and accuracy, which helps in minimizing the demand–supply gap for HCP.

III. **Early detection**

Early detection of any disease has its own advantages, and typically more when those diseases are the likes of sepsis and coronary artery disease (CAD) due to which millions of people are losing their lives every year.

With machine learning (ML) models, by analyzing clinical data, laboratory values, demographics, and sporadic data associated with patient treatment, sepsis can be detected with high degree of accuracy.

Similarly, with data analysis based on multimodal differential diagnosis of biomedical signals, patient demography, and disease history, CAD too can be detected when it is asymptomatic in early stages.

IV. **Diagnosis**

Data analytics using the computer vision domain of AI finds maximum leverage in diagnosing medical images, which includes (a) analysis of X-rays, computed tomography (CT) scans, magnetic resonance imaging (MRI) for landmark detection, information extraction, diagnostic aids, and reconstruction; (b) analysis of pathological images for histopathological findings, whole slide imaging, and high throughput cellular imaging; (c) Fundus image-based detection of glaucoma and damaged retina; (d) video analysis for annotation, dehazing, and gait/posture estimation and tumor detection; (e) 2-D/3-D image-based estimation of gait, range of motion (ROM), pose, and meta-learning for skin lesions; and (f) ultra-wideband (UWB) radar for human parameter estimation and in-body imaging and vital monitoring.

AI CONCEPTS: TRANSFER LEARNING AND META-LEARNING

Transfer leaning applies knowledge gained while solving one problem to solving different but related problem. For example, an AI model trained for detecting benign tumors can be leveraged to detect malignant tumors.

Meta-learning is about learning to learn. This feature can be leveraged, for example, to train a model to detect skin diseases having abundant data, then testing it against unseen or rare skin diseases for which there are very few examples.

V. Precautionary

In medical treatment, CT scans are quite common. Since they harm children and pregnant women, during their CT scan radiation dose is reduced, which leads to lower quality of the image. This is where AI-based image enhancement techniques come handy, which enhance these images to create the image quality to match the level to those CT scan images that were taken without any radiation dose reduction.

VI. Preventive measures

Wearables are very common these days. The data collected from these wearables can be analyzed in a cost-effective and rapid manner for enabling any preventive action. For example, photoplethysmogram (PPG) data collected from wearables worn by HCPs who are serving COVID-19 patients can be analyzed to see if they are infected by COVID-19.

VII. Digital twin of a human organ

Data collected from wearables, M-IoT devices, and other healthcare-related data can be leveraged to create a digital twin of a human organ. And when it is such a digital twin, doctors can do in silico simulation of a specific person to see how they would react to a heart-related treatment. This not only minimizes risk but also leads higher efficacy of treatment, as the digital twin can be personalized. For example, a digital twin of the heart can be created using data collected by from various cardiac-sensing devices, enabling the concepts of e-patient and e-medication.

VIII. Mass personalization

One of the major impact of data centricity, analytics, and AI is mass personalization, and it makes a greater impact when treating critical diseases such as cancer. The AI techniques are leveraged to model correlation between patient-specific omics data to clinical outcome. This is based on genome interpretation, functional analysis, and biological network analysis.

IX. Facility management

In the provider facility, especially the hospital facility, management is central to the healthcare services, as optimal and smooth functioning of these facilities is important to ensure ongoing quality service.

X. Hygiene management

Importance of hygiene is well understood by everyone. For hospitals, the highest level of cleanliness is of paramount importance. Using computer vision techniques, cleanliness in the hospital, be it in the hospital wards, hospital toilets, or hospital waste, can be managed.

Food in the hospital is another important aspect, as the type of food, and whether it is properly cooked, overcooked, or undercooked, is very important in the patient treatment. Again, using computer vision techniques, even food quality can be inspected.

XI. **Command center in a pocket**

In the smooth functioning of a hospital, doctors, nurses, facility managers, and operations managers have their specific role to play. Command center in a pocket is a solution based on augmented reality (AR), which assists these players with all the required information basis for the role they are playing, their task in hand, the time of day, and their current location. All that they have to do is point their mobile camera to the associated QR code and they get the contextual insights. Doctors will get details of patient illness, treatment, and diagnosis. Nurses get all the action items they need to work on. Operations managers see details of each and every operational aspect of hospital. Facility managers see the details of the status of the hospital's infrastructure aspects (such as electricity, water, and air conditioners).

XII. **Supply chain management**

Both inventory warehouse and just-in-time inventory are key considerations here.

The AI/ML algorithms enable arriving at optimized inventory levels (inventory cost, wastage of perishable goods, stock-out challenges) through accurate forecasting so that hospitals can get the best possible service from their network.

For just-in-time inventory, the AI/ML algorithms can help determine the most reliable service providers in their network.

1.3.4 Payers' Agility and Adaptiveness

Data centricity will enable payers to increase the scale of innovation to deliver anytime, anywhere care with the ability to offer higher quality at lower costs. This would cover a broad spectrum, from **personalized benefits and products** to **just-in-time contracts** (just-in-time-contracts provide the right care at the right time at the right cost by having insurance contracts between payers and providers for a specific case for an ascertained duration).

Data centricity, analytics, and AI would bring radical transformation to the payers' operations.

I. **Member experience management**

Identifying member pain points and providing recommendations to improve the patient's satisfaction and experience.

II. **Member engagement**

BOT (robot or internet bot) for contextual interaction and assisting the member (patient).

III. **Risk assessment**

Linking basis data to the patient's personal, social, and clinical profile and the patient's preferred provider profile. This can indicate knowledge of the medical condition under coverage as well as knowledge of treatment outcomes from the specific provider for the specific medical condition.

IV. **Benefit booklet validation and autocreation**

Automating the validation of the benefit booklet against the master plan and the CAPS database.

The next level would be automation of benefit booklet generation from the master plan and CAPS database.

V. **Medical coding**

Automating coding of healthcare diagnoses, procedures, medical services, and equipment into universal alphanumeric codes. Free-form text extracted from medical records (outpatient, lab records, radiology, same-day surgery, emergency care, inpatient) is automatically converted into ICD-10 codes.

VI. **Intelligent claims solutions**

Enhancing efficacy across claims cycle: preadjudication, adjudication, and postadjudication.

a. Claims pattern detection

Focusing on the higher propensity of overpayments or chances of incorrect payments.

b. Fraud management

Building the score for each claimant; setting cutoffs; establishing reasons for fraud trigger; establishing the relationship among payer, provider, and claimant; and analyzing data related to diagnosis codes, Current Procedural Terminology (CPT)/Healthcare Common Procedural Coding System (HCPCS) codes, revenue codes, and adjustment codes.

c. Claim denial reasoning

Covering eligibility verification/preinsurance verification, missing information, errors in medical billing codes, inappropriate time for claim file, duplicate claim or service, or out-of-network provider.

VII. **Revenue cycle management**

Analyzing the data points associated with the issues linked to claim denial, wrong code, timely response, and resource management.

VIII. **Effectiveness of care management**

Tracking medication errors, adherence to medication therapies, and adverse drug interactions.

IX. **Population care management**

Improving health outcome of groups, at reduced cost, by identifying potential risks, preparing relevant wellness programs, and monitoring patients with conditions.

X. **Network management**

Optimizing the provider network, including coverage of services, to ensure an appropriate mix of providers and adequate access to care, and to monitor provider performance in real time.

1.3.5 Higher Distributors' Efficacy

Distributors are vital link between manufactures of medicines and medical devices, healthcare providers (hospitals, nursing homes, clinics, pharmacists), and ultimately the patients. The delivery efficacy of distributors is very critical in ensuring timely and quality healthcare services while making sure that the associated costs are kept as minimal as possible.

Data centricity is key to enabling the delivery efficacy, as advanced analytics algorithms lead to better supply chain management cutting across demand forecast, optimal inventory levels, and transportation routing. It eases management of many-to-many relationships with manufacturers and healthcare providers with distributors in between, and it also significantly reduces the uncertainties associated with the number of unknowns in all operations of the distributor ecosystem.

The three key solutions that can bring radical change here are AI-driven supply chain management, the digital twin of the supply chain, and the data marketplace.

I. **AI-driven supply chain management**

In addition to traditional branded and generic drugs, the pharmaceutical market includes specialty products that are typically more expensive and developed to treat complex health issues affecting smaller patient populations. Distributors' have to offer both full-line and specialty products, so providers must consolidate orders rather than requiring separate distributors.

While the focus is on distributors, the AI-driven supply chain solution must consider the **entire ecosystem** to be effective right from **raw material suppliers** to the **customers**.

The AI solution would help address **challenges** linked to **scale,** which include stochasticity, dynamicity, and complex effects, while managing the **conflicting objectives** linked to inventory cost, wastage of perishable medicines, vehicle cost, stockout, and packaging.

For **manufacturers**, an AI solution would enable coordinated order placements managing aspects linked to variations in lead time and facility capacity constraints.

Next are the **warehouses**, where the focus is on integrated optimization of fulfillment node selection and routing. Solutions would be driven by the anticipatory pull to position products in the correct distribution nodes, that is, who should get how much, given limited stock and anticipated local demand.

Pharmacies are next in the value chain, where the focus is on multiproduct inventory replenishment with global supply chain awareness coupled with vehicle routing with capacity and delivery time window constraints. Here the decisions should be made with awareness of stocks upstream and demands in other pharmacies.

One of the **key examples** here is managing the **oxygen supply chain in a pandemic**, where the nuances are different than with typical medicines. Here the manufacturers could be large-scale, medium-scale, or captive plants, but ultimately they must reach the hospitals in right quantity within the right time frame. Medium-scale and captive plants, which directly produce oxygen, will typically work with a local distributor, whereas large-scale manufacturers have cryogenic oxygen plants that can store liquid oxygen in storage tanks, and have cryogenic tankers that can transport liquid oxygen to distributors, where it is converted to gaseous form, that is, in ready-to-use form.

II. **Digital twin of the supply chain**

Last mile delivery challenges are well known, such as the cost of last mile delivery, delivery location and address location, routing efficiency and route optimization, management of last mile delivery density, unpredictability in transit, availability of the customer, and meeting the fulfillment timeline. However, having the digital twin for the last mile, which would enable data-driven, justification-based, learning-aided, in silico simulation of the last mile delivery, along with what-if and if-what analysis, would lead to a number of benefits, such as reducing fleet operating and management cost, facilitating route planning, streamlining communication and data reporting, and speeding up deliveries.

III. **Data marketplace**

Distributors have access to data from both upstream and downstream partners, that is, data from both manufacturers and providers. This would lead distributors to develop deeper understanding of the needs and can thus provide more meaningful insights to increase efficiency, lower costs, and benefit the overall healthcare system.

IV. **Elevating the role of distributors**

Having a data marketplace solution in place is the first step for distributors to elevate their role in the healthcare ecosystem. With insights into the data, the **distributors** can actually **elevate** themselves to providers of **managed care services,** wherein they can enable **remote monitoring** for **patients** and **elder care**. By leveraging advancements in M-IoT and wearables devices, they can better provide all services from monitoring (from physical activity to medication) to taking timely corrective actions (involving right-time involvement and services of caregivers, pharmacy, ambulances, hospitals, and HCPs therein).

1.3.6 ECOSYSTEM COGNIZANT

Human life is full of uncertainty. The healthcare ecosystem is strongly impacted, as it must manage these uncertainties to ensure that timely, qualitative, and affordable healthcare services are provided to all.

During the COVID-19 pandemic, uncertainties were of the highest order. Historical data were not available to analyze this unprecedented pandemic and take corrective action, and as the pandemic progressed the data then collected were inadequate. Preparing for fighting the pandemic was all the more difficult, not only because of the nonavailability of the vaccine, but the heavy load on the healthcare ecosystem.

However, with technology advancements, using the concept of the digital twin, these uncertainties coupled by partial (inadequate) data can be managed. In midst of the COVID-19 pandemic, Tata Consultancy Services (TCS) scientists created the digital twin of Pune City (in India in state of Maharashtra), wherein they modeled the Pune City basis demographic information (such as age, gender, and profession) of people residing in Pune City; information about places, movements, and contacts; information about virus characteristics (such as transmissibility); and interventions (such as masks, social distancing, lockdowns, relaxation, and testing). This was an in silico simulation of Pune City. Using this simulation, recommendations on lock-down/unlockdown were provided to the city administration, as well as prediction of load on hospitals and institutional quarantining. It used COVID-19-related deaths to measure correctness of the digital twin. The digital twin recommendations were appreciated by the city administration for their accuracy, and the key reason for its success was data-based, justification-backed epidemic control.

Overall, the digital twin concept is about simulation-based, data-driven, justi-fication-based, learning-aided decision making in face of uncertainty. The health-care industry can be a big beneficiary of the digital twin, as this concept can be applied for the entire healthcare ecosystem to enable higher efficacy in healthcare services.

The digital twin of a city for the COVID-19 pandemic can be extended to create a **digital twin for all entities in the healthcare ecosystem** to understand the pre-paredness of the healthcare industry to manage the expectations from the industry for any healthcare scenario under consideration.

 I. **Location:** This amounts to first creating a digital twin of a specific location to get the data points about the healthcare services requirements of that location.
 II. **Provider:** Next, the digital twin of the provider can be created to simulate how it can manage the workload coming its way.
III. **Distributor:** Along similar lines, the digital twin of the distributor will help estimating how efficiently they can manage the ask from them in a timely and cost-effective manner.
IV. **Payer:** The digital twin for the payer too can be created, wherein they too can analyze the efficacy of the operations and benefits plan they offer to see if they can emerge as the payer of choice.
 V. **Patient:** For the most critical element in the value chain, the patient, the digi-tal twin of the patient results in giving personalized treatment to that patient.
VI. **Regulators:** Last but not least, the regulators too can use the digital twin to validate if their policies are indeed helpful or causing impediment to the much-needed smooth operations of the healthcare ecosystem.

Thus, in the ecosystem where performance of an entity depends on performance of other entities, having a digital twin–based approach leads to better preparedness for the healthcare industry to manage the expectations of them providing timely, qualitative, and affordable healthcare services.

1.3.7 COMPLIANT BY DESIGN

The healthcare industry has been paying huge penalties due to noncompliance to regulatory norms mandated by government, regulators, and policy makers. As per the data available in Violation Tracker, the healthcare industry has paid USD ~19 billion in penalties between year 2000 and year 2023.

Violation Tracker: https://violationtracker.goodjobsfirst.org/prog.php?major_industry_sum=healthcare+services

The top five offense groups leading to noncompliance are related to (1) government contracting, (2) employment, (3) competition, (4) financial, and (5) consumer protection.

The top five primary offense types leading to noncompliance are related to (1) false claims acts, (2) wage and hour violation, (3) kickbacks and bribery, (4) investor protection, and (5) labor relations.

A number of these violations are linked to having timely and right information about the regulations and both the effectiveness and efficiency with which those regulations are translated into the policies and standard operating procedures (SOPs) of the healthcare organization, and subsequently the efficacy with which the operations data are reconciled with the defined policies and SOPs.

Today managing the regulatory compliance is still typically a manual activity. It is effort intensive and prone to errors and thus is one of the key causes of noncompliance, and often such noncompliance results in paying a huge penalty. But beyond the financial penalty, noncompliance negatively impacts the company's brand reputation and competitive advantage.

AI-based automation solutions based on a natural language processing (NLP) technique can bring the following radical impact in enhancing the efficacy of managing regulatory compliance.

I. **Managing hygiene checks**

This is about ensuring that regulatory requirements are correctly understood. It focuses on:

a. Regulatory documents (*source: regulatory authorities*).
   i. Analyzing and understanding the contents written in natural language
   ii. Identifying the obligations stated in the regulatory document
b. Policy documents (*developed by the healthcare organization*)
   i. Analyzing and understanding the contents written in natural language
   ii. Identifying the obligations stated in the regulatory document
c. Matching of the obligations in the regulatory document vis-à-vis the policy document
   i. Highlighting close matches/partial matches/no match

The end user can then take the required corrective action so that the policy document is in complete alignment with the regulatory document.

II. **Managing compliance checks**

This is about ensuring that the healthcare organization's operational data are compliant with regulatory compliance norms. It focuses on:

a. Creation of business rules from the obligations (written in natural language)
   i. These are machine-executable rules
b. Executing those business rules against the enterprise transaction data
   i. Highlighting where the business rules execution is a success or a failure

This way, the end user can understand where the gaps in the business process execution are and initiate corrective action to manage regulatory compliance norms.

The automation in managing the regulatory compliance norms, a human-in-the-loop AI solution, would radically the transform management of regulatory compliance norms.

1.4 CONCLUSION

The transformation of healthcare industry from a fees-centric model to a patient-centric model will happen in an accelerated manner, with the industry treading on the path of data centricity. With data centricity, analytics and AI driving the 4-A(s) (affordability in medical treatment (MT), accuracy in MT, accelerated outcomes in MT, and augmenting the healthcare professionals for higher efficacy MT through AI) of the aspirational of goal #3 of the UN SDG, "Good Health and Well-being," will become the reality, wherein everyone on the planet, irrespective of the individual being rich or poor, living in an urban or rural area, literate or illiterate, male or female, child or aged, youth or adult, resident of a developed nation or a developing nation, will receive affordable and quality healthcare services.

2 AI-Based Healthcare
Top Businesses and Technologies

Dipali Ghatge[1] and K. Rajeswari[2]
[1]Department of Computer Science and Engineering,
Karmaveer Bhaurao Patil College of Engineering,
Satara, Maharashtra, India
[2]Department of Computer Engineering, Pimpri Chinchwad
College of Engineering, Satara, Maharashtra, India

CONTENTS

2.1   INTRODUCTION

Technology is essential in some aspects of healthcare systems because it makes the process of care smooth and quick for patients and the organization. The healthcare field should adapt to new and updated technology to improve patient care. Technology is the driving force for bigger and better things. We will talk about the evolution of technology in healthcare and the various companies and their efforts toward changing the face of the healthcare industry. It is a process, but the healthcare field is still improving and advancing for its patients to have the quality care they need.

DOI: 10.1201/9781003324430-3

19

Modern technology is the driving force behind advancements in healthcare. In the 1920s, the first medical records were produced. The history of the health information management sector can be traced back to the 1920s when healthcare professionals first began to record specifics, complications, and results of patient care in medical records. North America's Association of Record Librarians (ARLNA) was founded by the American College of Surgeons in 1928 to standardize medical records. The ARLNA specified how information was recorded and how medical records were used.

Computers and other technical advances opened up new possibilities and made it simpler to standardize and share medical records. At the time, the system allowed third-party facilities to confirm the diagnosis and provide clinicians access to a patient's medical history. The system of healthcare information systems was developed in 1965, together with Medicare and Medicaid. Using computers to gather and operate medical records was strange during this era but grew slowly. In around 73 hospitals, electronic medical records were in use by 1965. The cost of healthcare information technology was high. One of the founders and early adopters of such technology in this period was the Mayo Clinic in Rochester, Minnesota. Numerous healthcare information management systems were developed in the late 1960s and early 1970s as a result of these technological advancements. These included the Lockheed Corporation's 1971 development of Eclipsys, a computerized physician ordering system for California's El Camino Hospital; a clinical decision support system called Health Evaluation through logical processing by the University of Utah, 3M, Harvard University, and Latter Day Saints Hospital; and the Computer Stored Ambulatory Record by Massachusetts General Hospital and the Regenstrief Institute in Indianapolis.

The introduction of the desktop personal computer guided healthcare information technology in the 1980s, and Dragon Systems created a voice recognition prototype in 1982 to the delight of all medical assistants. Personal computers and Windows-based software were widely used in doctor offices by the late 1980s. However, they were generally utilized more for scheduling and invoicing than electronic medical records. Computerized registration improved check-in times and efficiency at the hospital level. The department's continued segmentation of hospital computer systems without communication capabilities is the only downside of the hospital.

Gradually, technology support kept increasing, and now it has reached the level of atomization and robotic support in diagnosis and treatment under the technological umbrella called artificial intelligence.

2.2   THE DEVELOPMENT OF AI IN HEALTHCARE

Understanding how artificial intelligence functions is helpful before discussing how it has evolved in healthcare. In 1955, a conference proposal from Dartmouth College was the first to mention the term "artificial intelligence." AI essentially refers to computer models and programs that mimic human intelligence to perform cognitive tasks like complicated problem solving and acquiring knowledge and experiences.

Most current AI tools are classified as "Narrow AI," meaning the technology can outperform humans at a task with a specific scope. Many modern methods are powered by machine learning algorithms, allowing computers to learn, carry out tasks, and adapt without human intervention.

AI applications for solving biomedical issues originally appeared in the 1970s. AI-powered apps have developed and evolved to revolutionize the healthcare sector by lowering costs, enhancing patient outcomes, and increasing productivity. However, the use of AI in healthcare did not begin until the early 1970s, when research led to the creation of MYCIN. This AI software assisted in the identification of medicines for blood infections. AI research continued to grow, and in 1979 the American Association for Artificial Intelligence was established (currently the Association for the Advancement of Artificial Intelligence, AAAI). The mission of AAAI is to promote artificial intelligence research and social application. Additionally, AAAI seeks to enrich the education and training of AI practitioners, broaden the public's awareness of AI, and encourage research funders and planners on the importance and potential of recent AI advancements.

In the 1980s and 1990s, faster data gathering and processing, assistance with more precise surgical treatments, in-depth DBA study and mapping, and a more thorough application of electronic health records were all made possible thanks to the construction of new AI systems.

AI and machine learning advancements have significantly impacted how healthcare services are delivered. The application of this cutting-edge technology, which started in the biomedical sciences, has evolved to include primary care, radiology, disease diagnosis screening, psychiatry, and telemedicine. AI in healthcare is now extensively used. In healthcare, AI primarily refers to software created to search enormous data sets and provide crucial patient information. Artificial neural networks are used in today's intelligent systems to enable computers to process raw data without explicit programming. The neurons in the human brain are analogous to these artificial neural networks in how they function.

The next sections discuss the contribution of the top businesses in developing AI-based modern healthcare technologies, which include IBM (Watson Health); AiCure; Atomwise, Inc.; Lifegraph; APIXIO, Inc.; Cyrcadia Health Inc.; and Welltok. Between 2017 and 2023, spending on AI in healthcare is anticipated to increase at an annualized rate of 48% [1, 2].

2.3 IBM WATSON

IBM Watson is AI for healthcare. Organizations may forecast future results with Watson, automate complicated tasks, and use staff time better.

2.3.1 MERGE CARDIO

The cardiology department aims to find, treat, and prevent heart and blood vessel diseases. This department is challenging to manage and busy, so physicians and staff work diligently daily to enhance patient outcomes and uphold stringent quality

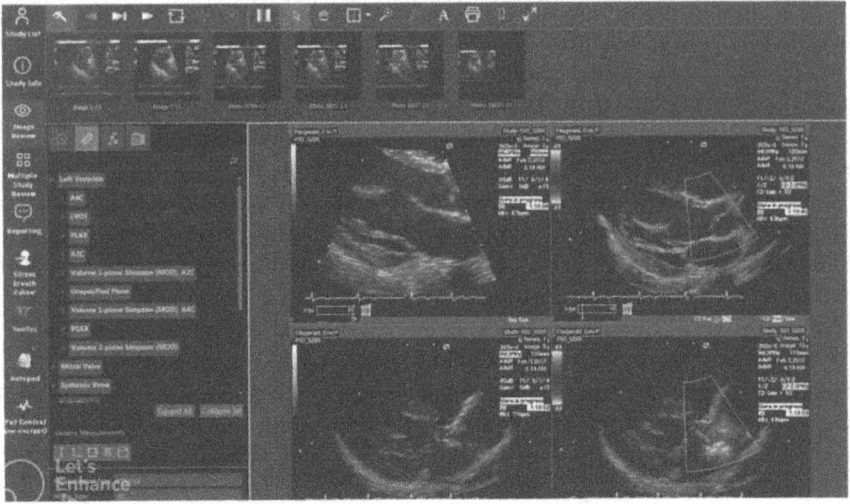

FIGURE 2.1   Merge Cardio.

standards despite tightening budgets. However, these challenges can put a massive burden on already constrained human and financial resources.

IBM devises, Merge Cardio, a cardiac imaging and information management that helps access, integrate, and manage patient records with a centralized, web-enabled system (see Figure 2.1). It allows medical professionals to access and manage patients' digitally integrated cardiovascular records from a centralized, web-enabled system, anywhere, any time. This award-winning cardiology solution improves patient management through a built-in report generation and distribution process.

The benefits of the system are as follows:

a. It is a centralized management system where patients' comprehensive cardiovascular records are accessed from a single point.

b. It leverages a robust imaging and diagnostic workstation that supports most imaging modalities.

c. Process for automated reporting data prepopulation from modality devices to the clinical report and Electronic Health Record (EHR) is a part of the automated workflow.

d. Reports are clinically organized:

   i.   Create structured clinical reports for most cardiology specialties, then examine and confirm them.

   ii. Integrate with 4D, echocardiography, nuclear medicine, CT angiography, and pediatric echo reporting applications.

e. It is used to obtain a comprehensive overview of a patient's cardiovascular record, an interactive, hierarchical timeline view, including pertinent past notifications, without switching screens or performing time-consuming searches.

Reimbursements are completed faster by automating the capture of professional and technical expenditures. Discover how to focus more on patient care and less on paper and process [3].

2.3.2 IBM IMAGING AI ORCHESTRATOR

The IBM Imaging AI Orchestrator is designed to simplify deployment and scale. The IBM Imaging AI Marketplace streamlines procurement, offering applications vetted for security and privacy. It intelligently routes applications to the correct applications and returns status in a single report. It even updates the work lists with the status of AI analysis while noting urgent cases. AI Orchestrator connects to the on-promise cloud or hybrid environments with every application strictly tested to meet IBM's privacy and security standards. The use of clouds offers less complexity and also fewer burdens on IT, and it results in confident diagnosis and greater productivity.

2.4 ATOMWISE, INC.

Atomwise is a technologically advanced pharmaceutical business, revolutionizing the search for small molecule drugs by harnessing the power of AI. The Atomwise team developed the technology that underpins Atomwise's best-in-class AI discovery engine, distinguished by its ability to identify and enhance novel chemical matter. Deep learning for structure-based drug design is a new application of deep learning that the Atomwise team created. By accomplishing over 185 projects covering a wide range of protein types and various "hard-to-drug" targets, Atomwise has proven its discovery engine in great detail. With three initiatives in lead optimization and more than 30 programs in discovery, Atomwise is developing a wholly owned pipeline of small-molecule therapeutic candidates.

The business has raised more than $174 million from prestigious venture capital firms to achieve its goal of producing better medications more quickly [4].

2.4.1 ATOMNET POSERANKER (ANPR)

ANPR is a convolutional graph network trained to recognize and rerank crystal-like ligand poses from an ensemble of protein conformations and sampled ligand poses. Unlike traditional virtual high throughput screening (vHTS) techniques that take receptor flexibility into account, a deep learning approach can internalize legitimate cognate and noncognate binding modes corresponding to various receptor conformations, teaching the learner to infer and account for receptor flexibility even on single conformations. The PDBbind v2019 data set's docking to cognate and noncognate receptors showed a dramatically improved pose quality due to ANPR. Improved pose rankings that more accurately reflect the experimentally reported ligand binding modes lead to higher hit rates in vHTS campaigns, which advance computational drug discovery – particularly for novel therapeutic targets or novel binding locations [5].

2.5 GOOGLE CLOUD'S HEALTHCARE APP

With the use of clinical decision support (CDS) services and other AI technologies, Google's Cloud Healthcare application programming interface (API) enables doctors to make better clinical judgments about their patients. Through machine learning, Google Cloud's AI uses data from customers' electronic health records to produce insights that help healthcare professionals make better clinical judgments. Google developed an AI system that forecasts the results of hospital visits in collaboration with the universities of California, Stanford, and Chicago. This helps to reduce the number of hospital stays for patients and prevent readmissions.

The Cloud Healthcare API allows easy and standardized data exchange between healthcare applications and solutions built on Google Cloud. With support for popular healthcare data standards such as HL7® FHIR®, HL7® v2, and DICOM®, the Cloud Healthcare API provides a fully managed, highly scalable, enterprise-grade development environment for building clinical and analytics solutions securely on Google Cloud. The Cloud Healthcare API also includes additional value-added capabilities, such as automated Digital Imaging and Communications in Medicine (DICOM) and Fast Healthcare Interoperability Resources (FHIR), to better prepare data for these solutions.

The Cloud Healthcare API provides a pathway to intelligent analytics and machine learning capabilities in Google Cloud with prebuilt connectors for streaming data processing in Dataflow, scalable analytics with BigQuery, and machine learning with Vertex AI.

Google Cloud's privacy backs the Cloud Healthcare API and security features that support HIPAA compliance and are in scope for Google Cloud's ISO/IEC 27001, ISO/IEC 27017, and ISO/IEC 27018 certifications. In addition, Google Cloud is HITRUST CSF certified [6].

2.6 LIFEGRAPH BIOMEDICAL

Lifegraph Biomedical Instrumentation Pvt. Ltd. is developing a tech-clinical solution via devices and instruments to minimize the problem of the health care sector faced by clinics, hospitals while caring and treating patients' health. An incubation center at IIT Patna supports this company. The product, called the Savitri IV bags monitoring and alarm system (see Figure 2.2), is developed by Lifegraph Biomedical. Savitri is an intelligent device that monitors IV bag status regularly and wirelessly monitors IV bag status in hospitals. Its dashboard feature and WiFi mode enable personnel to monitor every bag wirelessly.

2.7 APIXIO, INC.

Apixio, a cognitive computing company based in California, was established in 2009 to extract and make available therapeutic knowledge from digital medical records. With its team of healthcare experts, engineers, data scientists, and product experts, the company's current focus is on making it possible for healthcare professionals to adapt patient care based on practice-based evidence.

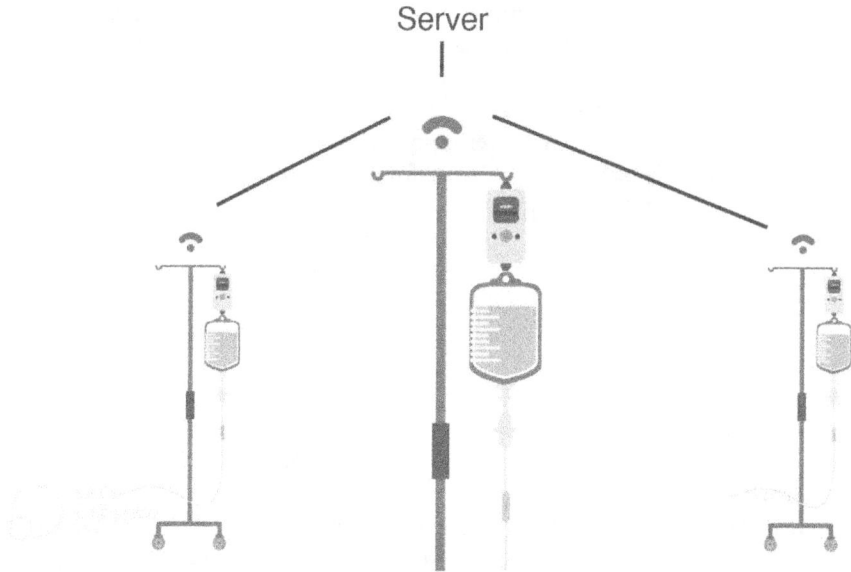

FIGURE 2.2   Savitri IV bags monitoring and alarm system.

Apixio works with the data using various methodologies and algorithms that are machine learning based and have natural language-processing capabilities. The data can be analyzed individually to create a patient data model. Gaining more knowledge about disease prevalence and treatment trends can also be aggregated throughout the population.

2.7.1   HEPATOCELLULAR CARCINOMA (HCC) PROFILER

The first product from Apixio's technology platform is the HCC Profiler. This product's two types of consumers are healthcare delivery networks and insurance companies. The HCC Profiler uses coded data found in electronic records and billing or administrative data sets. Apixio has demonstrated that computers enable coders to read two or three times as many charts per hour than manual review alone. In addition to speeding up the chart review process, Apixio has found that computers are more accurate. Compared to what a coder could find manually by reading the chart, there can be an accuracy boost of up to 20%. Finding gaps in patient paperwork with a computer is another advantage. For example, over nine months, within a population of 25,000 patients, Apixio discovered more than 5,000 instances of disorders that were not accurately and thoroughly reported.

Apixio works with structured and unstructured data, although most of its data are unstructured, typewritten clinical charts. These can include general practitioner (GP) notes, consultant notes, radiology notes, pathology results, and discharge notes from a hospital. They also work with information on diseases and procedures that are reported to the government.

Apixio's Big Data infrastructure comprises well-known infrastructure components, including nonrelational database technology like Cassandra and distributed computing platforms like Hadoop and Spark. Apixio has added its bespoke orchestration and management layer that automates a system that cannot be operated manually at the scale Apixio operates. Everything is operated on Amazon Web Services (AWS) in the cloud, which Apixio selected for its robustness, healthcare privacy and security, and regulatory compliance.

Apixio developed sophisticated technology to leverage and scale optical character recognition (OCR) to make machine-scanned medical charts readable by their algorithms. Sophisticated computational workflows that preprocess images, set parameters in the OCR engine, and correct output had to be developed to extract the text available in a scanned chart.

At Apixio, machine learning is used to predict medical conditions that patients most likely have based on clinical documentation and medical claims data. After ingesting, cleaning, and normalizing these data, they train models from which we make these predictions. They create a model or a function that, when given input x, produces one or more outputs that classify the input x. they use several computational techniques to create these functions, all of which involve three essential components: data points, features, and weights.

2.7.2 AI-POWERED RISK ADJUSTMENT PROGRAM

The traditional approach to auditing activities and coding involves manually reviewing patient charts and coding decisions, and is not struggling to scale up to the rising need for risk adjustment. Recent developments in AI have made it possible for risk adjustment (RA)teams to examine, code, and perform quality assurance (QA) on clinical audit evidence of HCCs in a much more effective and compliant way offering an alternate strategy. Your risk adjustment program may benefit from AI integration regarding reimbursements, operational effectiveness, and compliance. AI can benefit healthcare organizations if the appropriate technology is in place.

In order to conduct a thorough coding study in 2017, Apixio collaborated with a national health plan that provides services to over 4 million Medicare and Medicaid members. A collection of 284,000 Medicare Advantage (MA) charts were coded during the study utilizing two different methodologies: manual review and AI-assisted review. The study aimed to evaluate AI's impact on coding productivity and accuracy compared to traditional coding workflows. The results were conclusive: the AI-assisted coding team outperformed the manual coding team in every area, finding more HCCs, reducing chart review time, and increasing overall productivity. With Apixio's platform, the health plan could also capture where manual reviewers missed or rejected correct HCC codes found by AI algorithms to inform coder training efforts.

2.8   CYRCADIA ASIA

iTbra
Two cozy and clever patches called iTBra are worn under your clothes to detect variations in breast tissue's circadian temperature (see Figure 2.3). Anonymized data are

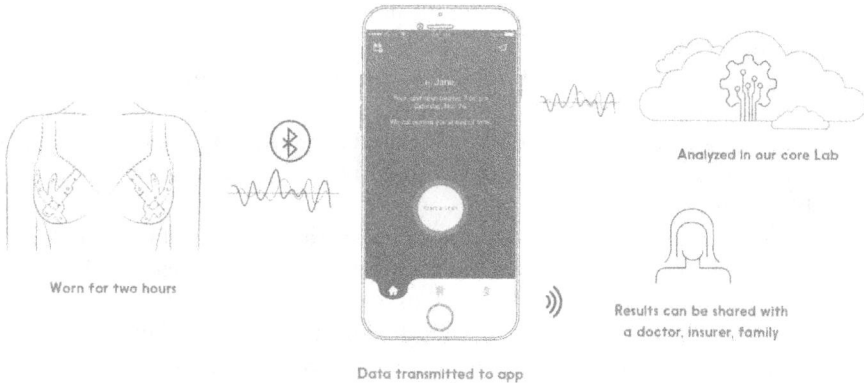

FIGURE 2.3 Working of iTBra.

communicated directly to Cyrcadia's core lab for analysis via your mobile device, and results are delivered to you in a matter of minutes. The iTBra allows women to keep track of their breast health and finds breast cancer in its earliest stages.

iTBra is designed to fit comfortably under our garments or sportswear. The user has to launch the iTBra app, which is connected to the device through Bluetooth. After wearing the iTBra for two hours, the results are sent to the physician and the user.

This technology is based on analyzing the human body's natural 24-hour circadian cycles. These circadian cycles are driven by specific genes in our cells that regulate our metabolism, and the cycles have distinct heat signatures and may be monitored metabolically. These circadian cycles are regulated by particular genes in our cells that are found in our cells. The metabolic profile is continuously monitored by technology. In just two hours, algorithms can discriminate between the metabolic traits of potentially cancerous and healthy people thanks to the predictive capacity of our artificial intelligence base. Our remarkable accuracy rate – beyond simple image interpretation – has been validated against actual patient pathology. Over image-based modalities like mammography and ultrasound, metabolic detection offers a breakthrough in cancer screening.

Many females are unaware that they have dense breast tissue and that their yearly mammograms can overlook the presence of cancer. Imaging is not a component of our technique. In order to give those women with dense tissue piece of mind, we obtain the same levels of accuracy in detection independent of breast tissue density, bringing peace of mind to those women with dense tissue.

2.9 VIRGIN PULSE

About Virgin Pulse

Virgin Pulse is the well-known leading global provider of health and well-being solutions discovered to drive outcomes and reduce costs by helping better decision-making across the entire care continuum – from prevention and well-being to pre-chronic and chronic disease management to episodic and acute care. Featuring the industry's only authentic Homebase for Health®, a personalized ecosystem where Virgin Pulse clients and members can access, navigate and interact with their health, well-being, and benefits in one trusted and familiar place, Virgin Pulse's solutions fuse high-tech, high-touch, predictive analytics, AI and data to unify and simplify health and well-being. Virgin Pulse is being used by over 14 million users and hundreds of organizations to transform lives and businesses for the better today in more than 190 countries.

The top international provider of technologically advanced solutions committed to enhancing its members' health and well-being. Today it was announced that the award-winning health activation firm Welltok had been fully acquired. For the combined 4,100 worldwide employers, health plan, and health system clients of the two firms, the integration of Virgin Pulse's daily engagement platform with Welltok's activation engine will improve health outcomes and result in cost savings.

According to Chris Michalak, CEO of Virgin Pulse, "This acquisition is the result of years of work to build a game-changing strategy to improving health and lowering costs for companies, health plans, and health systems." "By continuously engaging and activating millions of people, we will be able to improve their health, ultimately resulting in lower costs for customers, members, consumers, and patients. The personalization and analytics capabilities of Welltok will be integrated into Homebase for Health®, which will greatly increase the value for our clients and the people they serve. We will recognize quick wins for our clients and customers, scaling current programs, and launching a better activation engine shortly."

Virgin Pulse is well known for providing live and digital solutions that encourage long-term behavioral changes by encouraging people to develop daily routines that improve outcomes in all areas of their health and well-being. Welltok is renowned for empowering individuals by fusing social determinants of health data with powerful predictive analytics capabilities and utilizing a variety of communication channels (text/SMS, email, interactive voice response [IVR] calls, social media, etc.) to optimize reach. With the help of its unique activation engine, Welltok aims to persuade customers, staff, patients, and members to carry out specific tasks like enrolling in a mental health program, getting their prescriptions filled, or filling a care gap.

By making it simpler to start and finish essential actions that improve health and well-being, Virgin Pulse's Homebase for Health®, which offers these features, will improve user experience and speed up results and cost savings for clients and consumers.

Users of Virgin Pulse's Homebase for Health® practices small steps to build their resilience. They can engage with a coach's AI-powered nudge to help them start a new healthy habit. Users can receive health reminders to schedule the next blood test. Homebase for Health® delivers simplicity in a world of complexity, making it easy for you and your employees to achieve meaningful change that leads to measurable outcomes.

With this acquisition, Virgin Pulse will launch the first end-to-end engagement and activation platform in the market, supporting customers, members, and consumers throughout the entire health continuum by utilizing the most extensive consumer database in the market, consisting of 275 million individuals and more than 1,000 predictive analytics models that can target people with up to 90% accuracy based on risk, receptivity, and likelihood to act via various outreach methods. This extensive database is an effective tool that can assist employers, health plans, and health systems in generating social determinants of health insights to proactively address and reduce health disparities and close care gaps across diverse populations, including at-risk Medicare Advantage and Managed Medicaid members.

They provide individualized, digital-first health solutions that integrate technology, gamification, behavior science, live professional assistance, and a robust ecosystem into a unified, seamless experience to motivate people to improve their health and well-being daily.

Targeting activation across a wide range of people, including workers, patients, consumers, and health plan members, including Medicare Advantage and Managed Medicaid populations, to drive quantifiable health outcomes through multichannel outreach and inspire them with integrated incentives. When this "surround-sound" activation is enhanced through a platform that users frequently use, it serves as a multiplier for user engagement. It is a critical factor in the outcomes for health and well-being.

The transaction's financial specifics remain a secret. Virgin Pulse is supported by Marlin Equity Partners, a worldwide investment company that manages more than $7.7 billion in assets. Virgin Pulse received advice from Evercore, Lazard, and Kirkland & Ellis LLP in finance and law. Welltok was financially advised by UBS Securities LLC and Shearman & Sterling LLP legally.

2.10   CONCLUSION

AI can undoubtedly bring new efficiencies and quality to healthcare outcomes in the world. We have talked about what AI is and its application in healthcare. Many businesses are investing time and money for technological developments. These advancements will surely be accessible to common people at affordable rates in upcoming years.

REFERENCES

1. https://www.baytechit.com/history-healthcare-technology/The History of Healthcare Technology and the Evolution of HER, 2018.
2. https://www.ibm.com/watson/health/resources/artificial-intelligence-medical-imaging/
3. https://www.ibm.com/products/merge-cardio
4. https://www.atomwise.com/
5. Stafford, Kate A., Anderson, Brandon M., Sorenson, Jon, and van den Bedem, Henry, "AtomNet PoseRanker: Enriching Ligand Pose Quality for Dynamic Proteins in Virtual High-Throughput Screens," *Journal of Chemical Information and Modeling* 62 (5) (2022): 1178–1189. DOI: 10.1021/acs.jcim.1c01250
6. https://cloud.google.com/healthcare-api

3 Insights into AI, Machine Learning, and Deep Learning

Aditya Shinde[1] and Swati Shinde[2]
[1]Indian Institute of Information Technology,
Pune, Maharashtra, India
[2]Pimpri Chinchwad College of Engineering,
Pune, Maharashtra, India

CONTENTS

3.1 WHAT IS DEEP LEARNING?

Artificial intelligence (AI) is the branch of computer science that refers to the simulation of human intelligence in machines that are programmed to learn from experiences and can solve problems like humans do [1].

Artificial intelligence is the broad domain having machine learning (ML) as a subdomain that focuses on the study of different statistical algorithms that extract knowledge from the input data to bring intelligence in the machines [2]. There are many machine learning algorithms, like logistic regression, support vector machine, decision trees, naive Bayes, artificial neural networks (ANN), etc.. Among these, ANN is inspired by the structure and functioning of the human brain.

The branch of the machine learning that focuses on the study of artificial neural networks with many layers suitable for certain applications is called deep learning (DL) [3]. It is the fastest growing subject area and has applications in almost all fields.

The relationship among AI, ML, and DL is shown in Figure 3.1. In contrast to the artificial neural networks used in machine learning, deep learning uses artificial neural networks with many layers. These artificial neural networks with many layers are called deep neural networks, and the branch to study these deep neural networks is called deep learning.

DOI: 10.1201/9781003324430-4

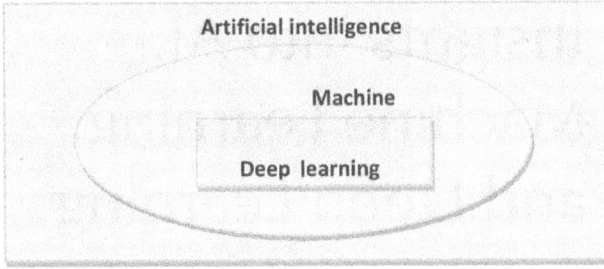

FIGURE 3.1   Relationship among AI, ML, and DL.

Recently deep learning has become the buzzword and is considered new fuel to drive human lives to the next level. Deep learning has existed for a long time, but it has gained momentum recently because of the following reasons:

1. An enormous amount of <u>Big Data</u> available over the Internet
2. Developments in computational power of graphics processing units (GPUs) with affordable costs
3. The effectiveness of deep learning models in image and video data modeling, language modeling. and sequential data processing

3.2   ARTIFICIAL NEURAL NETWORKS

ANNs are based on the functioning of the biological nervous system of the human brain [4]. Human brain consists of 10^{11} processing elements working together in parallel and in a distributed fashion toward a specific goal. These processing elements are called neurons. The structure of the biological neuron is given in Figure 3.2.

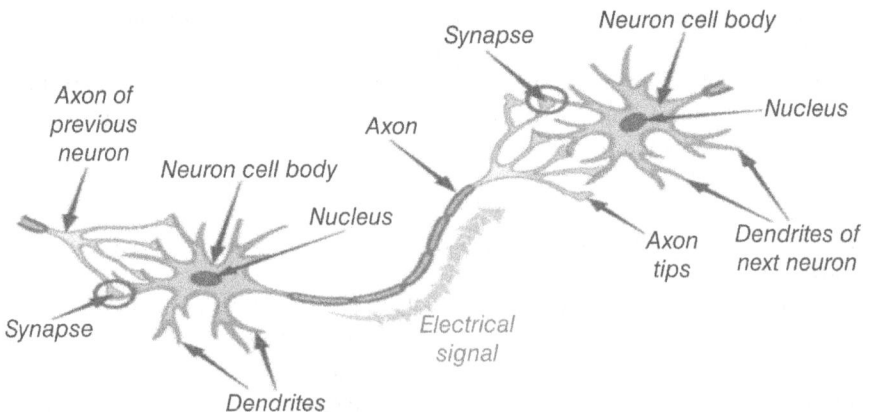

FIGURE 3.2   Structure of a biological neuron.

Each biological neuron consists of the main parts like dendrites, axon, synapses, and soma (cell body) [5]:

- **Dendrites** – These are tree-like branches around the cell body. These branches receive information from other neurons and are connected to axons of other neurons.
- **Soma** – It is the cell body of the neuron. It receives input though dendrites and is responsible for processing of input information and sending output signals to axon.
- **Axon** – It carries the output signal produced by soma and distributes it among other connected neurons through synapses.
- **Synapses** – These are the connection between the axon and other neuron dendrites. The amount of output signal transmitted to other neurons depends upon the strength of the connections.

In summary, every neuron receives input through dendrites. The input received through all dendrites is processed by the neuron cell to produce an output signal. This output signal is transmitted through the axon to other neurons, and other neuron's dendrites receive this output signal through synapses. In this manner, all neurons work collectively and produce the output of a brain. The collection of these biological neurons together is called a biological neural network.

Inspired by the working of the biological neural network, the concept of ANN came into existence. The ANN consists of a collection of artificial neurons functioning together to accomplish a certain task. These artificial neurons are the basic processing elements of the ANN [6]. The structure of each artificial neuron (which is henceforth simply referred to as neuron) is given in Figure 3.3.

Artificial neurons, as given in Figure 3.3, receive the inputs ($x_0, x_1, \ldots x_n$) through input links, and these inputs are multiplied by the strengths of connections called weights ($w_0, w_1, \ldots w_n$), and net i8put to the neuron is calculated [7]. Based on the strength of the net input, the neuron produces its output signal. Here the role of the activation function comes into the picture. The activation function receives the net input and produces the output signal of a neuron. There are different activation functions, such as Threshold, Sigmoid, Tanh, ReLu, and leaky ReLu. These different activation functions have their own merits and demerits. The analogy between a biological neuron and artificial neuron is given in Table 3.1.

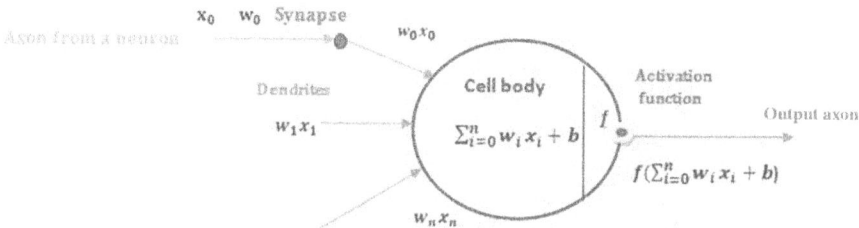

FIGURE 3.3   Structure of an artificial neuron ([6]).

TABLE 3.1

Analogy between a Biological Neuron and Artificial Neuron

Biological Neuron	Artificial Neuron
Dendrites	Inputs
Cell Nucleus/Soma	Node
Synapse	Weights
Axon	Outputs
Chemical diffusion or electrical impulses at synapses	Net input calculation and output signal using activation function

Figure 3.3 represents a single neuron. Multiple such neurons form a layer, and a multilayer neural network with many such layers are formed by connecting neurons in one layer to neurons in next layers. In multilayer neural networks, many such neurons do the processing in parallel and feed their output to the next layers [8, 9]. In this way, the overall output of the network is calculated and presented to the user through the output layer. The traditional artificial neural network with a limited number of layers is a machine learning technique, and the network with many layers stacked together is deep neural network architecture. Such deep neural networks are suitable for image, speech, and language applications where extraction of accurate spatial features is utmost important. In the case of machine learning, hand-crafted features are extracted and given as an input to machine learning algorithms. But in deep learning, features are not extracted explicitly; the deep neural network itself extracts the features. Simple data, such as an image, is given as an input, and earlier layers of the deep neural network do the job of feature extraction, and later layers do the machine learning tasks, like classification, clustering, etc. So in short, deep learning consists of feature extraction and machine learning together.

Example: Consider the example of an OR operation by using an artificial neuron shown in Figure 3.4.

Here the weights of two input links are given as $w_1 = 1$ and $w_1 = 1$. The threshold activation function with threshold value of $T = 0.5$ is used. The *net input* and *predicted output* values for different combinations of inputs features x_1 and x_2 are given in Table 3.2.

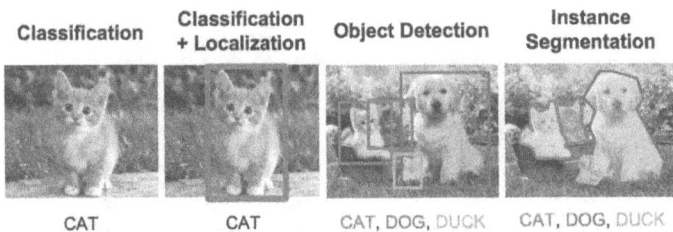

Classification	Classification + Localization	Object Detection	Instance Segmentation
CAT	CAT	CAT, DOG, DUCK	CAT, DOG, DUCK

FIGURE 3.4   Deep learning-based computer vision tasks.

TABLE 3.2

Logical OR Operation Using an Artificial Neuron

X_1	X_2	Actual Output	Net Input $(w_1 x_1 + w_2 x_2)$	Predicted Output If Net Input $> = T$, Then 1 Else 0
0	0	0	0	0
0	1	1	1	1
1	0	1	1	1
1	1	1	1	1

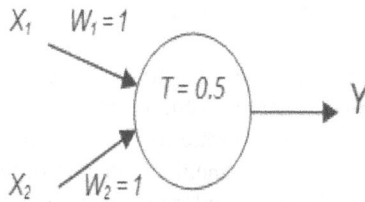

Python code for the preceding example is as follows.

```
w1=0.5
w2=0.5
x1=[0,0,1,1]
x2=[0,1,0,1]
predicted_output=[]
for i in range(0,4):
  net_input=x1[i]*w1+x2[i]*w2
  if net_input>=0.5:
    predicted_output=1
    print(predicted_output)
  else:
    predicted_output=0
    print(predicted_output)
Output:
0
1
1
1
```

3.3   BENEFITS OF DEEP LEARNING

Because of multiple benefits, deep learning is suitable for variety of applications, including speech recognition, speech processing and synthesis, natural language processing, image classification, object detection, gaming, autonomous vehicles, military, healthcare, agriculture, transports, etc. [10]. There are a number of deep learning architectures with specific characteristics suited to these applications, like convolutional neural networks, recurrent neural networks, long short-term memory, etc. [11]. Among these, convolutional networks are well suited for computer vision applications. Computer vision tasks include image classification, object localization, objects detection, and instance segmentation, as depicted in Figure 3.4. Image classification is the classification of the input images into predefined categories, for example classifying images of dogs and cats, cancerous and noncancerous, etc. Object localization is the finding of the location of an object in an image in terms of its surrounding bounded box dimensions, and object detection is locating the different objects and classifying those among classes. Instance segmentation is highlighting the object portions in contrast to its background.

The success of any computer vision task largely depends on accurate feature extraction from images. Before deep learning, hand-crafted features like shape, texture, edge, size, etc. were extracted by using separate image processing methods and then these extracted features were fed to machine learning algorithms. These hand-crafted features don't capture the optimal spatial information of the image, and the same set of features is not appropriate to represent all kinds of images, including images of animals, objects, cars, medical, etc. Also, this is a two-step process consisting of feature extraction followed by a machine learning task, as shown in Figure 3.5.

For these reasons, convolution neural networks have proved to be more efficient as they facilitate the extraction of optimal spatial features followed by machine learning tasks in a single step by the same neural network architecture.

Also, the traditional artificial neural networks used in machine learning suffer from the drawback of having a large number of parameters to learn. Due to the full connectivity between nodes, they suffer from the curse of dimensionality, and thus do not scale well to higher-resolution images. A $1,000 \times 1,000$ pixel image with RGB color channels has 3 million dimensions, so a single fully connected neuron in a first hidden layer of a regular neural network would have $1,000 \times 1,000 \times 3 = 3$ million weights. Thus, full connectivity of neurons is wasteful for purposes such as image recognition that are dominated by spatially local input patterns.

In addition, the full connectivity of neurons yields a large number of trainable parameters. Example: Consider the Modified National Institute of Standards and

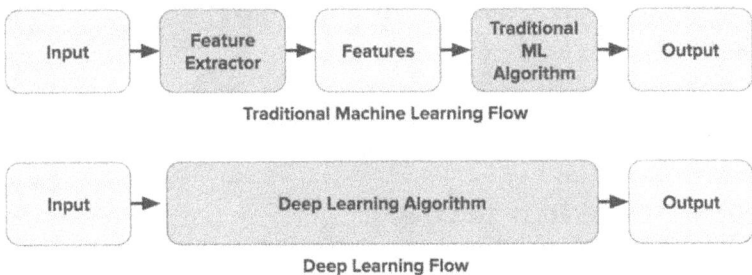

Traditional Machine Learning Flow

Deep Learning Flow

FIGURE 3.5 A machine learning algorithm requires feature extraction as a prior step while deep learning extracts the features by itself.

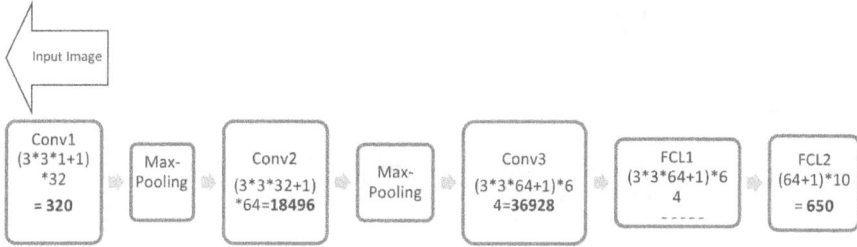

FIGURE 3.6   Trainable parameters in CNN.

$$\underline{\textbf{Total Parameters} = \textbf{320} + \textbf{18496} + \textbf{36928} + \textbf{36928} + \textbf{650} = \textbf{93322}}$$

Technology (MNIST) data set of digit recognition with 28 × 28 binary images as input and 10 total classes for digits from 0 to 9 [12]. The following description illustrates that even for small resolution images of size 28 × 28, the total numbers of parameters are 93,322 if we use convolutional neural networks (CNN), as given in Figure 3.6 and that of 101,770 parameters if we use a traditional feed-forward ANN as given in Figure 3.7. Because of sharing weights and biases, CNN has considerably reduced numbers of parameters compared to ANN.

Illustration of number of trainable parameters in CNN for MNIST digit classification problem:

In Figure 3.6, the input image size is 28 × 28 × 1, where the width and height of the image is 28 each and 1 represents the number of channels for binary image. In RGB images, instead of 1, the number of channels is 3. There are a total three convolution layers (Conv), two max pooling, and two fully connected layers (FCL) shown in rectangles. The trainable parameters for each convolution layer are represented in the form $(a+b) \times c$, where a is filter size, b is number of bias parameters, and c represents the number of filters. The trainable parameters for each fully connected layer are represented in the form $(a+b) \times c$, where a is the input size of each neuron, b is the number of bias parameters, and c represents number of neurons in that layer. The max-pooling layer does not have any parameters. Forthcoming chapters provide more details about CNN.

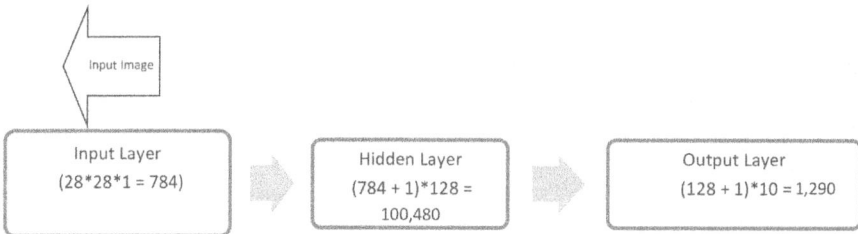

FIGURE 3.7   Trainable parameters in ANN.

$$\textbf{Total Parameters} = \textbf{784} + \textbf{100480} + \textbf{1290} = \textbf{101770}$$

Following is the python implementation of the CNN architecture shown in Figure 3.6.

```
[ ]    model = Sequential([
           Conv2D(32, 3, activation='relu', input_
           shape=(28, 28, 1)),
           MaxPooling2D( ),
           Conv2D(64, 3, activation='relu'),
           MaxPooling2D( ),
           Conv2D(64, 3, activation='relu'),
           Flatten( ),
           Dense        ( 64, activation= 'relu'),
           Dense(10, activation= 'softmax')
           ])
```

Illustration of a number of trainable parameters in ANN for the MNIST digit classification problem:

Consider the ANN as shown in Figure 3.7 with 28 * 28 * 1 input size flattened into a vector of size 784 elements with 784 input neurons in the input layer, a fully connected single hidden layer with modest count of 128 neurons, and a fully connected output layer with 10 neurons, which is equal to 10 classes in the MNIST data set. The number of trainable parameters for the hidden layer and output layer is estimated as $(a+b) * c$, where a is the number of inputs to each neuron in the layer, b represents number of bias parameters to that neuron, and c represents the number of neurons in the layer.

Following is the python implementation of the ANN architecture shown in Figure 3.7.

```
[ ]    model = Sequential([Flatten(input_shape=(28, 28)),
           Dense        ( 128, activation= 'relu'),
           Dense        ( 10, activation= 'softmax'),
           ])
```

Another important deep learning architecture called recurrent neural network is more suited to sequence data like speech, text, signals, weather, where predictions not only depend on current data items but also past data. In such applications understanding a data item along with its context is necessary. For example, to understand the meaning of a particular word in a paragraph, we need to understand the preceding and following sentences. Other different architectures of the same category are LSTM, GRU, etc. These are the extensions to the basic recurrent neural network architecture [13].

Deep learning also has a benefit of a concept called transfer learning. Transfer learning allows using pretrained models to new problems, thereby saving on computational cost and reducing the need for large data to some extent [14].

In summary, deep learning has following benefits:

- Deep learning is applicable to a wide range of applications based on image, video, text, and speech processing, such as autonomous vehicles, military, healthcare, agriculture, and transports.
- Deep learning architectures can extract optimal features, thus reducing the need of explicit feature engineering.
- It provides different architectures that are suited to different research problems, such as convolutional neural networks, recurrent neural networks, and long short-term memory.
- Existing trained models can be made available for public use and extension through transfer learning without losing earlier knowledge.

DL is employed in several situations where machine intelligence would be useful (see Figure 3.4):

- In the absence of a human expert (navigation on Mars).
- When humans are unable to explain their expertise (speech recognition, vision, and language understanding).
- When the solution to the problem changes over time (tracking, weather prediction, preference, stock, price prediction).
- Where solutions need to be adapted to the particular cases (biometrics, personalization).
- When the problem size is too vast for our limited reasoning capabilities (calculation webpage ranks, matching ads to Facebook, sentiment analysis).

Disadvantages of deep learning include the following:

- Deep learning requires a large amount of data to get trained.
- It is computationally expensive in terms of training the model, but inferences from the trained model are less expensive
- Deep neural networks are considered black boxes because their decisions are not easily interpretable.
- Fine-tuning of different hyperparameters is needed.

3.4   HISTORY

The history is classified into the history of deep learning (Table 3.3) [15, 16], history of convolutional neural networks (Table 3.4) [17, 18], history of recurrent neural networks (Table 3.5) [19, 20].

3.5   APPLICATIONS OF DEEP LEARNING

Different deep neural networks have specific designs suitable to a particular set of applications. Among these, CNNs are good at recognizing images and objects in the images, RNNs are good for continuous time series data, while generative adversarial

TABLE 3.3

History of Deep Learning

Year	Contribution	Researchers	Detailed Contribution
1943	McCulloch model	McCulloch (neurologists) and Piits (logician)	• Proposed an oversimplified computational/ mathematical model that receives binary input, processes it, and gives a binary decision.
1957–58	Perceptron model	Rosenblatt	• Able to learn, make decisions, translate languages.
1965–1968	First-generation multilayer perceptron	Ivakhneko	• The first time proposed, the neural network with multiple layers was arranged in a deep architecture. • So Ivakhneko is considered a founding father of deep learning.
1969	Limitations of perceptron	Minsky and Papert	• The researchers outlined the limitations of perceptron: that it cannot even solve simpler problems like XOR classification. • In their work, they have mentioned this limitation of perceptron and not of the multilayer perceptron, • But they are misquoted, and connectionist AI underwent a lot of criticism and loss of interest in it.

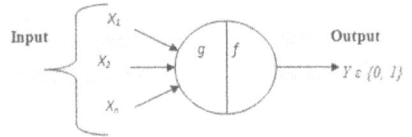

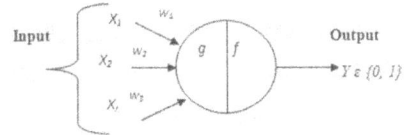

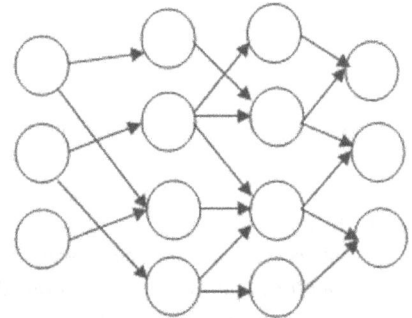

(Continued)

TABLE 3.3 *(Continued)*
History of Deep Learning

Year	Contribution	Researchers	Detailed Contribution
During 1969–1986: Downtime of Connectionist AI, Which Is Called "Winter AI"			
1986	Backpropagation algorithm	Rumelhart	• This algorithm can train a multilayer neural network. • Although discovered long ago, it is still being used for training current deep neural networks.
1989	Universal approximation theory	N/A	• A multilayered neural network with single hidden layer can approximate any continuous function with desired precision. • Still, computing power issues, and the limitation of backpropagation to train a very deep neural network, have resulted in loss of interest in AI.
During 1989–2006: Again Downtime in AI, Which Is Called "Slow Winter AI"			
2006	Deep revival	Hinton and Salakhutdinov	• Proposed effective way of initializing weights that allows deep autoencoder networks to learn low-dimensional representation of data. • It has sparked again the interest in training deep neural networks.
2007–2009	Enhancements in neural networks		• More investigations were made into effectiveness of unsupervised pretraining. • Researchers started finding solutions to the issues during this period. • Interest in AI started rising.
2009 onward	Series of successes		Many practical applications, such as handwritten recognition (2009), speech recognition (2010), the MNIST data set with GPUs, and visual pattern recognition (2011).
2012–16	ImageNet challenge	Google	• The ImageNet challenge involves classifying a given image in one of the 1,000 classes. • The following convolutional neural network implementations successively have given benchmark performance:

Network	# of Layers	Error %
AlexNet	8	16.0
ZFNet	8	11.2
VGGNet	19	7.3
GoogLeNet	22	6.7
Ms ResNet	152	3.6 (better than human!)

• This has created a lot of interest in deep learning.
• Many companies started investing in deep learning.

TABLE 3.4
History of CNNs

Year	Contribution	Researchers	Detailed Contribution
1959	Hubel and Wiesel experiment	Hubel and Wiesel	• Different neurons in the brain fire to different types of visual stimuli, i.e., all neurons are not fired to all visual stimuli. • This is roughly the idea behind convolutional neural networks.
1980	Neocognitron	Fukushima	• Primitive CNN. • Used for handwritten character recognition and pattern recognition.
1989	CNN	Lecun et al.	Handwritten digit recognition in the context of postal services to read pin codes.
1998	LeNet-5	Lecun et al.	Introduced the famous MNIST data set with CNN.
2012–16	ImageNet challenge		• Many implementations of CNN, including AlexNet, ZFNet, VGGNet, GoogleNet, and ResNet, have made CNN popular • Currently it is actively adopted all over the world.

TABLE 3.5
History of Recurrent Neural Networks (RNNs)

Year	Contribution	Researchers	Detailed Contribution
1986	Jordan network	Jordan	• This is the first recurrent neural network proposed. • The output state previous time step is fed to the next time step, thereby allowing interactions between time steps in the sequence.
1990	Elman network	Elman	• The hidden state of each time step is fed to the next time step, thereby allowing interaction between time steps in the sequence.
1991–94			Exploding and vanishing gradient problems.
1997	Long short-term memory	N/A	It can solve complex long time lag tasks that could never be solved before.
2014	Sequence-to-sequence learning	N/A	• Initial success in using RNNs/LSTMs for large-scale sequence-to-sequence learning problems. • Introduced the attention mechanism, which inspired a lot of research over the next two years.
2014	Reinforcement learning for attention	Schmidhuber and Huber	• This proposed RNN uses reinforcement learning to decide where to look. • Attention basically tells that what elements of the large sequence to look for. • Currently RNNs are used for many natural language processing and other sequence data applications.

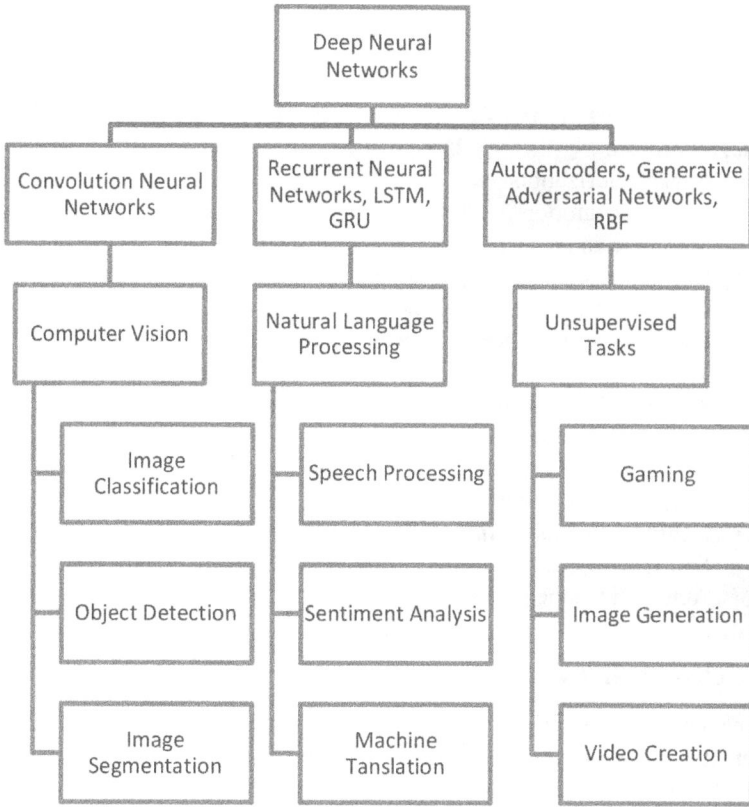

FIGURE 3.8 Deeps neural networks and their application domains.

networks (GANs) are mainly designed for unsupervised tasks such as clustering. This is depicted in Figure 3.8.

At present, DL is being applied in almost all areas. As a result, this approach is often called a universal learning approach. Deep learning is a key technology that supports areas such as driverless cars, traffic controls, and disease predictions, and learning to perform classification tasks directly from images, text, sound, etc. Its models can achieve state-of-the-art accuracy, sometimes exceeding human-level performance and previous methods. Models are trained by using a large set of labeled data and deep neural network architectures with many layers.

In the current scenario, machine learning is entrusted to solve complex problems by using deep learning supports [21–23]. This is getting more optimized as the algorithms continue to learn via the infusion of data. The following are some practical examples of deep learning:

- **Natural language processing**
  - Virtual assistants
  - Machine translations

- Chatbots and service bots
- Adding sounds to silent movies
- Text sentiment analysis
- **Computer vision: image classification, object detection, and image segmentation**
  - Image colorization
  - Facial recognition
  - Medicine and pharmaceuticals
  - Object classification in photographs
  - Medical image classification and object detection in medical images like all types of cancers, diabetic retinopathy, lung disease, etc.
  - Video surveillance and diagnostics
- **Unsupervised applications**
  - Automatic handwriting generation
  - Character text generation
  - Image caption generation
  - Neural networks in finance
  - Self-driving cars
  - Automatic game playing

3.6 CONCLUSION

This chapter has summarized the correlation among AI, ML, and DL. It also has differentiated between the traditional artificial neural network and deep neural network and its computational parameters. In today's world of the Internet and social media, a large amount of data in the form of images, videos, and text is generated. To analyze this data, deep neural networks are preferred over the traditional neural networks. Deeps neural networks seem complex, but the number of trainable parameters is less than that of artificial neural networks. Due to the complex architecture, training time for CNN is more than traditional neural networks, but testing time is less. Therefore, deep neural networks are becoming more popular in almost all the applications and opened up many research directions.

REFERENCES

1. Somvanshi, Madan, et al. "A review of machine learning techniques using decision tree and support vector machine." *2016 International Conference on Computing Communication Control and Automation (ICCUBEA)*. IEEE, Pune, India, 2016, pp. 1–7.
2. Alpaydin, Ethem. *Introduction to Machine Learning*. MIT Press, Cambridge, MA, 2020, 02142.
3. Goodfellow, Ian, Bengio, Yoshua, and Courville, Aaron. *Deep Learning*. MIT Press, Cambridge, MA, 2016, 02142.
4. Viera-Martin, E., et al. "Artificial neural networks: A practical review of applications involving fractional calculus." *The European Physical Journal Special Topics* 231 (2022): 2059–2095.
5. Yamazaki, Kashu, et al. "Spiking neural networks and their applications: A review." *Brain Sciences* 12(7) (2022): 863.

6. Zhu, Li, et al. "Artificial neuron networks enabled identification and characterizations of 2D materials and van der Waals heterostructures." *ACS Nano* 16(2) (2022): 2721–2729.

7. Agatonovic-Kustrin, S., and Beresford, R. "Basic concepts of artificial neural network (ANN) modeling and its application in pharmaceutical research." *Journal of Pharmaceutical and Biomedical Analysis* 22(5) (2000): 717–727, https://doi.org/10.1016/S0731-7085(99)00272-1

8. Shinde, S. V., and Kulkarni, U. V. "Mining classification rules from fuzzy min-max neural network." *Fifth International Conference on Computing, Communications and Networking Technologies (ICCCNT)*, 2014, pp. 1–7, https://doi.org/10.1109/ICCCNT.2014.6963079

9. Swati, S., and Uday, K. "Extended fuzzy hyperline-segment neural network with classification rule extraction." *NeuroComputing* 260 (2017): 79–91.

10. Buduma, Nithin, Buduma, Nikhil, and Papa, Joe. *Fundamentals of Deep Learning.* O'Reilly Media, Inc., Newton, MA, 2022.

11. Shwartz-Ziv, Ravid, and Amitai Armon. "Tabular data: Deep learning is not all you need." *Information Fusion* 81 (2022): 84–90.

12. Salman, Odai S., and Salman, Ammar S. "Addressing challenging problems using optimized deep learning classification algorithms on the MNIST dataset." *Future of Information and Communication Conference.* Springer, Cham, 2022, pp. 78–89.

13. Genzel, Martin, Jan Macdonald, and Marz, Maximilian. "Solving inverse problems with deep neural networks-robustness included." *IEEE Transactions on Pattern Analysis and Machine Intelligence* 45(1) (2022): 1119–1134.

14. Dombrowski, Ann-Kathrin, et al. "Towards robust explanations for deep neural networks." *Pattern Recognition* 121 (2022): 108194.

15. Schmidhuber, Jürgen. "Deep learning." *Scholarpedia* 10(11) (2015): 32832.

16. Kelleher, John D. *Deep Learning.* MIT Press, Cambridge, MA, 2019, 02142.

17. Chen, Qiming, and Wu, Ren. "CNN is all you need." *arXiv preprint arXiv:1712.09662* (2017).

18. Zarándy, Ákos, et al. "Overview of CNN research: 25 years history and the current trends." *2015 IEEE International Symposium on Circuits and Systems (ISCAS).* IEEE, Lisbon, Portugal, 2015, pp. 401–404.

19. Wang, Haowen, et al. "Video emotion recognition using local enhanced motion history image and CNN-RNN networks." *Chinese Conference on Biometric Recognition.* Springer, Cham, 2018, pp. 109–119.

20. Xiao, Jianqiong, and Zhou, Zhiyong. "Research progress of RNN language model." *2020 IEEE International Conference on Artificial Intelligence and Computer Applications (ICAICA).* IEEE, Dalian, China, 2020, pp. 1285–1288.

21. Deng, Li, and Yu, Dong. "Deep learning: Methods and applications." *Foundations and Trends® in Signal Processing* 7.3–4 (2014): 197–387.

22. Ahmad, Jamil, Farman, Haleem, and Jan, Zahoor. "Deep learning methods and applications." *Deep Learning: Convergence to Big Data Analytics*, Springer, Singapore, 2019, pp. 31–42.

23. Shinde, S. V., and Mane, D. T. "Deep learning for COVID-19: COVID-19 detection based on chest X-ray images by the fusion of deep learning and machine learning techniques." In Nayak, J., Naik, B., and Abraham, A. (eds.). *Understanding COVID-19: The Role of Computational Intelligence. Studies in Computational Intelligence*, vol. 963, Springer, Cham, 2022. https://doi.org/10.1007/978-3-030-74761-9_21

Part II

Medical Image Processing Using Deep Learning Algorithms

4 Deep Learning for Visual Perceptual Brain Decoding as Image Classification

Saumya Kushwaha, Priyanka Jain, and N. K. Jain
Centre for Development of Advanced Computing (C-DAC),
Delhi, India

CONTENTS

4.1 INTRODUCTION

Brain decoding for visual perception skills like behavior, perception, or cognitive tasks is explored in this proposed work using neural signals. Our brain has a distinct pattern of electrical activity that comes from the aggregate firing patterns of billions of individual neurons. Depending on the person's visual perception skills, these electrical impulses can be recognized. Further, these impulses can be processed to infer a discriminative brain activity over a wide range of visual categories in an attempt to read people's minds. In addition to clinical uses, this capability is useful for brain-machine interaction, among other things. Interaction with machines can often exceed the capabilities of the natural human experience, because of the availability of sensors that collect data that the human body cannot.

This research better focuses to extract information (features) from electroencephalography (EEG) signals to classify or differentiate them based on the images used to trigger brain activity. The key contribution is on implementing and comparing several deep learning methods so as to accomplish higher classification accuracy of EEG signals. In this structured proposed pipeline, a defined exploratory data analysis (EDA) and data preparation methodologies were carried out for the purpose of the same. A comparative study is presented on the evaluation of the various applied algorithms. The proposed research work is supported by a focused literature survey in the related domain.

The remainder of this chapter is organized as follows. A brief presentation of the background concepts related to the present work along with the description of the related work is provided in Section 4.2. The proposed works are discussed in Section 4.3, with the details of all the intermediate components. The implementation part is discussed in Section 4.4, and evaluation with discussion of the results is carried out in Section 4.5. Finally, Section 4.6 concludes the chapter by shining a light on the future scope.

4.2 BACKGROUND

Here we have presented a literature survey on more than 20 research papers to find the study gap in EEG-based decoding mechanisms. Perceptual brain decoding (PBD) is an emerging subdomain that includes detecting an external perceptual (e.g., visual, audio) stimulus using brain responses (evoked by such stimuli). This is the understanding of any person's cognitive processes, like seeing, perceiving, attending to, or remembering by analyzing their brain activity patterns [3]. Both cognitive and therapeutic benefits can be found in perceptual brain decoding. The activity patterns in early visual areas can be predicted with remarkable accuracy by using brain imaging as presented by [4]. Several neurocognitive studies [5–9] have been carried out by combining features from event-related potential (ERP) components, utilizing implicit human processing to classify images, predicting variations of perceptual performance, and organizing the human object vision pathway on the neural basis of perceptual learning. To explain cortical responses at ventral-stream areas, image recognition on static pictures is presented by [10] using a convolutional neural network (CNN) on functional magnetic resonance imaging data from humans watching natural movies. A deep learning architecture on EEG classification for visual brain decoding via metric learning was presented by [11], using 1-D CNN (on the time axis) followed by 1-D CNN (on the channel axis) and Siamese network (for metric learning). Visual stimuli classification for Alzheimer's disease subjects using deep convolutional neural network-based EEG signals was reported by [12].

On the same data set, the proposed framework is benchmarked against EEG-based image classification algorithms [13, 14], which are the most recent deep learning approaches, and the baseline method, representational similarity-based linear discriminant analysis (RS-LDA) [15]. Some research also shows how CNNs can be used to decode information in the brain. Schirrmeister et al. [16] investigate different

CNN topologies for deciphering imagined stimuli from EEG data. A very recent work [17] presented a pipeline for EEG decoding based on convolutional neural networks CNNs. Changing discriminant features on a trial-by-trial level shows the accurate classification of single-trial EEG outperforming existing multi-variate pattern analysis (MVPA). With the use of topology-preserving multispectral pictures and LSTM-based features, Bashivan et al. [18] describe a unique approach for learning appropriate representations of EEG signals from raw EEG data. The brain activity of a person executing a visual task has also been studied in recent studies [19, 20]. However, only a few approaches [21, 22] have been devised to address the difficulty of decoding EEG data linked with visual perception tasks. On the ThoughtViz data set, Tirupattur et al. [23] suggested a deep learning network for the classification of long-duration EEG signals while executing a visual perception task.

One of the popular works in this direction is on preparing the Mind Big data IMAGENET data set [1, 2]. It was constructed utilizing the stimulus of seeing a random image from the ImageNet ILSVRC2013 [24] train data set [25] (14,012 so far) and thinking about it on a computer while attempting to focus on the digit for two seconds. The experiments are all run on the ImageNet-EEG data set, which is the industry standard for EEG-based image classification. Spampinato et al. [13] presented this data set as a freely available EEG data set for brain imaging categorization. The authors [26] proposed an LSTM-based deep learning network for EEG classification based on digits-based visual stimuli on a short-duration data set from the same source (Mind Big data) that we employed in this study. The authors of [27] offered another method using a GRU-based deep network on the same data set. As a result, the Mind Big data is recorded using four devices, with EEG signals from a four-channel MUSE device being used by the authors of both [26] and [27] (details are in the subsequent section). The classification accuracy for these works, however, ranges between 11% and 30%. Our present work uses Mind Big data, and we have chosen to use the EEG signal acquired with the Emotiv Epoc device, which has 14 channels, because there is a lot of room for growth in terms of classification performance on this data set. The contribution of the proposed work is for seeking decent accuracy on Mind Big data by applying three ML models (DNN, CNN, and LSTM) with the combinations of three optimizers (Adam, RMSprop, and AdaGrad).

4.3   PROPOSED WORK

To begin the process of image classification by EEG analysis, data sets and documents related to MindBigData IMAGENET are studied. This data set is preprocessed, and the required features are extracted for deep learning approaches for classification. The pipeline of the proposed work in as shown in Figure 4.1. Further, componentwise detailed information is provided in this section subsequently.

4.3.1   DATA SET

IMAGENET of the brain recorded EEG data from a single subject viewing 14,012 stimulus presentations spanning 13,998 ILSVRC 2013 training images and 569 classes, each for 3 s, over a one-year period [1]. The number of images per class ranged

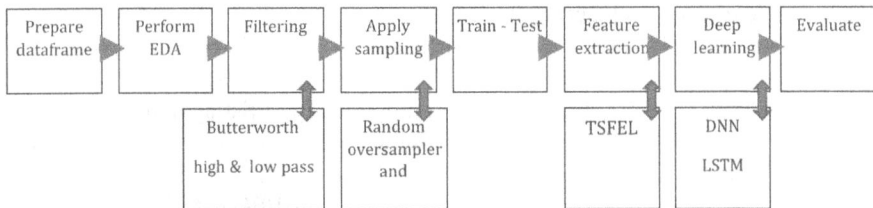

FIGURE 4.1 Pipeline of deep learning implementation for EEG signals classification.

from 8 to 44. Fourteen images were presented as stimuli twice. It was recorded by the subject themselves with a single consumer-grade EEG recording device (Emotiv Insight) with five electrodes. (The number of "brain signals" reported by Vivancos [1, 2] differs from the above due to the multiplication of the stimulus presentations by the number of electrodes.)

For each EEG data point associated with a single image, there is one comma-separated values (CSV) file that is kept in a plain text format. We used the file "Mind Big data Imagenet Insight n09835506 15262 1 20.csv" as an example of the naming convention.

- "MindBigData Imagenet Insight" is only concerned with EEG headset utilized by Insight at the time.
- n09835506 corresponds to the ILSVRC2013 synsent image category. For this instance, n09835506 is "ballplayer, baseball player." A WordReport-v1.04.txt file is also provided that has three files for each row, separated by a tab for each category name, EEG image recorded count, and synsent ID respectively.
- 15262 relates to the specific image from the aforementioned category. This image, for example, is n09835506 15262.jpeg from the ILSVRC2013 trainn09835506 folder, and all of the images are from the ILSVRC2013 train data set.
- _1_ refers to the number of EEG sessions recorded for this image. Normally it is only one, but several brain recordings for the same image are conceivable. The second one will be two, and so on.
- _20 refers to a global session number where the EEG signal for this image was recorded. Just five images are shown in each session, in order to avoid long recording durations with intervals of 3 s of visualization and 3 s of the black screen between them.

Each EEG channel recorded is represented by five lines of plain text, ending with a new line escape character in each CSV file. For the Insight Headset, channel values such as AF3, AF4, T7, T8, and PZ can be used to identify the signal's 10/20 brain region.

4.3.2 Data Preparation

The data set has 70,060 EEG signals of the brain recorded in three-second intervals with the brain stimulus by looking at a random image. These are saved in a CSV file with a unique name identifying the image category and session ID. A sample

TABLE 4.1
WordReport-v104.txt

Index	Category	eeg_image_count	Synsent ID
0	Felis catus, Felis domesticus, house cat, domestic cat	24	n02121808
1	Python sebae, rock snake, rock python,	29	n01744401
2	Chihuahua	32	n02085620
3	Flute, transverse flute	28	n03372029
4	Urocyon cinereoargenteus, gray fox	25	n02120505
5	Bassinet	29	n02804414
...	...	...	...
...	...	...	...
564	Keeshond	19	n02112350
565	Corkscrew, bottle screw	23	n03109150
566	Angora, Angora rabbit	21	n02328150
567	Coffee maker	28	n03063338
568	Pot, flowerpot	25	n03991062

is presented in Table 4.1. Signals from five channels are included in each file (AF3, AF4, T7, T8, and PZ). To reduce noise in signals, we used EDA and experimented with several filters.

The followed broad steps are mentioned here, and a detailed description of these is mentioned in the subsequent section.

- Step 1: 140,072 data files are merged resultant 70,060 rows and 450 columns are made up.
- Step 2: On the basis of data from WordReport-v1.04, categories are merged with the merged.csv file.
- Step 3: Exploratory data analysis is performed to study attributes of features and signals.
- Step 4: Sampling techniques are used to remove the imbalance in the data set.
- Step 5: High-pass and low-pass filtering methods are used to reduce noise in signals.
- Step 6: The data model was produced by train-test-split after shuffling the data to remove bias in classification.
- Step 7: Different deep learning models are developed.
- Step 8: The results are compiled with the Adam optimizer and fit the model on the test data set.
- Step 9: Performance of the model is evaluated using the train, test accuracies, and loss.

4.3.3 Exploratory Data Analysis (EDA)

Exploratory data analysis is the crucial process of using summary statistics and graphical representations to undertake preliminary investigations on data in order to uncover patterns, spot anomalies, test hypotheses, and verify assumptions. To study attributes of categorical features and signals, we used the matplotlib package to visualize data features, plot histograms, and pie charts. The EDA steps are as follows:

- Check the shape
- Check and fill null values
- Retain columns with at least 90% data
- Check data types of columns
- Drop unnecessary columns
- Reduce class density
- Perform multivariate analysis (correlation matrix)
- Perform univariate analysis (signals after and before filtering)

4.3.4 FILTERING BUTTERWORTH HIGH AND LOW PASS

A Butterworth filter is a signal processing filter with a frequency response in the pass-band that is as flat as possible. As a result, the Butterworth filter is sometimes referred to as a "maximally flat magnitude filter." We applied a Butterworth filter of order 2, i.e., the scipy.signal.butter() function for noise reduction in signals, using high-pass and low-pass filtering methods, with a low cut at 20 Hz and a high cut at 50 Hz. A sampling frequency of 128 Hz is given for our EEG data. The standard filtering paradigm is followed by removing the DC (0 Hz frequency) parameter from the data. We have used a backward-forward filter using scipy.signal.filtfilt(). To extract the relevant EEG bands (alpha band, beta band, and theta band), an additional bandpass filter (3–30 Hz) is applied. The sample signal before and after filtering is presented in Figure 4.2 (a and b).

The observations noticed by EDA indicate that there are too many target classes in the data set that may lead to significantly less accuracy. The data set is highly unbalanced and has too many classes distribution. To correct these observed anomalies from the data set, we have introduced subcategories to replace these classes to reduce the class distribution and target class problem in the data set.

The unique image_category is 569, and this unique image_category belongs to the unique 29 category, i.e., 569 image_category target classes are replaced with

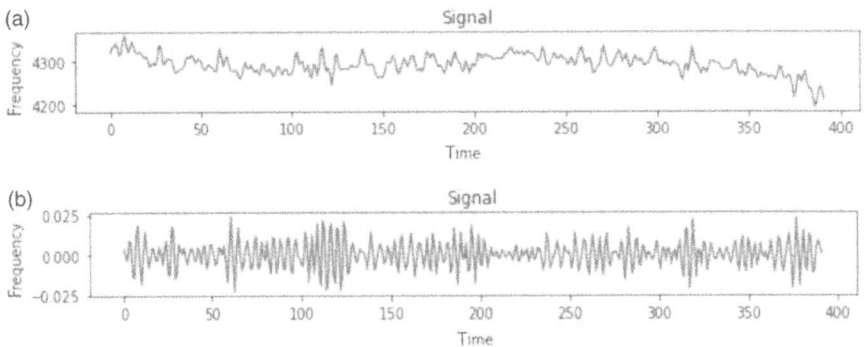

FIGURE 4.2   (a) Before filtering; (b) after filtering.

29 category target classes. These 29 target classes are further replaced with nine target classes, as follows:

- 9 Target classes are replaced with one Target class, Animals: Mammals, Bird, Reptile, Fish, amphibian, Asteroidea, Arthropods, arachnids, Insect.
- 4 Target classes are replaced with one Target class, Tool: Tool, MusicInstrument, Medical Instrument, Stationary.
- 2 Target classes are replaced with one Target class, Fashion: Clothe, Cosmetics.
- 3 Target classes are replaced with one Target class, Home_Appliances: KitchenWare, Electronics, Furniture.
- 2 Target classes are replaced with one Target class, Transport: Vehicle, shipboat.
- 1 Target class is replaced with one Target class, Sports: Sports
- 4 Target classes are replaced with one Target class, Place: Road, Place, Airport, Event.
- 3 Target classes are replaced with one Target class, Food: Fruit, Food, Vegetable.
- 1 Target class is replaced with one Target class, Human: Human.

4.3.5 HANDLING IMBALANCED DATA

The original distribution of target columns was highly unbalanced, as shown in Figure 4.3.

Sampling techniques were used to handle unbalanced data. Sampling is a technique for obtaining information about a population based on statistics from a portion of the population (a sample) rather than having to analyze each individual. Two types of sampling techniques are used: random oversampling and random undersampling.

- Random undersampling is the process of removing examples from the majority class from the training data set at random. The number of examples in the majority class in the modified version of the training data set is reduced as a result of this. This method can be repeated until the desired class distribution, such as an equal number of samples for each class, is attained.

```
Class=0, n=38675 (55.203%)
Class=2, n=3190 (4.553%)
Class=5, n=2695 (3.847%)
Class=7, n=5045 (7.201%)
Class=3, n=8565 (12.225%)
Class=8, n=5895 (8.414%)
Class=6, n=2905 (4.146%)
Class=4, n=745 (1.063%)
Class=1, n=2345 (3.347%)
```

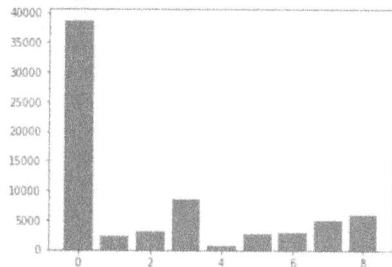

FIGURE 4.3 Class distribution before sampling.

```
Class=0, n=9668 (23.550%)
Class=1, n=2345 (5.712%)
Class=2, n=3190 (7.770%)
Class=3, n=8565 (20.863%)
Class=4, n=745 (1.815%)
Class=5, n=2695 (6.565%)
Class=6, n=2905 (7.076%)
Class=7, n=5045 (12.289%)
Class=8, n=5895 (14.359%)
```

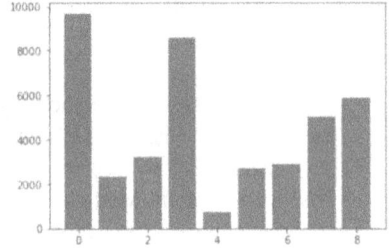

FIGURE 4.4   Class distribution after random undersampling.

- Random oversampling entails duplicating minority class instances and adding them to the training data set at random. Replacement is used to select examples from the training data set at random. This means that minority class examples can be selected and introduced to the new "more balanced" training data set repeatedly; they are selected from the original training data set, added to the new training data set, and then returned or "replaced" in the original data set, allowing them to be selected again.

  Firstly, if we undersample the majority of classes by using RandomUnderSampler(), we get the class distribution shown in Figure 4.4.

  Then we oversample the minority classes by using RandomOverSampler(), and we get the class distribution as shown in Figure 4.5.

  Figure 4.6(a) shows the class distribution of 29 previously described Target (category) classes before sampling procedure. Figure 4.6(b) shows the class distribution after the sampling procedure classes, which are further replaced with nine Target (sub_category) classes. The prepared data frame with shape size before (70,060, 392) and (87,012, 392) after sampling is presented in Figure 4.3.

- We have also employed the synthetic minority oversampling technique (SMOTE) to handle an unbalanced data set. SMOTE is an oversampling technique that differs from traditional oversampling. The minority data

```
Class=0, n=9668 (11.111%)
Class=1, n=9668 (11.111%)
Class=2, n=9668 (11.111%)
Class=3, n=9668 (11.111%)
Class=4, n=9668 (11.111%)
Class=5, n=9668 (11.111%)
Class=6, n=9668 (11.111%)
Class=7, n=9668 (11.111%)
Class=8, n=9668 (11.111%)
```

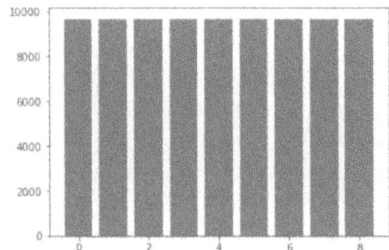

FIGURE 4.5   Class distribution after random oversampling.

(a)

(b)

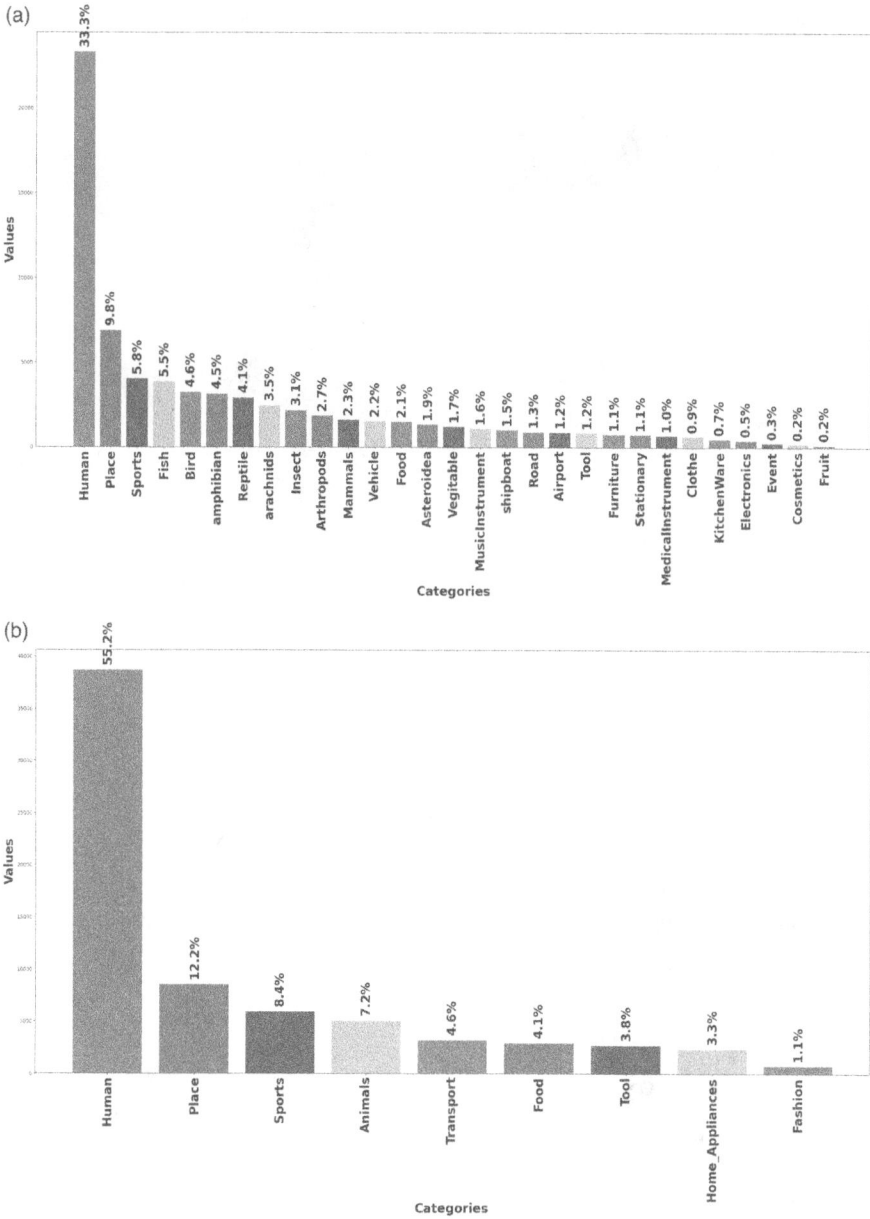

FIGURE 4.6   (a) Class distribution before sampling; (b) class distribution after sampling.

population is duplicated in traditional oversampling techniques like random oversampling. While it increases the amount of data, it does not
provide the machine learning model with any additional knowledge or
variation. While SMOTE generates synthetic data using the k-nearest-
neighbor technique. SMOTE begins by selecting random data from the

```
Before OverSampling, counts of label '0': 38675
Before OverSampling, counts of label '1': 2345

Before OverSampling, counts of label '2': 3240

Before OverSampling, counts of label '3': 8565

Before OverSampling, counts of label '4': 745

Before OverSampling, counts of label '5': 2695

Before OverSampling, counts of label '6': 2905

Before OverSampling, counts of label '7': 5045

Before OverSampling, counts of label '8': 5895

After OverSampling, the shape of X: (348075, 392)
After OverSampling, the shape of y: (348075,)

After OverSampling, counts of label '0': 38675
After OverSampling, counts of label '1': 38675
After OverSampling, counts of label '2': 38675
After OverSampling, counts of label '3': 38675
After OverSampling, counts of label '4': 38675
After OverSampling, counts of label '5': 38675
After OverSampling, counts of label '6': 38675
After OverSampling, counts of label '7': 38675
After OverSampling, counts of label '8': 38675
```

FIGURE 4.7 SMOTE result analysis.

minority class, after which the data's k-nearest neighbors are determined. The random data and the randomly chosen k-nearest neighbor would then be combined to create synthetic data. We can see the result of smote analysis in Figure 4.7 and the EEG signal data frame with 5 rows × 450 columns in Figure 4.8.

4.4 IMPLEMENTATION

4.4.1 CLASSIFICATION ALGORITHMS

After filtering, we split and prepare data for the final model. First, we shuffle the data frame to remove bias in classification and split data using sklearn.model_selection import train_test_split, where test size is 30% of the data frame and

	category	global_session_id	number_of_sessions	image_id	image_category	channels	t_1	t_2	t_3	t_4
0	Mammals	2602	1	4823	n02077923	AF3	4320.000000	4332.307692	4334.871795	4342.564103
1	Mammals	2602	1	4823	n02077923	AF4	4294.871795	4305.128205	4298.974359	4307.179487
2	Mammals	2602	1	4823	n02077923	T7	4187.692308	4200.000000	4208.717949	4199.487179
3	Mammals	2602	1	4823	n02077923	T8	4203.076923	4224.615385	4249.743590	4231.794872
4	Mammals	2602	1	4823	n02077923	Pz	4145.128205	4138.461538	4145.128205	4142.051282

5 rows × 450 columns

FIGURE 4.8 EEG signal data frame.

remaining for the training data set, i.e., X_train.shape, X_test.shape, y_train. shape, and y_test.shape ([60,908, 392], [26,104, 392], [60,908, 9], [26,104, 9]). Out of the various classification algorithms available, we have applied deep learning algorithms for this task. Unlike typical machine learning methods, deep learning necessitates the use of high-end equipment. Deep learning algorithms have the biggest advantage over machine learning algorithms in that they strive to learn high-level features from data incrementally. This reduces the need for domain expertise and the extraction of hard-core features. For in-depth learning, the DNN, RNN(LSTM), and CNN are three basic neural network topologies that perform well on various types of input.

- Deep Neural Network (DNN): The primary purpose of a neural network is to receive a set of inputs, do more complex computations on them, and then output results to solve real-world problems like categorization. We are only interested in neural networks that feed information forward. There is an input, an output, and a continuous flow of data in a deep network. To be trained, deep learning models rely substantially on data sets. Backpropagation is the most common way to train DL models. Deep learning is the study of how to train huge neural networks with complicated input–output transformations.
- Long Short-Term Memory (LSTM): The LSTM network captures data in a sequential fashion, which helps to keep a sentence's word order. LSTMs are a form of RNN. They were made to deal with the problem of long-term reliance. In a conventional RNN, the problem frequently emerges when connecting old knowledge to new information. This problem is known as *long-term dependency*.
- Convolutional Neural Network (CNN): CNNs are frequently utilized in computer vision, and they have also been used in speech recognition acoustic modeling. Convolutional neural networks work with the idea of a "moving filter" that moves across an image. This moving filter, also known as convolution, is applied to a group of nodes, such as pixels, where the filter is 0.5 times the node value. CNNs are a type of multilayer neural network. The input data are supposed to be photographed, and the layers can be as many as 17 or more. When using CNNs, the number of parameters that need to be modified is significantly decreased. As a result, CNNs are capable of handling raw images with high dimensionality.

Training a deep learning model is computationally complicated where we have implemented DNN, 3-D CNN, and 3-D LSTM models in this research. There are many internal hyperparameters that demand a well-planned fine-tuning, such as, number epoch, number batches, loss, optimizers, etc. For this purpose, we implemented 3-D models, as these models use 3-D kernels to make segmentation predictions for a volumetric patch of a scan. The ability to leverage interslice context can lead to improved performance; therefore, we tried different epochs and batches. The loss function in our case was categorical cross-entropy, a common choice when classifying between different classes. The dropout technique is used to minimize overfitting. The three optimizer methods are worked upon to use the loss and calculate the new possible value. We have used three optimizers in our research: Adam, root mean squared propagation (RMSProp), and the adaptive gradient algorithm (AdaGrad). In our architecture, we have tuned some hyperparameters and performed early stopping. On training a model, if the validation accuracy did not increase in 50 epochs, it stopped the training. The next three sections explain the implementation of DNN, LSTM, and CNN.

4.4.1.1 DNN

Figure 4.9 presents the architecture of the DNN model, and Figure 4.10 presents the DNN layers structure along with the detailed pipeline subsequently.

Input: merged data.
Output: Fully trained DNN model.
Process:

1. Load the data set using the read_csv() function.
2. Check for null values and drop unnecessary columns.
3. The shape of this data frame is 70,060 rows and 393 columns.
4. Apply the Butterworth filter with a 128 Hz sample rate and a 20 Hz low cut and 50 Hz high cut for low pass and high pass with 64 Hz of Nyquist frequency.
5. Use random oversampling and random undersampling to balance these filtered data.
6. Split this balanced data into 70% training and 30% testing.
7. The DNN model is constructed with 13 layers in total: eight are dense layers, and five are dropout layers.
8. The Relu activation function is used in the dense layer.
9. The Softmax activation function is used in the output dense layer.
10. By using Adam optimizer and 0.2 dropout, we get the highest test accuracy at 72.39%.

4.4.1.2 LSTM

The LSTM architecture is presented in Figure 4.11, with the LSTM layers structure in Figure 4.12. The detailed pipeline is presented subsequently.

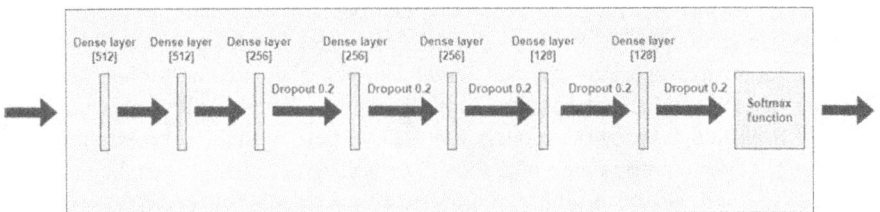

FIGURE 4.9 DNN architecture.

```
Layer (type)                    Output Shape                    Param #
=================================================================
dense (Dense)                   (None, 512)                     201216

dense_1 (Dense)                 (None, 512)                     262656

dense_2 (Dense)                 (None, 256)                     131328

dropout (Dropout)               (None, 256)                     0

dense_3 (Dense)                 (None, 256)                     65792

dropout_1 (Dropout)             (None, 256)                     0

dense_4 (Dense)                 (None, 256)                     65792

dropout_2 (Dropout)             (None, 256)                     0

dense_5 (Dense)                 (None, 128)                     32896

dropout_3 (Dropout)             (None, 128)                     0

dense_6 (Dense)                 (None, 128)                     16512

dropout_4 (Dropout)             (None, 128)                     0

dense_7 (Dense)                 (None, 9)                       1161
=================================================================
Total params: 777,353
Trainable params: 777,353
Non-trainable params: 0
```

FIGURE 4.10   DNN layers structure.

Input: merged data.
Output: fully trained LSTM model.
Process:

1. Load the data set using the read_csv() function.
2. Check for null values and drop unnecessary columns.
3. The shape of this data frame is 70,060 rows and 393 columns.
4. Apply the Butterworth filter with 128 Hz sample rate and 20 Hz low cut and 50 Hz high cut for low pass and high pass with 64 Hz of Nyquist frequency.

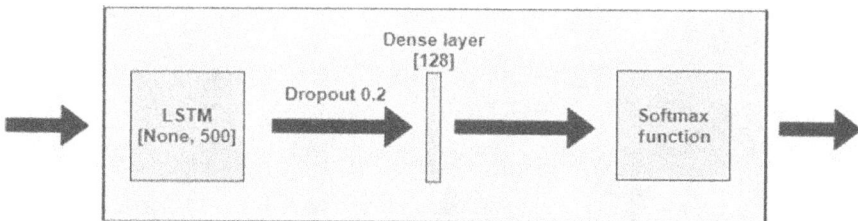

FIGURE 4.11   LSTM architecture.

```
Layer (type)                  Output Shape               Param #
=================================================================
lstm (LSTM)                   (None, 500)                1786000

dropout_3 (Dropout)           (None, 500)                0

dense_1 (Dense)               (None, 128)                64128

dense_2 (Dense)               (None, 9)                  1161
=================================================================
Total params: 1,851,289
Trainable params: 1,851,289
Non-trainable params: 0
```

FIGURE 4.12 LSTM layers structure.

5. Use random oversampling and random undersampling to balance these filtered data.
6. Split these balanced data into 70% training and 30% testing.
7. LSTM model is constructed with 4 layers in total, 1 LSTM layer, 2 are Dense layers and 1 is a Dropout layer.
8. Relu activation function is used in Dense Layer.
9. Softmax activation function is used in Output Dense Layer.
10. By using Adam optimizer and 0.2 Dropout we get the highest accuracy Test accuracy at 72.91%

4.4.1.3 CNN

Figure 4.13 is the architecture of the CNN model, and Figure 4.14 is the CNN layers structure.

Input: Merged data
Output: Fully trained CNN model
Process:

1. Load the dataset using read_csv() function.
2. Check for Null values and drop unnecessary columns.
3. Shape of this data frame is 70060 rows and 393columns.
4. Apply Butterworth filter with 128hz sample rate and 20 Hz lowcut and 50 Hz high-cut for Low pass and High pass with 64hz of Nyquist frequency.

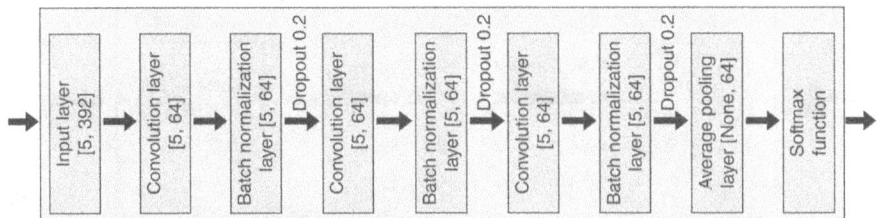

FIGURE 4.13 CNN architecture.

```
Layer (type)                    Output Shape            Param #
=================================================================
input_1 (InputLayer)            [(None, 5, 392)]            0

conv1d (Conv1D)                 (None, 5, 64)            75328

batch_normalization (BatchNo    (None, 5, 64)              256

dropout (Dropout)               (None, 5, 64)                0

re_lu (ReLU)                    (None, 5, 64)                0

conv1d_1 (Conv1D)               (None, 5, 64)            12352

batch_normalization_1 (Batch    (None, 5, 64)              256

dropout_1 (Dropout)             (None, 5, 64)                0

re_lu_1 (ReLU)                  (None, 5, 64)                0

conv1d_2 (Conv1D)               (None, 5, 64)            12352

batch_normalization_2 (Batch    (None, 5, 64)              256

dropout_2 (Dropout)             (None, 5, 64)                0

re_lu_2 (ReLU)                  (None, 5, 64)                0

global_average_pooling1d (Gl    (None, 64)                   0

dense (Dense)                   (None, 9)                  585
=================================================================
Total params: 101,385
Trainable params: 101,001
Non-trainable params: 384
```

FIGURE 4.14   CNN layers structure.

5. Use Random Oversampling and Random Undersampling to balance this filtered data.
6. Split these balanced data into 70% training and 30% testing.
7. CNN model is constructed with 15 layers in total, one Input layer, three convolution layers, three BatchNormalization layers, three dropout layers, and one AveragePooling layer.
8. The Relu activation function is used in the dense layer.
9. The Softmax activation function is used in the output dense Layer.
10. By using Adam optimizer and 0.2 dropout, we get the highest test accuracy at 73.54%.

4.5   EVALUATION AND RESULTS DISCUSSION

The experiments were performed with different algorithms and with hyperparameter tuning. In this section, we discuss the metric used for evaluation purposes as well as the results produced using the recommended methodology.

1. Metrics for evaluation
   - **Accuracy**
     We have used accuracy metrics, which are critical for assessing a model's performance. It would be necessary to grasp these measures in order to do so. The term *accuracy* refers to the ratio of the number of right predictions to the total number of input samples in classification accuracy. It only works when there is an equal number of samples in each class.
     - Accuracy rate = TP + TN/TP + FP + FN + TN
     - Error rate = FP + FN/TP + FP + FN + TN
   - **Precision**
     Precision refers to the number of true positives divided by the total number of positive predictions (i.e., the number of true positives plus the number of false positives).
   - **Recall**
     The number of correct positive predictions produced out of all possible positive predictions is referred to as recall.
   - **F1-Score**
     F1-Score is a precision and recall metric. It's commonly referred to as the harmonic mean of the two.

The loss function in our case was categorical cross-entropy, a common choice when classifying between different classes. Dropout is a technique to minimize overfitting. We have tried different dropouts, such as 0.2, 0.3, and 0.5. We got the best accuracy in 0.2 dropouts: 72.39% in DNN, 73.25% in CNN, and 72.81 in LSTM. The optimizer is the method to use the loss and calculate the new possible value. We tuned the hyperparameter to use 100–500 epochs and with batch size 32. Too many epochs can lead to overfitting of the training data set, whereas too few may result in an underfit model. We also added early stopping to stop training at the point when performance on a validation data set starts to degrade. If we were training a model and the validation accuracy did not increase in 50 epochs, it stopped the training.

We compared our best results of DNN, LSTM, and CNN models in Tables 4.2–4.4.

TABLE 4.2
DNN, LSTM, and CNN Models Results for EEG Signals Classification

Models	Dropout	Train Accuracy	Test Accuracy
DNN	0.2	96.28	72.39
	0.3	92.60	70.90
	0.5	61.11	52.33
CNN	0.2	99.25	73.25
	0.3	95.97	70.86
	0.5	79.09	67.47
LSTM	0.2	98.71	72.81
	0.3	97.76	70.03
	0.5	99.51	67.47

TABLE 4.3
DNN, LSTM, and CNN Models Results on Different Optimizers

Models	Dropout	Optimizer	Train Accuracy	Test Accuracy
DNN	0.2	Adam	96.28	72.39
		RMSprop	56.37	48.62
		AdaGrad	62.18	51.34
CNN	0.2	Adam	99.25	73.54
		RMSprop	93.72	70.22
		AdaGrad	100	73.25
LSTM	0.2	Adam	98.71	72.91
		RMSprop	99.36	72.81
		AdaGrad	12.76	11.01

Figures 4.15–4.17 show the output graphs of accuracy and loss for training and validation. The epochs run were 500 with early stopping. The training and validation losses were comparable in the graphs for the CNN, DNN, and LSTM models.

In DNN architecture, we experimented with dropout layers and optimizers. We found that we get the highest test accuracy of 72.39% with precision of 0.72 and recall of 0.71, giving an F1-Score of 0.71, while taking 0.3 dropout we get accuracy of 70.92% by using 0.2 dropout and the Adam optimizer. At the same time, we see a significant drop in accuracy at 52.33% when we take 0.5 dropout with the Adam optimizer.

We experimented on the LSTM architecture because this approach takes less time to train and is less expensive computationally. In this architecture, we experimented with dropout layers and optimizers. Here we found that by using 0.2 dropout and the Adam optimizer, we get the highest test accuracy of 72.91% with precision of 0.73 and recall of 0.72, giving an F1-Score of 0.72, while taking 0.3 dropout we get accuracy of 70.03% and we see a significant drop in accuracy at 67.47% when we take 0.5 dropout with the Adam optimizer.

TABLE 4.4
Metrics of DNN, LSTM, and CNN Models Results on Different Optimizers

Models	Dropout	Optimizer	Precision	Recall	F1-Score
DNN	0.2	Adam	0.72	0.71	0.71
		RMSprop	0.45	0.36	0.31
		AdaGrad	0.47	0.39	0.42
CNN	0.2	Adam	0.74	0.73	0.73
		RMSprop	0.68	0.61	0.64
		AdaGrad	0.75	0.72	0.74
LSTM	0.2	Adam	0.73	0.72	0.72
		RMSprop	0.74	0.71	0.72
		AdaGrad	0.14	0.12	0.12

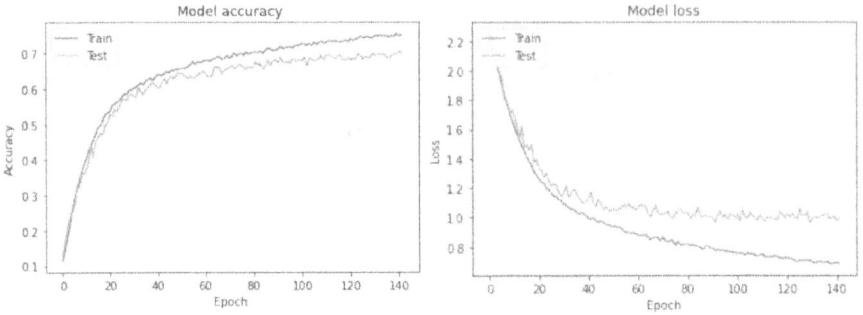

FIGURE 4.15   Accuracy and loss graph for CNN.

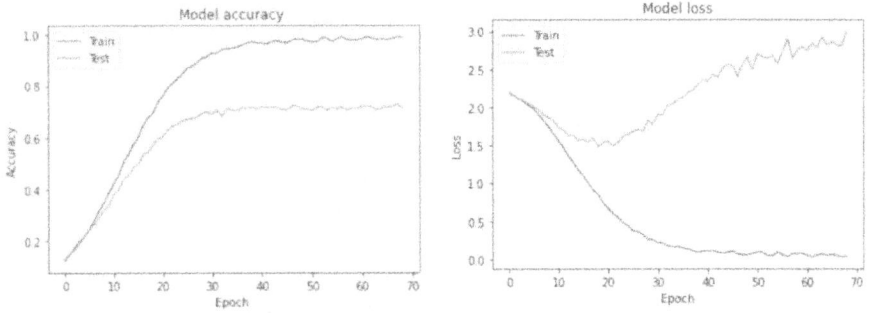

FIGURE 4.16   Accuracy and loss graph for LSTM.

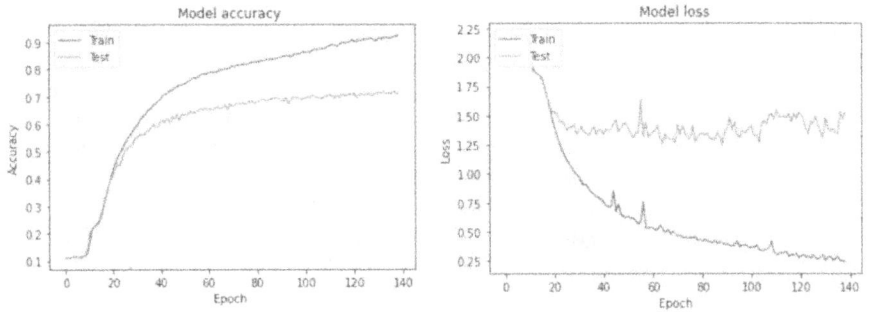

FIGURE 4.17   Accuracy and loss graph for DNN.

We experimented with dropout layers and optimizers in CNN architecture. By using 0.2 dropout and the Adam optimizer, we get the highest test accuracy of 73.54% with precision of 0.74 and recall of 0.73, giving an F1-Score of 0.73, while taking 0.3 dropout we get accuracy of 70.86% and see a significant drop in accuracy at 67.47% when we take 0.5 dropout with the Adam optimizer.

We conclude our result that CNN architecture yields best accuracy of 73.54%. LSTM is a close second with 72.91% being computationally easy, and third is DNN architecture with 72.39%.

1. **AUC-ROC curve for evaluation**

   The area under the curve (AUC)–receiver operating characteristic (ROC) curve is a performance statistic for classification issues at various threshold levels. AUC represents the degree or measure of separability, whereas ROC is a probability curve. It indicates how well the model can distinguish between classes. The AUC indicates how well the model predicts 0 classes as 0 and 1 courses as 1. The higher the AUC, the better the model predicts 0 classes as 0 and 1 classes as 1. By analogy, the higher the AUC, the better the model distinguishes between people who have the condition and those who do not.

   The ROC curve is a graph with the true positive rate (TPR) on the y-axis and the false positive rate (FPR) on the x-axis, as we can see in Figure 4.18.

   Following are the formulas of TRP and FPR:

   $$TPR/Recall/Sensitivity = TP/TP + FN$$

   $$FPR = 1 - Specificity$$

   $$= FP/TN + FP$$

   Figures 4.19–4.21 present the ROC curve for the CNN pipeline.

   As we can see in Figures 4.19–4.21, the cases of CNN for the Adam optimizer and RMSprop optimizer are giving good results in comparison with

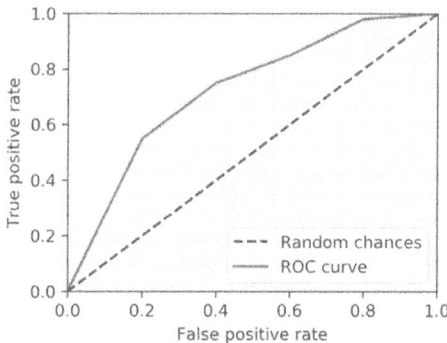

FIGURE 4.18   Example of the ROC curve and AUC.

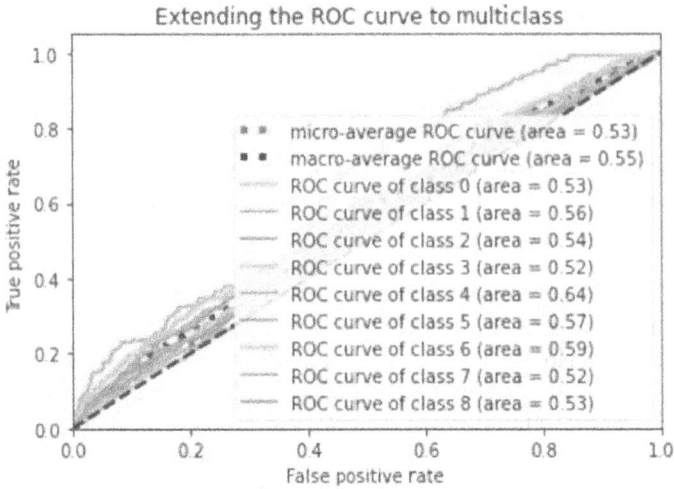

FIGURE 4.19 ROC curve for CNN with the AdaGrad optimizer.

the AdaGrad optimizer. This result suggests that the Adam and RMSprop optimizers are doing good job of classification of different classes compared to the AdaGrad optimizer. This study concludes that the Adam or RMSprop optimizer is better suited for these types of tasks.

ROC curve evaluation with the DNN pipeline is presented in Figures 4.22–4.24 with the AdaGrad, Adam, and RMSprop optimizers.

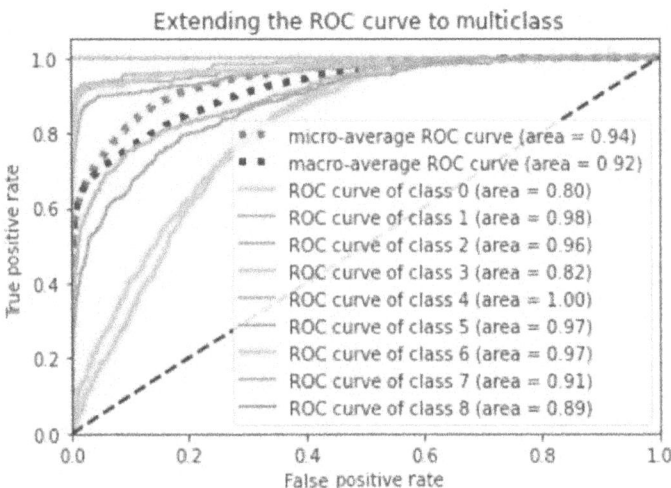

FIGURE 4.20 ROC curve for CNN with the Adam optimizer.

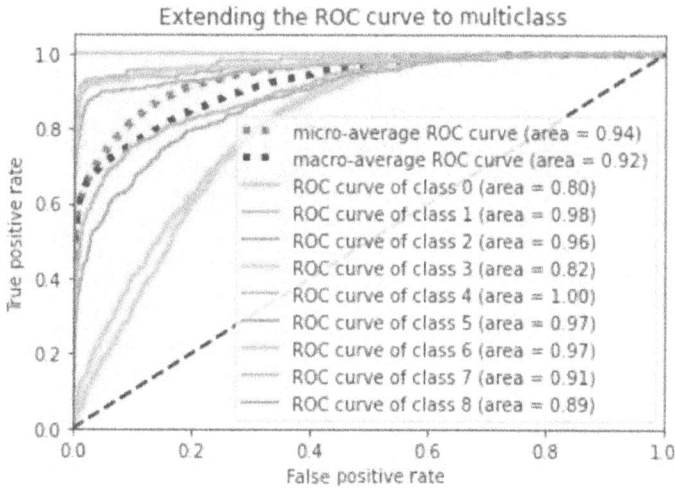

FIGURE 4.21 ROC curve for CNN with the RMSprop optimizer.

As we can see in the case of DNN in Figures 4.22–4.24, the Adam optimizer outperforms both the AdaGrad and RMSprop optimizers. This result suggests that the Adam optimizer is doing the best job of classification of different classes compared to the RMSprop optimizer, which is giving relatively good results compared to AdaGrad. This study concludes that the Adam optimizer is best suited for these types of tasks.

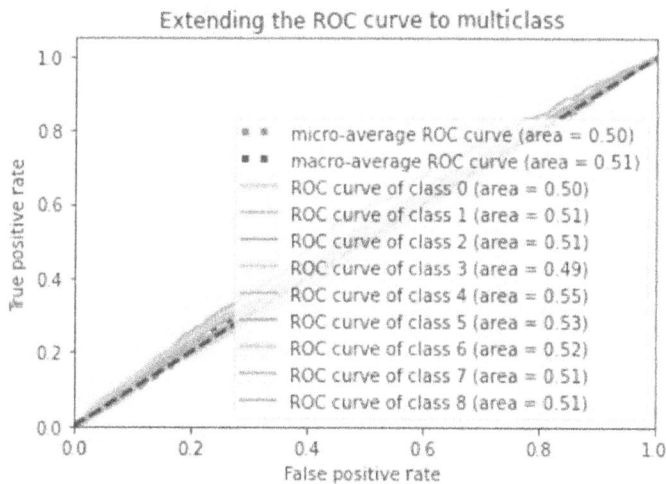

FIGURE 4.22 ROC curve for DNN with the AdaGrad optimizer.

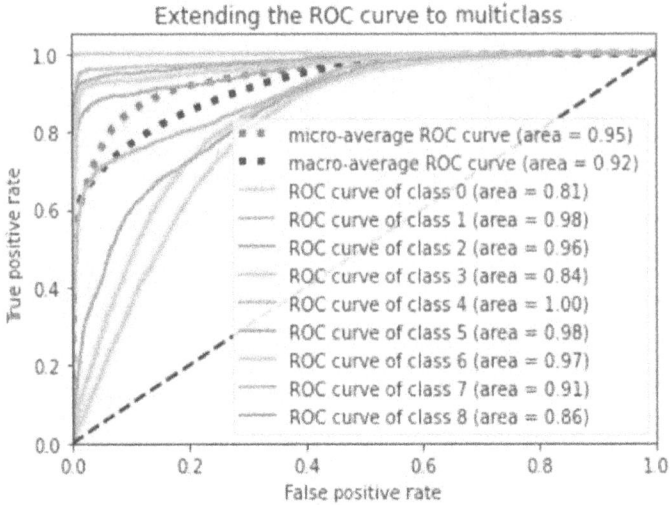

FIGURE 4.23   ROC curve for DNN with the Adam optimizer.

2. ROC curve evaluation with LSTM architecture

As we can see in Figures 4.25–4.27, the case of LSTM for the Adam optimizer and RMSprop optimizer are giving good results in comparison with the AdaGrad optimizer. This result suggests that the Adam and RMSprop optimizers are equally good in classification of different classes compared to the AdaGrad optimizer. This study concludes that the Adam optimizer or RMSprop optimizer are better suited for these types of tasks compared

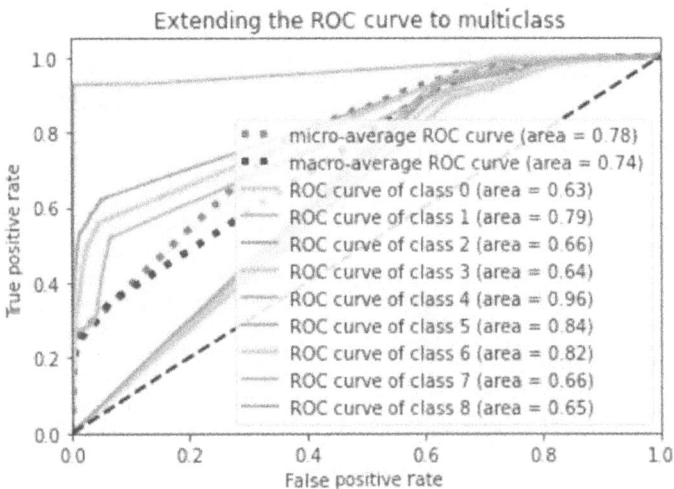

FIGURE 4.24   ROC curve for DNN with the RMSprop optimizer.

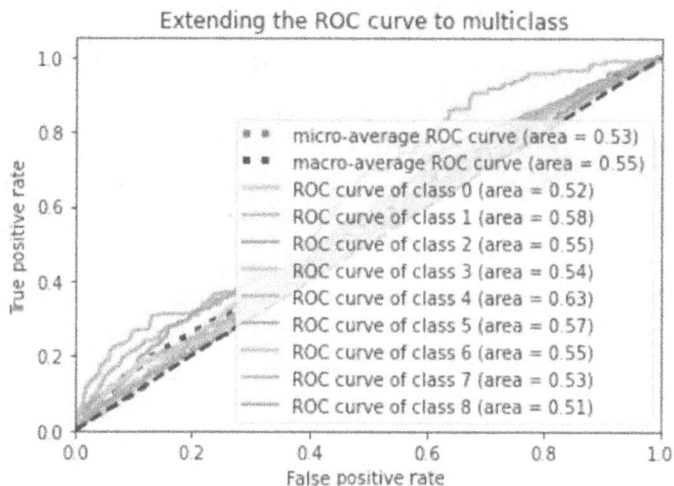

FIGURE 4.25 ROC curve for LSTM with the AdaGrad optimizer.

to AdaGrad as both the Adam and RMSprop optimizers perform equally well in this case.

4.6 CONCLUSION AND FUTURE SCOPE

A standard EEG-based image classification data set ImageNet-EEG is extensively used for experiment in research. This chapter proposed three deep learning models for EEG-based image classification along with their implementation and comparison.

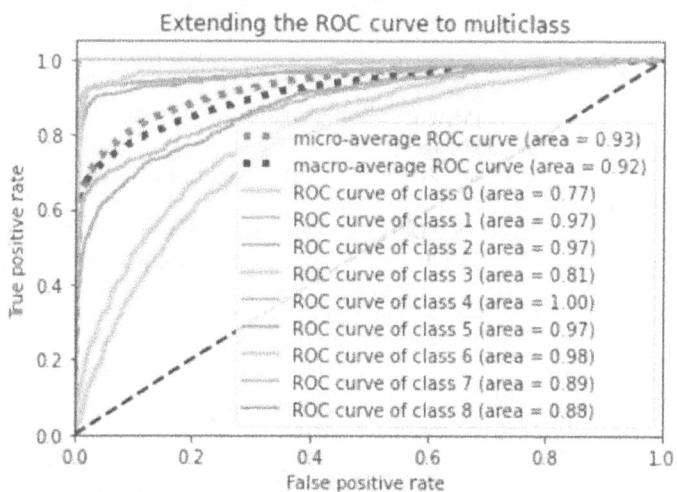

FIGURE 4.26 ROC curve for LSTM with the Adam optimizer.

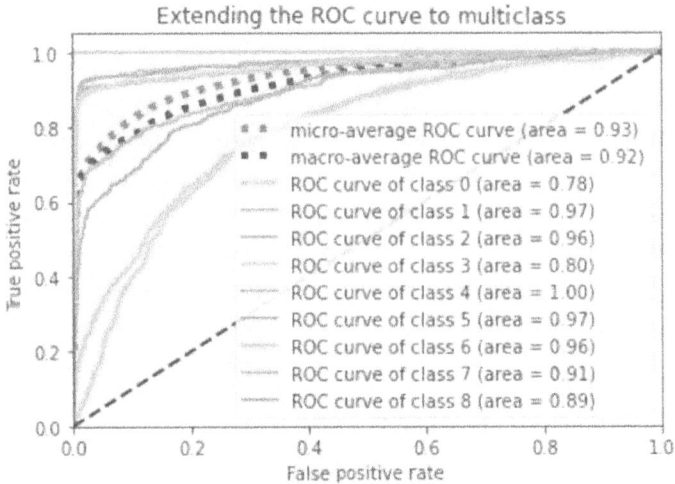

FIGURE 4.27 ROC curve for LSTM with the RMSprop optimizer.

We have accessed the effective accuracy of the proposed pipelines and validated the results under experimental setups.

As we have seen, CNN can perform efficiently to classify EEG signals generated by seeing random images. We can increase the model's performance by adjusting the number of epochs, layers, data resampling, and signal noise reduction. Hyperparameter tuning and modifications to the CNN model can improve the accuracy with which researchers can read spectrograms and help us anticipate the proper label. It motivates us to further extend the research in two aspects: (i) utilizing spectrogram images of EEG brain signals by the CNN classifier and (ii) applying various filtering and sampling techniques to get better accuracy.

REFERENCES

1. Vivancos, D. (2018). "IMAGENET" of the brain. Retrieved from http://www. Mindbigdata.com/opendb/imagenet.html
2. Vivancos, D. (2019). The "MNIST" of brain digits. Retrieved from http://www. Mindbigdata.com/opendb/
3. Tong, F., and Pratte, M. S. "Decoding patterns of human brain activity." *Annual Review of Psychology* 63 (2012): 483–509. https://doi.org/10.1146/annurev-psych-120710-100412
4. Kamitani, Y., and Tong, F. "Decoding the visual and subjective contents of the human brain." *Nature Neuroscience* 8 (2005): 679–685. [PMC free article] [PubMed] [Google Scholar].
5. Op de Beeck, H. P., Torfs, K., and Wagemans, J. "Perceived shape similarity among unfamiliar objects and the organization of the human object vision pathway." *Journal of Neuroscience* 28, 40 (2008): 10111–10123. https://doi.org/10.1523/JNEUROSCI.2511-08.2008. [PMC free article] [PubMed] [CrossRef] [Google Scholar].
6. Gilbert, C. D., Sigman, M., and Crist, R. E. "The neural basis of perceptual learning." *Neuron* 31, 5 (2001): 681–697. https://doi.org/10.1016/S0896-6273(01)00424-X

7. Das, K., Giesbrecht, B., and Eckstein, M. P. "Predicting variations of perceptual performance across individuals from neural activity using pattern classifiers." *Neuroimage* 51, 4 (2010): 1425–1437. https://doi.org/10.1016/j.neuroimage.2010.03.030

8. Wang, C., Xiong, S., Hu, X., Yao, L., and Zhang, J. "Combining features from erp components in single-trial EEG for discriminating four-category visual objects." *Journal of Neural Engineering* 9, 5 (2012): 056013. https://doi.org/10.1088/1741-2560/9/5/056013

9. Shenoy, P., and Tan, D. (2008). Human-aided computing: Utilizing implicit human processing to classify images. Retrieved from https://www.microsoft.com/en-us/research/publication/human-aided-computing-utilizing-implicit-human-processing-to-classify-images/

10. Wen, H., Shi, J., Zhang, Y., Lu, K.-H., Cao, J., and Liu, Z. "Neural encoding and decoding with deep learning for dynamic natural vision." *Cerebral Cortex* 28, 12 (2017): 4136–4160. https://doi.org/10.1093/cercor/bhx268

11. Mishra, R., and Bhavsar, A. "EEG classification for visual brain decoding via metric learning." *Proceedings of the 14th International Joint Conference on Biomedical Engineering Systems and Technologies (BIOSTEC 2021) – Volume 2: BIOIMAGING*, pages 160–167, https://doi.org/10.5220/0010270501600167, ISBN: 978-989-758-490-9, SCITEPRESS, Setúbal – Portugal, 2021.

12. Komolovaitė, D., Maskeliūnas, R., and Damaševičius, R. "Deep convolutional neural network-based visual stimuli classification using electroencephalography signals of healthy and Alzheimer's disease subjects." *Life* 12, 3 (2022): 374. https://doi.org/10.3390/life12030374

13. Spampinato, C., Palazzo, S., Kavasidis, I., Giordano, D., Souly, N., and Shah, M. "Deep learning human mind for automated visual classification." *Proceedings of the IEEE Conference on Computer Vision and Pattern Recognition*, 2017, pp. 6809–6817.

14. Palazzo, S., Spampinato, C., Kavasidis, I., Giordano, D., and Shah, M. (2018). Decoding brain representations by multimodal learning of neural activity and visual features. Abs/1810.10974. Retrieved from http://arxiv.org/abs/1810.10974

15. Kaneshiro, B., Perreau Guimaraes, M., Kim, H. S., Norcia, A. M., and Suppes, P. "A representational similarity analysis of the dynamics of object processing using single-trial EEG classification." *Plos One* 10, 8 (2015): e0135697. [PMC free article] [PubMed] [CrossRef] [Google Scholar].

16. Schirrmeister, R. T., Springenberg, J. T., Fiederer, L. D. J., Glasstetter, M., Eggensperger, K., Tangermann, M., Hutter, F., Burgard, W., and Ball, T. "Deep learning with convolutional neural networks for EEG decoding and visualization." *Human Brain Mapping* 38, 11 (2017): 5391–5420.

17. Aellen, F. M., Göktepe-Kavis, P., Apostolopoulos, S., and Tzovara, A. "Convolutional neural networks for decoding electroencephalography responses and visualizing trial by trial changes in discriminant features." *Journal of Neuroscience Methods* 364 (2021): 109367. ISSN 0165-0270. https://doi.org/10.1016/j.jneumeth.2021.109367

18. Bashivan, P., Rish, I., Yeasin, M., and Codella, N. (2015). "Learning representations from EEG with deep recurrent-convolutional neural networks." arXiv preprint arXiv:1511.06448.

19. Nishimoto, S., Vu, A. T., Naselaris, T., Benjamini, Y., Yu, B., and Gallant, J. L. "Reconstructing visual experiences from brain activity evoked by natural movies." *Current Biology* 21, 19 (2011): 1641–1646.

20. Huth, A. G., De Heer, W. A., Griffiths, T. L., Theunissen, F. E., and Gallant, J. L. "Natural speech reveals the semantic maps that tile human cerebral cortex." *Nature* 532, 7600 (2016): 453–458.

21. Kapoor, A., Shenoy, P., and Tan, D. "Combining brain computer interfaces with vision for object categorization." *IEEE Conference on Computer Vision and Pattern Recognition*. IEEE, Alaska, USA, 2008, pp. 1–8.

22. Bigdely-Shamlo, N., Vankov, A., Ramirez, R. R., and Makeig, S. "Brain activity-based image classification from rapid serial visual presentation." *IEEE Transactions on Neural Systems and Rehabilitation Engineering* 16, 5 (2008): 432–441.

23. Tirupattur, P., Rawat, Y. S., Spampinato, C., and Shah, M. "Thoughtviz: Visualizing human thoughts using generative adversarial network." Association for Computing Machinery, New York, 2018. [Online]. Retrieved from https://doi.org/10.1145/3240508.3240641

24. Deng, J., Dong, W., Socher, R., Li, L. J., Li, K., and Li, F. F. *IEEE Conference on Computer Vision and Pattern Recognition, 2009. CVPR 2009.* ImageNet: A large-scale hierarchical image database, Miami, FL, 2009, pp. 248–255. [Google scholar].

25. Russakovsky, O.*, Deng, J.*, Su, H., Krause, J., Satheesh, S., Ma, S., Huang, Z., Karpathy, A., Khosla, A., Bernstein, M., Berg, A. C., and Fei-Fei, L. (* = equal contribution). (2015). ImageNet Large Scale Visual Recognition Challenge. IJCV. paper | bibtex | paper content on arxiv.

26. Bird, J. J., Faria, D. R., Manso, L. J., Ekart, A., and Buckingham, C. D. "A deep evolutionary approach to bioinspired classifier optimization for brain-machine interaction." *Complexity* 2019 (2019): 4316548:1–4316548:14

27. Jolly, B. L. K., Aggrawal, P., Nath, S. S., Gupta, V., Grover, M. S., and Shah, R. R. "Universal EEG encoder for learning diverse intelligent tasks." *IEEE Fifth International Conference on Multimedia Big Data (BigMM).* IEEE, Singapore, Singapore, 2019, pp. 213–218.

5 Automatic Brain Tumor Segmentation in Multimodal MRI Images Using Deep Learning

Seyyed-Mahdi Banan-Khojasteh
and Mohammad-Ali Balafar
Department of Computer Engineering,
University of Tabriz, Tabriz, Iran

CONTENTS

5.1 INTRODUCTION

Abnormal cell growth inside the brain might cause a tumor. These tumors of the brain are divided into benign and malignant categories. The former ones have a uniform structure, but the latter ones have active cells of cancer with a structure that is not uniform [1]. Meningioma and glioma tumors are examples of low-grade tumors. The appearance of these tumors is similar to that of the normal ones, and their growth is fairly slow. On the contrary, astrocytoma and glioblastoma (GBM) tumors are malignant ones that have faster growth in contrast to the former ones. Gliomas are broadly classified as glioma with high grade and as glioma with low grade. The gliomas that are in the high-grade class grow faster than low-grade gliomas. Magnetic resonance imaging (MRI) is used to find out whether these tumors are invasive or noninvasive,

DOI: 10.1201/9781003324430-7

as well as to analyze them. MRI is an effective method to help diagnose these tumors and for detecting tumors with soft tissue and is, therefore, a famous technique for imaging of the brain [2, 3, 4].

The MRI scan is a noninvasive anatomic imaging approach that is used for detecting and keeping the track of the disease. This method is based on an advanced technology that changes the alignment of liquid protons. To image organs, structures using MRI magnetic fields are used. In many cases, an MRI scan provides different information about the internal structure of the body compared to what is observed with an X-ray, ultrasound, or CT scan. This approach is also being used to detect issues that cannot be seen with other imaging methods. By detecting the released energy of the radio frequency on the body organs, MRI scans are built. The amount of returned energy and the taken time reveals the chemical structure of the scanned organ. Based on these magnetic properties, doctors can tell the difference between various classes of tissue. The MRI image is obtained by placing the patient inside a magnetic field, and sometimes, to increase contrast and the brightness of the imaging, contrastive materials are injected into the patient [5]. The modalities of magnetic resonance images are categorized as Flair, T2, T1, and T1ce. During magnetic resonance imaging, the period when two energy pulses are sent one after another is the repetition time, and the delay of the sent and the received pulse is the reflection time. By changing the values of repetition time and reflection time, different magnetic resonance imaging modalities are obtained. T1 modality has the lowest repetition time and reflection time, and the Flair modality has the highest repetition time and reflection time. The T1c modality has better contrast than the T1 modality. The reason why the contrast of the T1c modality is better than T1 is the injection of gadolinium contrast agent to the person before the start of imaging. This material makes the vessels brighter in the form of magnetic resonance and thus improves the contrast of the scan. The brightness intensity of different tissues in magnetic resonance imaging modalities is different, and each modality has its applications [6].

Image segmentation is the most crucial stage of the analysis of biomedical images, which aims to gather information in the images like edges, shapes, and the identity of each region. In this process, through the description of features, areas are identified and prepared to reduce them in a suitable form for computer processing and recognition of each area. The desired segmentation results will have a crucial effect on the accuracy of image analysis. Segmentation is generally referred to as the procedure of dividing the shape into its main parts and localizing the desired areas. One of the most difficult steps in image processing is the segmentation task, which is very effective in the success of the image analysis process. For the segmentation of 2-D images, various methods are available, which are divided into some general categories: methods based on histogram or thresholding, methods based on region analysis, and methods based on classification. The important point is that each of these three general methods also has methods in its subset. In methods based on histograms, images are segmented based on how the pixels of the image are distributed. The main part of histogram methods is to identify a suitable threshold level to apply to the scans. In the region analysis methods, the neighborhoods of each pixel are examined to find common features and attributes such as edges. In methods based on classification, likenesses and connections between scans are utilized to classify the data. In these methodologies, the data are grouped so that those placed in the same group have the maximum similarity to each other [7].

The glioma brain tumor segmentation is still a challenge because these tumors can be diagnosed anywhere in the brain with an unknown appearance with fuzzy and blurry boundaries with healthy tissue [3].

5.2   RELATED WORKS

Brain tumor segmentation studies have been categorized into supervised, and unsupervised learning bases [8–11]. The combination of region growing and fuzzy clustering methods in the segmentation task using T2 and T1 was done by Hsieh et al. [12]. Using fuzzy c-mean for segmenting the tumors, Wu et al. [13] reached solid results even though the used data set was sparse. Balafar et al. [14, 15] used fuzzy c-mean for medical image segmentation. To initialize seed points, region growth methodologies are used. Mainly, when the initialization is inappropriate, their segmentation is not accurate. As a result, we are going to need better methods.

Convolutional neural networks (CNNs) are widely used to extract rich features from input data [16]. CNNs have been designed to obtain hierarchical contextual features from input tensors [14]. Pereira et al. [16] used a 2-D CNN-based model to automatically segment brain tumor scans and achieved compelling results in the BRATS 2013 challenge. With the advent of dense prediction networks, the prediction of voxel labels in the input patch became more accurate and faster. Shen et al. [1] used a fully convolutional network (FCN) to do segmentation of brain tumors. The fully connected layer is replaced with a convolutional layer in FCNs and has up-sampling layers to retrieve its initial shape. To do an effective segmentation of the glioma tumors, Zhao et al. [4] used a mixture of FCN with conditional random fields (CRF).

U-Net was primarily designed and used for the segmentation of biomedical scans. Its architecture is built on an encoder block followed by a decoder block. U-Net is an important model and acquires satisfactory results in biomedical image segmentation because encoding features with contextual information and decoding features consisting of semantic information are combined in hierarchical order [17]. U-Net is used by Caver et al. [18] in BRATS 2018 and got 87.8% in dice score. Abd-Ellah et al. [19] used two U-Nets in parallel with each other to do the segmentation. The segmentation accuracy improved by utilizing both parallel paths. Wang et al. [20] proposed the WRN-PP-Net model using a concatenation of the global features at different stages of the network, so DSC is enhanced, which denotes network soundness. A 3-D patch-based U-Net was presented by Cabezas et al. [21], which utilizes 3-D information in MRI scans. Hu et al. [22] used 3-D-dilated U-Net, which got 86% in the dice score. For efficient learning of the representations in deep neural networks, a detachable 3-D U-Net was proposed by Chen et al. [23]. Three-dimensional meshes can easily handle 3-D MRI scans.

However, there are some issues when segmentation is done using the U-Net model. As an example, there are a significant number of discrete points in MRI images. In addition, the blurred border of the tumor area and the uneven distribution of unhealthy tissue and healthy tissue make it difficult to learn the features of the tumor area. To improve the problem caused by discrete points, postprocessing is suggested [19, 24]. These postprocessing methods are not efficient due to being separated from the segmentation process. To efficiently decrease the aforementioned problem, multistage cascaded deep neural networks [25, 26] are used in multimodal MRI segmentation of gliomas [27]. In these methods, first the segmentation of the tumor area is done, and then the infrastructure segmentation is limited within this region.

We propose a methodology for the segmentation of these tumors based on MRI scans. Our contributions are threefold in this chapter: (1) to do the glioma brain tumor segmentation, we utilized a modified version of the U-Net model; (2) second, we introduce a block of two-path structures with a residual connection; and finally (3) we propose three new modified U-Net models to get higher performance in the segmentation task using these blocks.

The rest of this chapter is organized as follows: the proposed method is introduced in Section 5.3. Then the experimental results are explained in Section 5.4. And finally, we conclude this research in Section 5.5.

5.3   THE PROPOSED METHOD

This section introduces the proposed method to segment brain tumors. According to Figure 5.1, the input images are enhanced through a preprocessing pipeline, and then modified U-Net-based architectures are used to do the segmentation of the brain tumor scans. All four modalities of MRI images are used to determine the tumor.

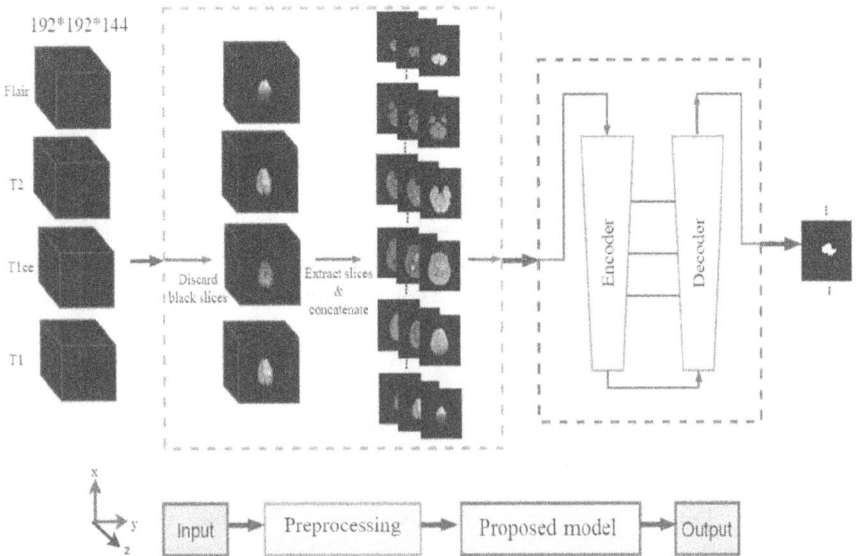

FIGURE 5.1   The overall structure of the proposed methodology.

5.3.1 PREPROCESSING

Data normalization is crucial to be sure that all input parameters have the same distribution. By performing the normalization, the convergence of the network becomes faster. To normalize the data, we subtracted the mean from the value of each pixel and then divided it by the standard deviation. The normalized data's distribution is a Gaussian curve, in which its center is zero. The pixel numbers to be used as input of the model must be positive, so we choose the normalized data scale in the range 0 and 1. Figure 5.2 shows the initial and normalized form of the MRI scan.

Each of the four modalities in our data set is a NIFTY image with a tensor size of [240,240,155] containing a black area with zero-pixel values in the border region, which practically does not affect network training, and their existence increases the computational overhead of the network. In the preprocessing stage, it is cut symmetrically from each side so that the size of the output tensor becomes [192,192,144], which reduces the computational complexity and increases the learning speed. In Figure 5.3, the effect of cropping pixels with zero values around the image is shown.

The segmentation map of the images in the data set is of shape [240,240,155]. Each of the pixels in the segmentation map could take four values in 0, 1, 2, and 4, where pixel values of 0 correspond to the background area of the image, pixel values of 1 correspond to the necrosis and nonenhanced area, pixels with a value of 2 correspond to the edema area, and finally pixel values of 4 correspond to the enhanced region of the glioma tumor. The values of the segmentation map are reencoded to the range of 0–3 for the sake of convenience.

The One-Hot coding method is one of the most widely used approaches and its performance is very good except in cases where the categorical variable takes too many values (usually this method is not suitable for variables that take more than 15 different values). In some cases where the number of variables is less, this method may not be a suitable option. One-Hot encoding creates new binary columns, each

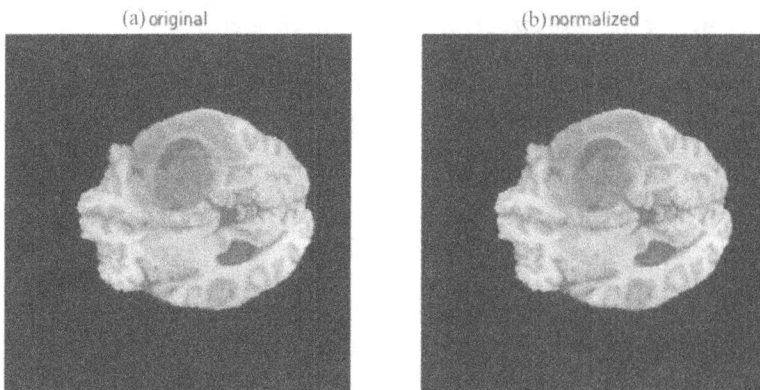

(a) original   (b) normalized

FIGURE 5.2 The effect of Gaussian noise on images: (a) the original image; (b) the image with Gaussian noise.

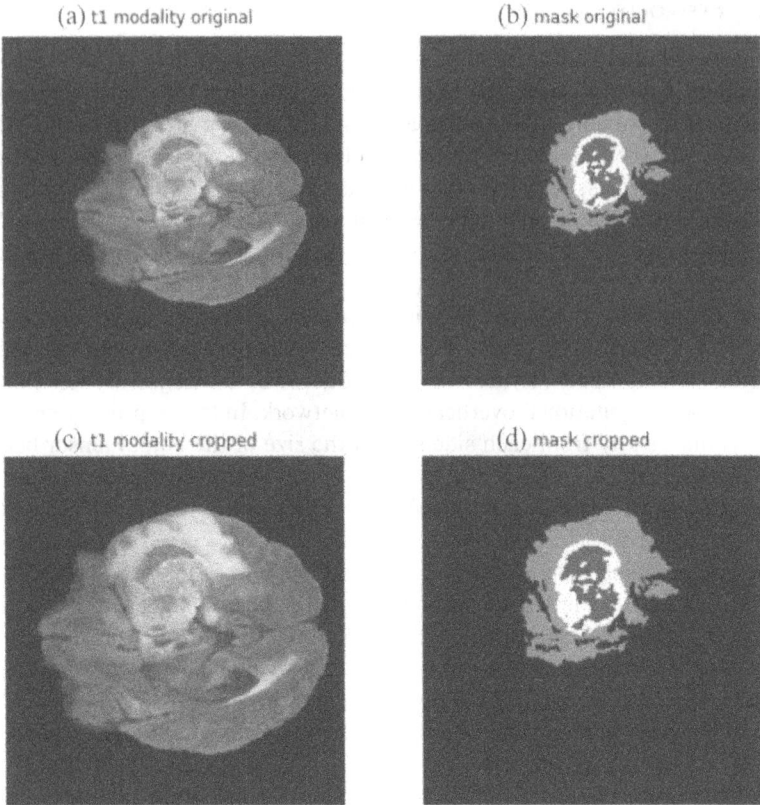

FIGURE 5.3   Cropping operations on images: (a) the original brain MRI image, along with (b) its segmentation map; (c) the cropped image; (d) the cropped segmentation map.

corresponding to one of the values that the variable takes. At this step, the segmentation map's tensor size is of size [192,192,144], which after applying One-Hot encoding becomes [4,192,192,144].

The BRATS 2020 data set consists of 3-D MRI scans of the axial, coronal, and sagittal views. We only used 2-D slices from the axial view that have sufficient contextual features to train the model. Among these MRI images, some of them are black, which adds no value for training the model, so they are discarded in this step of the preprocessing pipeline. Also, those images in which the brain-to-segmentation map ratio was larger than 20% are selected to be fed to the model in the training phase.

For data augmentation, we applied some transformation techniques such as rotation, zooming, sharpening, elastic transformation, and drop out. An example of rotation on the image and segmentation map is shown in Figure 5.4.

Images can be augmented by flipping them horizontally or vertically. The image horizontal and vertical flipping operation with a probability of 50% is done in the preprocessing step, which is shown in Figures 5.5 and 5.6 respectively.

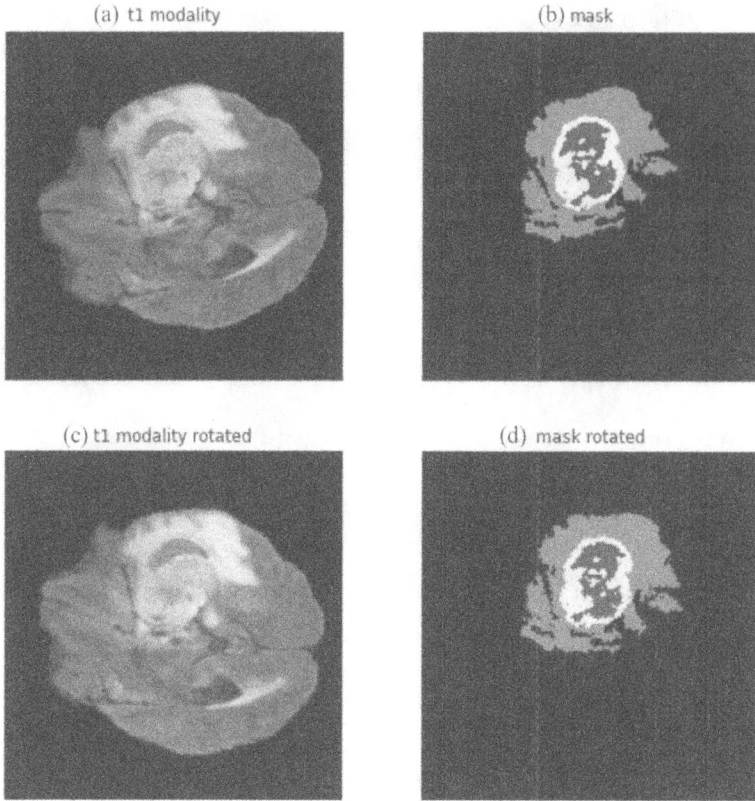

FIGURE 5.4 Rotation operations on images: (a) the original brain MRI image along with (b) its segmentation map; (c) the rotated image and (d) the rotated segmentation map.

5.3.2 Modified U-Net Architecture

In the U-Net architecture, the encoding path of the network consists of a batch of double 3×3 convolutional blocks, ReLU activation functions, and 2×2 max-pooling blocks. Through the encoding path, the number of feature channels is doubled, and the size of the tensor is halved. The decoding path contains a sequence of transposed convolutional blocks, double 3×3 convolutional blocks, and ReLU activation functions. As with FCNs, high-resolution features from the compression path are combined with the up-sample output, which is then fed into a series of convolutional layers. The main difference with FCN is that there are many feature channels in the up-sample part, which allows the network to pass contextual features to higher-resolution layers. Furthermore, the network does not contain fully connected layers but only uses convolutional blocks.

Brain tumor segmentation using U-Net architecture has some weaknesses, such as the size of the tumor is usually very small compared to the whole image, so as the depth of the network increases, due to the presence of max-pooling blocks at the end of each layer, some small tumors disappear in deeper layers, so the power of

(a) t1 modality

(b) mask

(c) t1 modality horizontal flip

(d) mask horizontal flip

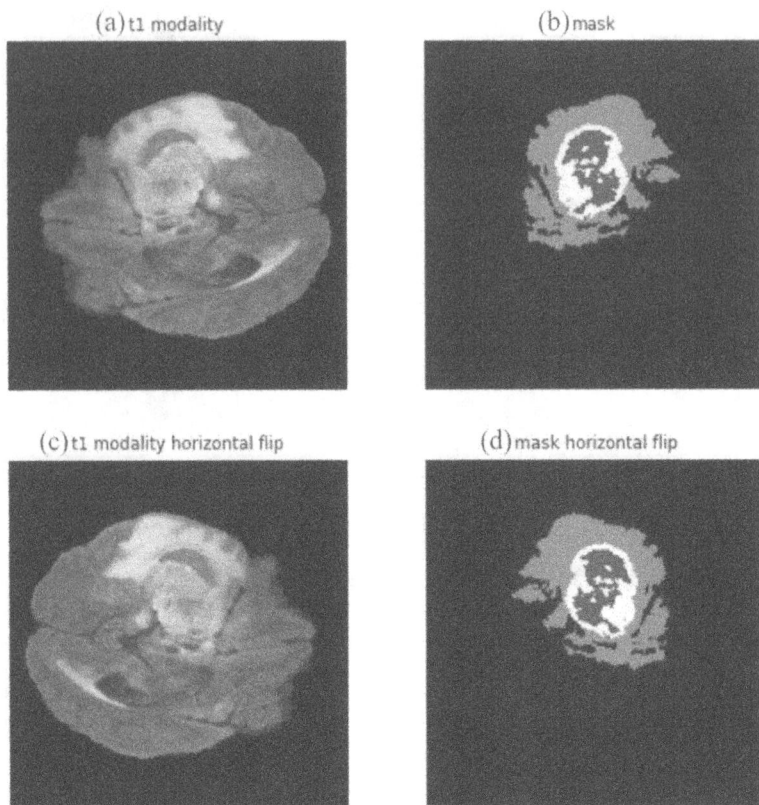

FIGURE 5.5   Horizontal flip operations on images: (a) the original brain MRI image along with (b) its segmentation map; (c) the horizontal flipped image and (d) the horizontal flipped segmentation map.

the next layers to identify tumors is reduced. In addition, the size of the filter in the initial network layers of the U-Net is small, which limits to learning of the local features. These problems reduce the capability of these networks to distinguish tumors precisely. To better learn the global contextual features of the images, as shown in Figure 5.7, we propose a block that consists of two paths: the first path consists of a 3 × 3 convolutional block followed by a residual block, and the second path includes a 5 × 5 convolutional block with padding of size 2 and stride of size 1 followed by batch normalization and the ReLU activation function. The residual block itself contains two paths: one residual connection, and the other one containing double blocks of batch normalization and ReLU alongside with a 3 × 3 convolutional block in which output of these paths are added together before applying another batch normalization plus the ReLU activation function. Finally, in the proposed block output of each path is concatenated together to be passed on to the next layer. The proposed model consists of three layers and is based on the U-Net model and has been obtained by modifying the blocks and layers of the U-Net architecture. In the encoder-modified model, which is shown in Figure 5.8, the proposed block is used on the encoder

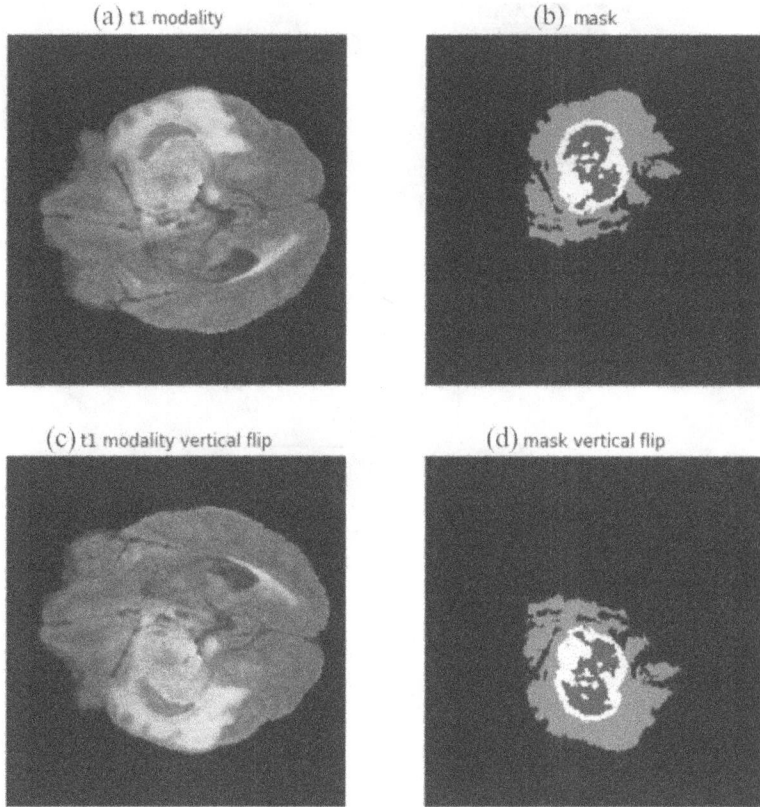

FIGURE 5.6 Vertical flip operations on images: (a) the original brain MRI image along with (b) its segmentation map; (c) the vertical flipped image and (d) the vertical flipped segmentation map.

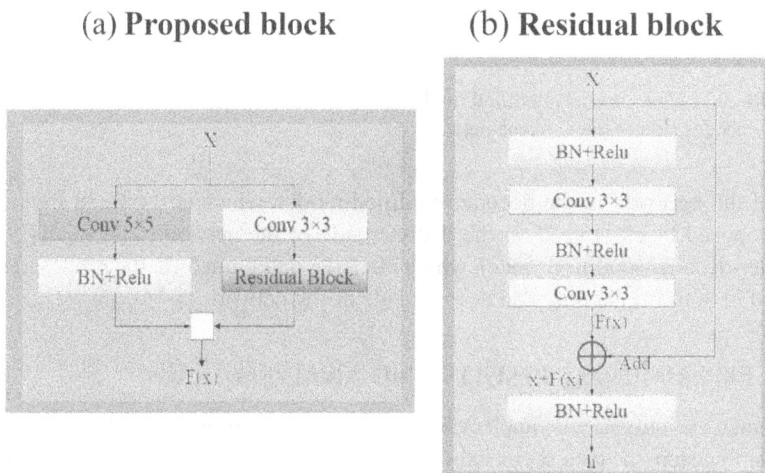

FIGURE 5.7 (a) The proposed block structure; (b) the residual block structure.

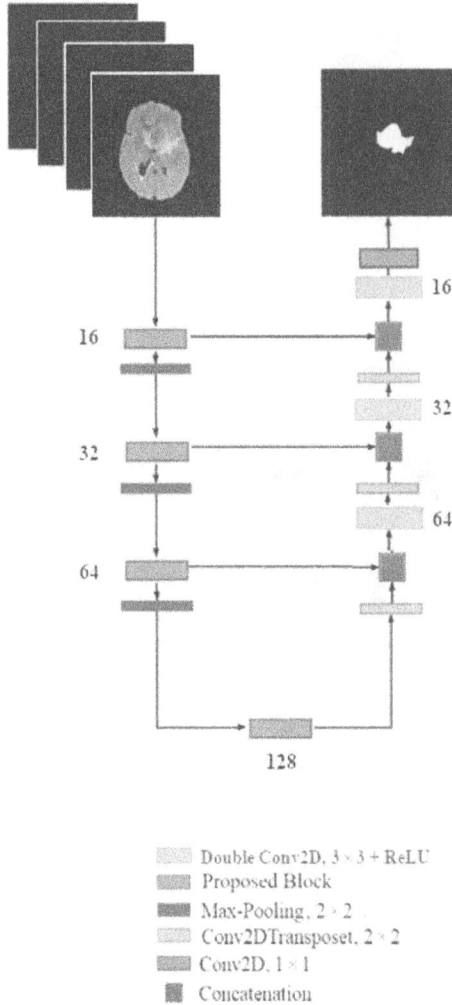

Double Conv2D, 3 × 3 + ReLU
Proposed Block
Max-Pooling, 2 × 2
Conv2DTransposet, 2 × 2
Conv2D, 1 × 1
Concatenation

FIGURE 5.8   The encoder-modified model is shown in which the proposed blocks are used on the encoder side of the U-shape network.

side of the network; in the decoder-modified model, which is shown in Figure 5.9, the proposed block is used on the decoder side of the network; and finally, in the encoder-decoder-modified model, which is shown on Figure 5.10, the proposed block is used in both the encoder and decoder side of the network.

5.4   EXPERIMENTAL RESULTS AND ANALYSIS

Here, first, we introduce the implementation details of the proposed method. Second, in the training step, the data set including 3-D images around the axial axis is converted into 2-D images. After that preprocessing is done on the images, data augmentation is

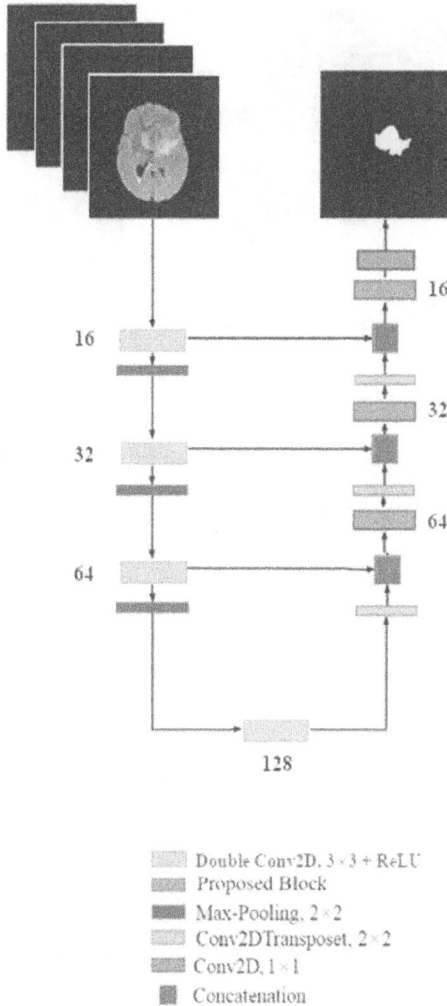

FIGURE 5.9 The decoder-modified model is shown in which the proposed blocks are used on the decoder side of the U-shape network.

performed to improve the learning capability of the proposed network on the data set. We start training the network on the BRATS 2020 data set with the specified number of iterations. After completing the training phase, the proposed models are evaluated.

5.4.1 DATA SET

In this research, the BRATS 2020 data set is used for multimodal brain tumor segmentation. Multiple, clinically common, preoperative multimodality MRI scans of high-grade GBM (HGG) and low-grade glioma (LGG) are used. Here we have 293 patients for HGG and 76 patients for LGG and a total of 369 four-channel 3-D MRI

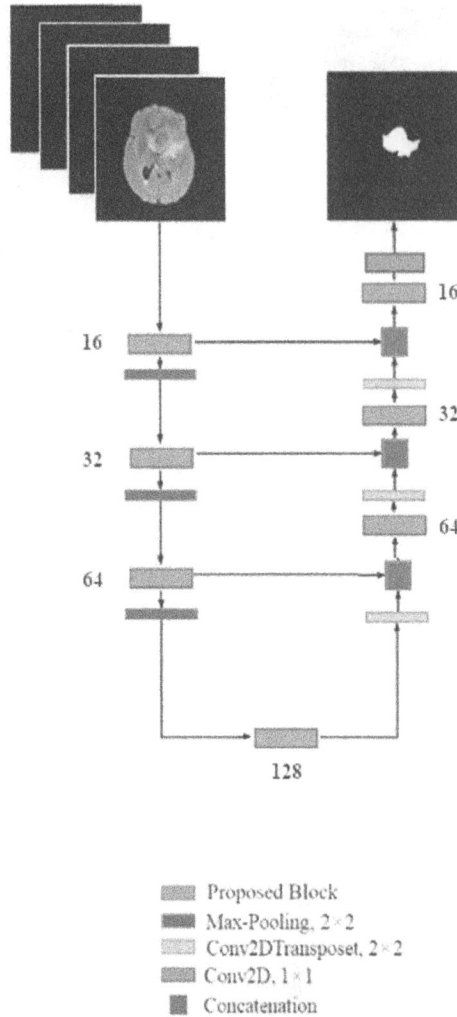

FIGURE 5.10   The encoder-decoder-modified model is shown in which the proposed blocks are used both on the encoder and the decoder side of the U-shape network.

images. Each patient includes four channels – T1, T2, T1ce, and Flair – and segmentation ground truth.

5.4.2   HYPERPARAMETERS OF THE TRAINING

To train the proposed models, we used the Google Colab service and PyTorch library. All four imaging modalities have been trained together, and the hyperparameters in this experiment are:

- Input tensor shape is $(32 \times 4 \times 192 \times 192)$.
- Segmentation map shape is $(4 \times 192 \times 192)$.

- The Softmax is used as last layer activator function.
- Batch_size is with the size of 32.
- The Adam optimizer with lr of 0.003.
- Intersection Over Union (IOU) and Dice SCore (DSC) are used as evaluation metrics.
- The epoch number is 30.

The cross-validation with the fivefold method is used to separate the data set into the training and validation parts, class weights were used in the Dice loss function, and class weights were assigned to each class in proportion to the frequency, for example for class 0, which is healthy or background tissue. The image ratio of the number of pixels of 1 is assigned as the class weight.

5.4.3 EVALUATION CRITERIA

In this research, we will use two main criteria to evaluate the obtained results, considering that TP is the number of positive samples that are correctly labeled, TN is the number of negative samples that are correctly labeled, FP is the number of positive samples that are mislabeled, and FN is the number of negative samples that are mislabeled. In the formulas that follow, "A" represents the shape segmented by the model, and "B" represents the correct map. The total count of pixels in the segmentation region with |A| and the number of correct map pixels with |B| is shown. The evaluation criteria shown in Equation (5.1) and Equation (5.2) are defined as follows:

$$DSC = \frac{2|A \cap B|}{|A| + |B|} \tag{5.1}$$

$$J(A,B) = \frac{|A \cap B|}{|A| + |B| - |A \cap B|} \tag{5.2}$$

5.4.4 CONVERGING OF THE NETWORK

The average value of the cost function is calculated for the train, and the validation steps are calculated to the number of epochs, in 10 iterations of training, as shown in Figure 5.11. The increase in the number of epochs in the training of the proposed models causes an increase in the validation loss. As a result, an optimal value of epochs is chosen to be 30.

5.4.5 PROPOSED MODELS EVALUATION

Table 5.1 indicates the evaluation metrics obtained in the validation step from the BRATS 2020 data set. In the encoder-decoder-modified U-Net, where the proposed block is used on both the encoder and decoder side of the network, the Dice score coefficient and the intersection over the union ratio have increased significantly. In addition to showing the segmentation performed by the proposed models, Figure 5.12 shows

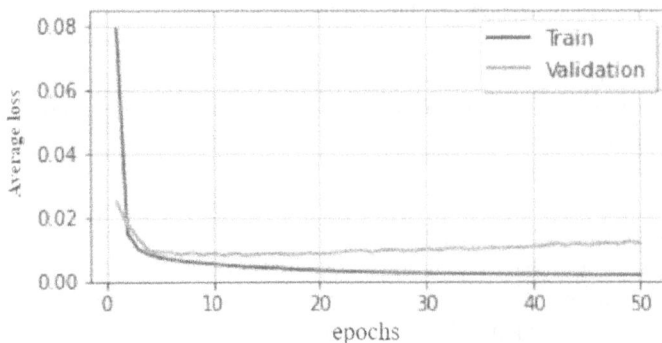

FIGURE 5.11 Average cost function to the number of epochs.

TABLE 5.1
Comparing the Results of Measuring Quantitative Criteria

Models	DSC	IOU
U-Net	90.76	84.25
Encoder-modified U-Net	91.08	84.83
Decoder-modified U-Net	91.48	86.24
Encoder-decoder-modified U-Net	**94.16**	**89.21**

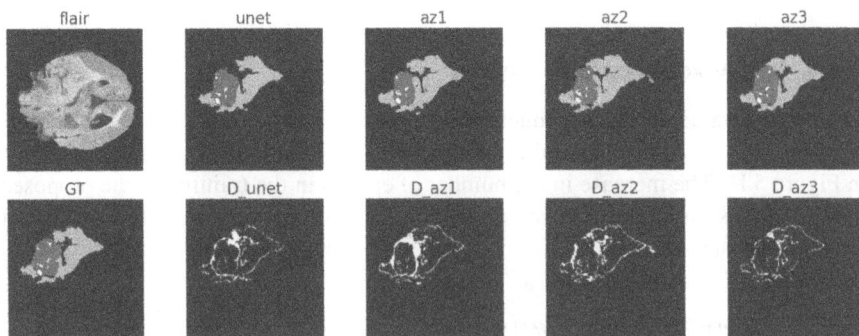

FIGURE 5.12 Difference between predicted and grand truth segmentation. In the first row, flair modality along with predicted segmentation from U-Net, encoder-modified U-Net, decoder-modified U-Net, and encoder-decoder-modified U-Net are shown, and in the second-row the grand truth segmentation map and difference between predicted and grand truth are shown.

the difference between the segmentation map and the predicted segmentation. As is clear from the figure, in the encoder-decoder-modified model, the difference between the grand truth segmentation map and the predicted segmentation decreased compared to other methods. The obtained value of the Dice score for the segmentation results of the encoder-decoder-modified U-Net methodology shows the effectiveness of proposed models in segmenting tumors efficiently.

5.5 CONCLUSION

In this research, we investigated tumor segmentation in brain MRI images using the deep convolutional network. The data set used in this research consists of BRATS 2020 images. Despite the high ability of deep learning methods in learning hierarchical features and automatically extracting features in segmentation, there are problems such as low generalization power. But considering that the feature extraction stage is done automatically, the feature extraction speed is much higher than is the case where the feature extraction is done manually. First, preprocessing operations are performed to increase the data quality for use in the learning phase on MRI images. Then the proposed model is used for brain tumor segmentation. In the proposed model, by using blocks with different filter sizes in the U-Net structure, in addition to local features, global features in MRI images are used simultaneously. With the change made in the structure of U-Net, not only the evaluation criteria such as DSC and IOU have been improved, but also the number of parameters of the proposed model has been reduced in proportion to the U-Net network so that there is no need to perform postprocessing operations in this method.

REFERENCES

1. Shen, H., Zhang, J., and Zheng, W. "Efficient symmetry-driven fully convolutional network for multimodal brain tumor segmentation." *2017 IEEE International Conference on Image Processing (ICIP)*, IEEE, Beijing, China (2017), pp. 3864–3868.
2. Bahadure, N., Kumar Ray, A., and Pal Thethi, H. "Image analysis for MRI based brain tumor detection and feature extraction using biologically inspired BWT and SVM." *International Journal of Biomedical Imaging* 2017 (2017): 1–12.
3. Chena, S., Dinga, C., and Liu, M. Dual-force convolutional neural networks for accurate brain tumor segmentation. Preprint submitted to *Pattern Recognition* (2018): 88. 10.1016/j.patcog.2018.11.009
4. Zhao, X., et al. "A deep learning model integrating FCNNs and CRFs for brain tumor segmentation." *Medical Image Analysis* 43 (2018): 98–111.
5. Wong, K-P. "Medical image segmentation: Methods and applications in functional imaging." In Suri J. S., Wilson D. L., and Laxminarayan S. (eds.). *Handbook of Biomedical Image Analysis.* Topics in Biomedical Engineering International Book Series. Springer, Boston, MA (2005). https://doi.org/10.1007/0-306-48606-7_3
6. Derraz, F., Beladgham, M., and Khelif, M. "Application of active contour models in medical image segmentation." *Proceedings of the International Conference on Information Technology: Coding and Computing* 2 (2004), pp. 675–681.
7. Amin, J., Sharif, M., Yasmin, M., and Fernandes, S. L. "A distinctive approach in brain tumor detection and classification using MRI." *Pattern Recognition Letters* 139 (2017): 118–127.

8. Mei, P. A., de Carvalho, C. C., Fraser, S. J., Min, L. L., Reis, F. "Analysis of neoplastic lesions in magnetic resonance imaging using self-organizing maps." *Journal of Neurological Science* 359 (1–2) (2015): 78–83.

9. Götz, M., Weber, C., Bloecher, J., Stieltjes, B., Meinzer, H-P., and Maier-Hein, K. "Extremely randomized trees based brain tumor segmentation." *Proceedings of BRATS Challenge-MICCAI* (2014), pp. 006–011.

10. Balafar, M. A., Ramli, A. R., and Mashohor, S. "Brain magnetic resonance image segmentation using novel improvement for expectation maximizing." *Neurosciences Journal* 16 (3) (2011): 242–247.

11. Balafar, M. A. "New spatial based MRI image de-noising algorithm." *Artificial Intelligence Review* 39 (3) (2013): 225–235.

12. Hsieh, T. M., Liu, Y-M., Liao, C-C., Xiao, F., Chiang, I-J., and Wong, J-M. "Automatic segmentation of meningioma from non-contrasted brain MRI integrating fuzzy clustering and region growing." *BMC Medical Informatics and Decision Making* 11 (1) (2011): 54.

13. Wu, W., Chen, A. Y., Zhao, L., and Corso, J. J. "Brain tumor detection and segmentation in a CRF (conditional random fields) framework with pixel-pairwise affinity and superpixel-level features." *International Journal of Computer Assisted Radiology and Surgery* 9 (2) (2014): 241–253.

14. Balafar, M. A., Rahman Ramli, A. B. D., Saripan, M. I., Mashohor, S., and Mahmud, R. "Medical image segmentation using fuzzy c-mean (FCM) and user specified data." *Journal of Circuits, Systems and Computers* 19 (01) (2010): 1–14.

15. Balafar, M. A., Ramli, A. B. D. R., Saripan, M. I., and Mashohor, S. "Improved fast fuzzy C-mean and its application in medical image segmentation." *Journal of Circuits, Systems and Computing* 19 (01) (2010): 203–214.

16. Pereira, S., Pinto, A., Alves, V., and Silva, C. A. "Brain tumor segmentation using convolutional neural networks in MRI images." *IEEE Transactions on Medical Imaging* 35 (5) (2016): 1240–1251.

17. Havaei, M., Davy, A., Warde, D., Biard, A., Courville, A., Bengio, Y., and Larochelle, H. "Brain tumor segmentation with deep neural networks." *Medical Image Analysis* 35 (2017): 18–31.

18. Caver, E., Liu, C., Zong, W., Dai, Z., and Wen, N. "Automatic brain tumor segmentation using a U-Net neural network." *International MICCAI BraTS Challenge in Conjunction with the Medical Image Computing and Computer-Assisted Interventions Conference*, Granada, Spain (2018), p. 63.

19. Abd-Ellah, M. K., Khalaf, A. A. M., Awad, A. I., and Hamed, H. F. A. "TPUAR-Net: Two parallel U-Net with asymmetric residual-based deep convolutional neural network for brain tumor segmentation." In Karray, F., Campilho, A., and Yu, A. (eds.). *Image Analysis and Recognition – 16th International Conference, ICIAR 2019, Proceedings* (Lecture Notes in Computer Science (including subseries Lecture Notes in Artificial Intelligence and Lecture Notes in Bioinformatics); Vol. 11663 LNCS), Springer Verlag (2019), pp. 106–116. https://doi.org/10.1007/978-3-030-27272-2_9

20. Wang, Y., Lia, C., Zhua, T., and Zhang, J. "Multimodal brain tumor image segmentation using WRN-PPNet." *Computerized Medical Imaging and Graphics* 75 (2019): 56–65.

21. Cabezas, M., Valverde, S., Gonzalez-Villa, S., Clerigues, A., Salem, M., Kushibar, K., et al. "Survival prediction using ensemble tumor segmentation and transfer learning." *Pre-Conference Proceedings of the 7th MICCAI BraTS Challenge* (2018), p. 54.

22. Hu, X., and Piraud, M. "Multi-level activation for segmentation of hierarchically-nested classes on 3D-UNet." *Pre-Conference Proceedings of the 7th MICCAI BraTS Challenge, International MICCAI BraTS Challenge in Conjunction with the Medical Image Computing and Computer-Assisted Interventions Conference*, Granada, Spain (2018), p. 188.

23. Chen, W., Liu, B., Peng, S., Sun, J., and Qiao, X. "S3D-UNet: Separable 3D U-Net for brain tumor segmentation." *International MICCAI BraTS Challenge in Conjunction with the Medical Image Computing and Computer-Assisted Interventions Conference*, Granada, Spain (2018), p. 91.

24. Kamnitsas, K., Ledig, C., Newcombe, V., Simpson, J., Kane, A., Menon, D., and Glocker, B. "Efficient multi-scale 3D CNN with fully connected CRF for accurate brain lesion segmentation." *Medical Image Analysis* 36 (2017): 61–78.

25. Li, X., Luo, G., and Wang, K. Multi-step cascaded networks for brain tumor segmentation. arXiv:1908.05887 (2019).

26. Zhou, C., Ding, C., Lu, Z., Wang, X., and Tao, D. "One-pass multi-task convolutional neural networks for efficient brain tumor segmentation." *21st International Conference*, Granada, Spain, September 16–20, 2018, Proceedings, Part III (2018). 10.1007/978-3-030-00931-1_73

27. Long, J., Shelhamer, E., and Darrell, T. "Fully convolutional networks for semantic segmentation." *IEEE Transactions on Pattern Analysis and Machine Intelligence* 39 (2014): 640–651.

6 Automated Prediction of Lung Cancer Using Deep Learning Algorithms

S. Das[1], P. Kumar[2], S. Pal[3], and S. Majumder[4]
[1]Ramthakur College, Agartala, Tripura, India
[2]NERIST, Itanagar, Arunachal Pradesh, India
[3]Calcutta University, Kolkata, West Bengal, India
[4]Tripura University, Tripura West, Tripura, India

CONTENTS

DOI: 10.1201/9781003324430-8

6.1 INTRODUCTION

Nowadays, lung carcinoma is considered one noxious cancer for human beings glob-
ally. Each year, we get novel reports of a huge number of people suffering from lung
cancer. Smoking of tobacco is one reason of pulmonary cancer, and this relationship
between lung cancer and smoking is strongly supported by several studies. In comparison to non-smokers, smokers are 30% more vulnerable to suffering from cancer.
The well-timed detection and accurate recognition of lung cancer is very important
for successful treatment of patients suffering from lung cancer. However, classification of large numbers of computed tomography (CT) images by doctors is tough and
tedious. Therefore, the automated detection of lung cancer is a significant research
area, and this remarkably enhances the efficiency of lung cancer detection architectures. In this chapter, we have made the following contributions:

1. We have described the main types of lung cancer currently found in world.
2. We have discussed about traditional CAD system in brief.
3. Different deep learning networks are highlighted with their application areas.
4. Nodule detection systems and false positive reduction systems are analysed
   on the basis of different parameters.
5. We have implemented a simple CNN model and the InceptionV3 CNN
   Model for detection of lung cancer on the IQ-OTH/NCCD and Kaggle open
   database.
6. We have discussed methods used for detection of lung cancer in smokers.
7. Recent applications of deep learning in lung cancer diagnostics are presented and their pros and cons are compared.

6.2 CLASSIFICATION OF PULMONARY CANCER

Two groups of lung cancer exist:

I. **Non-small cell lung cancer (NSCLC):** This is the regularly diagnosed sort
   of lung cancer. From studies, we have found that, 80–85% of cases identified with pulmonary cancer are NSCLC. Usually, NSCLC grows at a slower
   pace in comparison to SCLC and generally shows no or few symptoms until
   it reaches advanced stage. There are three main subtypes of NSCLC:
   a. **Adenocarcinoma:** Adenocarcinoma occurs commonly in both younger
      men and women. Adenocarcinoma is mostly diagnosed in patients with
      current or previous smoking records. Radiologists can detect adenocar-
      cinoma before it spreads in the larger region of lungs. For this reason,
      the outlook is much better compared to other types of lung cancer, when
      radiologists locate atypical cells in glandular tissue that lines the lungs.
   b. **Squamous cell carcinoma:** This subtype of NSCLC usually accounts
      for 10–15% of cases of NSCLC and can be robustly linked with ciga-
      rette smoking.
   c. **Large cell (undifferentiated) carcinoma:** Similarly, large cell carci-
      noma tumors can also be sturdily correlated with smoking. Treatment

of this sort of pulmonary cancer is difficult, as it may grow faster and spread quickly compared to other classes of cancer.

II. **Small cell lung cancer (SCLC):** About 10–15% of cases identified with lung cancer have SCLC. Generally, SCLC is known as oat-cell cancer. Unfortunately, this type of lung cancer grows and spreads faster than NSCLC and therefore immediate treatment is required. Categorization of small lung cancer is as follows:

    a. **Small cell carcinoma (oat-cell cancer):** Small cell lung cancer grows fast and develops in the tissues of the lungs. When a patient is diagnosed with this disease, lung cancer has already spread outside of lungs.

    b. **Combined small cell carcinoma:** Combined small cell carcinoma can be diagnosed by a pathologist. These cancer cells contain components of SCLC and one or more components of NSCLC.

6.2.1 SOME UNCOMMON TYPES OF LUNG CANCER

A rare type of lung cancer that usually grows at a slower pace in comparison to other kinds of lung cancer is known as lung carcinoid tumors, or lung carcinoids. This type of lung cancer is responsible for only 1–2% of cases of lung cancer. Typically, these occur in lung cells called neuroendocrine cells.

There are mainly two types of lung carcinoids:

- **Typical carcinoids:** About 90% of lung carcinoid cases are typical carcinoids, and this type of cancer develops at a slow rate. Typical carcinoids often spread inside the lung area and do not have any relation to smoking.
- **Atypical carcinoids:** This type of cancer grows quicker and may spread to other organs, and they have a relation to smoking habits of patients. There is a smaller number of cases with atypical carcinoids than typical carcinoids.

6.3 TRADITIONAL CAD MODEL FOR LUNG CANCER

Recently, CAD systems have been a point of interest for researchers, as such systems assist doctors in analyzing biomedical images and categorizing detected nodules as malignant or benign. CAD systems have five significant steps, as shown in Figure 6.1 and as follows:

  I. Database acquisition: this step involves collection of CT images from online databases viz. LIDC-IDRI, RIDER or real-time databases from different hospitals.

 II. Preprocessing of images: this step improves the biomedical image by elimination of noises. Examples of preprocessing methods are adaptive median filter and top-hat filter.

III. Segmentation operation: segmentation of the biomedical image is done with standard segmentation techniques. In the recent years, many lung segmentation models have been developed for nodules, which can be classified as thresholding technique, morphological technique, graph cut method,

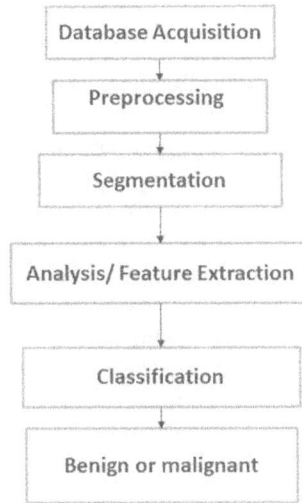

FIGURE 6.1 Steps in a CAD model.

deformable model, clustering technique, Markov random field, and histogram-based method. In this manner, pulmonary nodules are marked in the CT images.

IV. Analysis: during this step, characteristics are extracted from nodule, viz. area and perimeter.

V. Classification: during this step, the nodule structure from the CT images is either classified as benign or malignant using an artificial network like CNN. SVM, ANN, and CNN are commonly utilized for classification.

6.4 VARIOUS DEEP LEARNING NETWORKS FOR LUNG CANCER RECOGNITION

Different deep neural networks are used in detection of lung cancer and include the following:

6.4.1 CONVOLUTIONAL NEURAL NETWORKS (CNNs)

In deep neural networks, CNN is the most powerful network famous and commonly used algorithm. CNNs are dominant in image processing and execute both generative and explanatory jobs. They are generally used in machine vision, including image recognition and natural language processing (NLP). Two key processes of CNN algorithm are convolution and sampling. A convolutional neural network has five layers, as shown in Figure 6.2:

1. Convolutional layer: extraction of several features from CT-scans is done in this phase.

Simple CNN

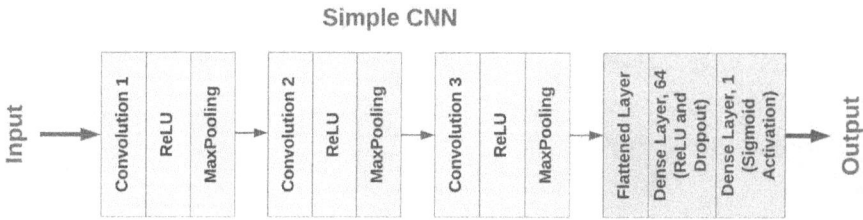

FIGURE 6.2   Architecture of CNN.

2. Pooling layer: dimension of a convolved feature map is shrunk in this layer, which in turn reduces the computational costs. Pooling layer connects the convolutional layer and the fully convolutional network.
3. Fully connected layer: this layer has weights, biases, and neurons and connects the neurons between two layers.
4. Dropout: a dropout layer is used to alleviate the trouble of overfitting in the training data set. During training process, some neurons are eliminated from the network, and in this manner the dimension of the model is shrunk.
5. Activation functions: it determines which data of the system move in the forward direction and which data do not move to the last part of the network. ReLU, Softmax, tanH, and the sigmoid functions are some of the important activation functions.

6.4.1.1   InceptionV3 CNN Architecture

One variant of CNN is the InceptionV3 CNN Architecture. Before we start with the architecture of Inception version 3, we should know about Inception version 1. In CNN models, utilization of multiple deep convolution layers leads to data overfitting. This can be avoided in the InceptionV1 model with the use of several filters of diverse sizes at the matching level. Therefore, we can say that the inception model is wider than deep.

The Inception V3 model as shown in Figure 6.3. Several mesh optimization techniques are used to better fit the model. InceptionV3 has the following features:

1. It is more efficient.
2. It is deeper in mesh, but its speed is not conceded.
3. Cheaper computations are found in this model.
4. In this model, auxiliary classifiers are used as regularizer.

The Inception v3 model came in 2015 with 42 layers and a low error rate. The optimizations made in the initial V3 model that made it better than other versions of itself include the following:

1. Factorization into smaller convolutions
2. Spatial factoring into irregular convolutions
3. Usefulness of auxiliary classifiers
4. Effective grid size reduction

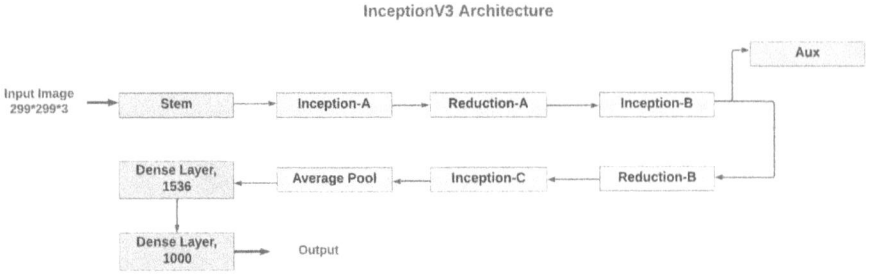

FIGURE 6.3   InceptionV3 architecture.

The InceptionV3 architecture is built one layer over another, as follows:

1. Factorized convolution: this helps in reduction of computational efficiency by reducing the number of parameters in the network. Network efficiency is controlled.
2. Smaller convolutions: this model replaces larger convolutions with smaller convolutions and thus training is faster. Say a 5×5 filter has 25 parameters; the two 3×3 filters replacing the 5×5 convolution have only 18 (3×3 + 3×3) parameters instead.
3. Asymmetric convolution: the 3×3 convolution could be replaced by a 1×3 convolution followed by a 3×1 convolution. If the 3×3 convolution is replaced by a 2×2 convolution, the number of parameters would be slightly higher than the proposed asymmetric convolution.
4. Auxiliary classifier: this is a small CNN inserted between the layers during training, and the resulting loss is added to the loss of the main network. In InceptionV3, the auxiliary classifier acts as a regularizer.
5. Grid size reduction: Pooling operations reduce grid size.

6.4.1.2 VGG16 CNN Architecture (16 Layers)

In VGG16 architecture, we have 16 layers with weights. In total, there are 21 layers, in which 13 layers are convolutional layers, five layers are max-pooling layers, and three are dense layers, but it only has 16 weight layers, i.e., the learnable parameter layer. The model has an input image size of 224×244 with three color channels. The first convolution layer has 64 filters, the second layer has 128, the third has 256, and the fourth and fifth have 512 filters.

After applying the VGG16 architecture, which is shown in Figure 6.4, the output tries to generate 1,000 results but, in our research work, we want only two results, i.e., either the image is cancerous or noncancerous, so we add an extra sigmoid activation layer at the end with the defined number of outputs as one. So, the final output will be a single value that will be between 0 and 1.

ImageNet Large-Scale Visual Recognition Challenge (ILSVRC) is a task to classify a lot of images from a large image data set containing various images into 1,000 possible object categories. This task serves as the standard benchmark for deep learning.

VGG16 Architecture

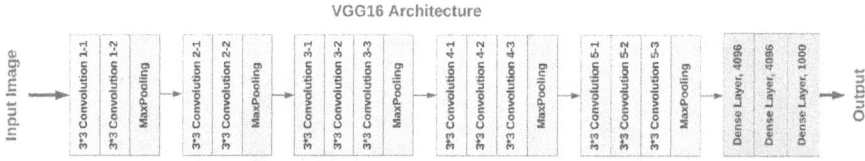

FIGURE 6.4   VGG16 architecture.

6.4.1.3   VGG19 CNN Architecture (19 Layers)

In the VGG19 Architecture a variant of VGG16 model as shown in Figure 6.5, there are 19 layers that have weights. Sixteen of them are convolution layers, three are fully connected dense layers, five are max-pooling layers, and lastly one is a Softmax layer.

The model takes an input image of fixed size of 224×224 with three color channels, which means the image matrix is of shape (224,224,3). Its kernel is of size 3×3 with a stride of 1 pixel, which enables the model to cover the entire details of the image. Spatial padding was used to preserve the spatial resolution of the image. After the convolution layers, the max-pooling layer was used with a filter size of 2×2 with stride of 2, which was followed by a ReLU layer to introduce nonlinearity to the model to make its classifications better and improve computation time, as previous models used sigmoid functions, and those performed badly compared to the ReLU function.

The VGG network was created with the main goal to win the ILSVRC, but ever since it has been used in many other ways. It is used as a classification architecture for many data sets, and since the authors of the model made them publicly available, they can be used as they are or with modification for other similar tasks. It is used in facial recognition tasks also, and the pretrained weights are easily available with other frameworks like keras, so the weights can be adjusted according to the user's need and can be used however they please.

6.4.1.4   ResNet-50 CNN Architecture (50 Layers)

In the ResNet-50 convolutional neural network architecture, as shown in Figure 6.6, there are 50 layers that have weights. Forty-eight of them are convolutional layers, one max-pooling layer and one average pool layer. ResNet, short for Residual Networks, is a neural network that is used as a standard for many computer vision tasks.

The main advantage of ResNet architecture was that it allowed the users to train extremely deep neural networks with more than 150 layers. Convolutional neural

VGG19 Architecture

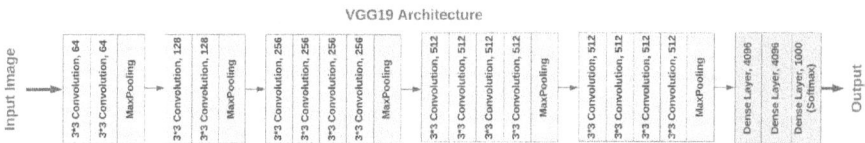

FIGURE 6.5   VGG19 architecture.

RESNET50 Architecture

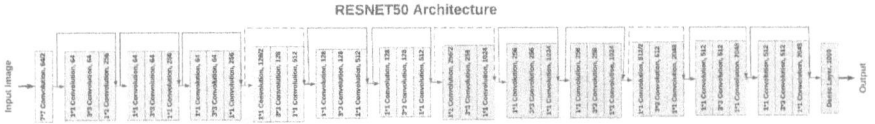

FIGURE 6.6 ResNet-50 architecture.

networks have a major problem of "vanishing gradient." During backpropagations, the value of the gradients decreases significantly, therefore no visible changes are seen in the weights. ResNet uses a method called "skip connections" that solves the problem of vanishing gradient, which makes it a very useful CNN architecture.

Skip connection is a method of adding the original input to the output of the convolution block. It is a direct connection that skips some layers of the model. The output is not the same due to this connection. Figure 6.7 shows that, without the skipped connection, the X input is multiplied by the layer weights, and a bias term is added to the result.

The first convolution layer of ResNet50 has a kernel size of 7×7 with feature map dimension 64 with a stride of size 2. Next, there is a max-pooling layer with stride of 2. The next convolution layer has a kernel of size 1×1 with feature map dimension 64, and following that layer there is a 3×3 kernel with feature map dimension 64. Finally, there is a kernel of size 1×1 with feature map dimension 256. These three layers are repeated three times in total, giving us nine layers in this step.

After that, there is a kernel of size 1×1 with feature map dimension 128, followed by a kernel of size 3×3 with feature map dimension 128, and at last a kernel of size 1×1 with feature map dimension 512. This step was repeated four times, giving us 12 layers in this step.

After that, there is a kernel of size 1×1 with feature map dimension 256 and two more kernels with filter size 3×3 and feature map dimension 256, followed by kernel of size 1×1 with feature map size of 1,024. This is repeated six times, giving us a total of 18 layers. Again, after that there was a kernel of size 1×1 with feature map dimension 512 followed by a kernel of size 3×3 with feature map dimension 512, and kernel size 1×1 with feature map dimension 2,048. This was repeated three times, giving us a total of nine layers. After that, we do an average pool and end it with a fully connected layer containing 1,000 nodes and at the end a Softmax function, so this gives us one layer.

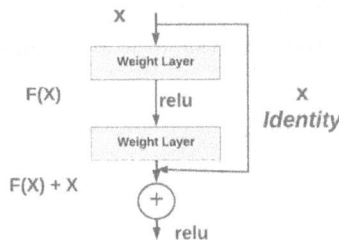

FIGURE 6.7 A skip connection.

We don't actually calculate activation functions and maximum or average pooling layers. So, in total it gives $1 + 9 + 12 + 18 + 9 + 1 = 50$ layers of deep convolutional network. The ResNet architecture can be used for computer vision tasks such as image classification, object localization, and object detection, and this framework can also be used for noncomputer vision tasks to give them the advantage of depth and also reduce the computational cost.

6.4.1.5 MobileNet CNN Architecture (28 Layers)

In the MobileNet convolutional neural network architecture, as shown in Figure 6.8, there are 28 layers that have weights. Twenty-seven of them are convolution layers, which includes 13 depthwise convolution layers, one fully connected layer, one average pool layer, and one Softmax layer.

The MobileNet model is suitable for mobile applications, and it is the first TensorFlow mobile computer vision model. It uses depth-separable convolutions. It significantly reduces the number of parameters compared to a regular convolution network with the same depth in the networks. The result is a lightweight deep neural network. A depthwise separable convolution is created from two operations, first a depthwise convolution followed by a pointwise convolution.

Depthwise separable convolution is a process where one convolution is split into two convolutions based on the depth and spatial dimensions of the image.

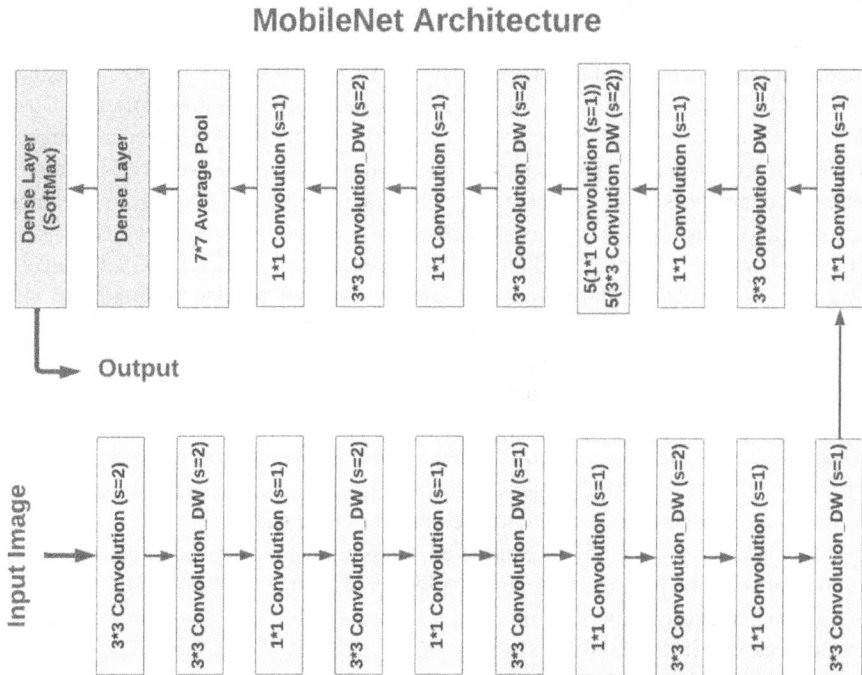

FIGURE 6.8 MobileNet architecture.

6.5   CAD SYSTEM FOR DETECTION OF LUNG CANCER USING DEEP LEARNING

Deep learning can be utilized for classification of pulmonary nodules from CT images. Lung nodule detection systems are as follows:

1. Detection of lung nodules
2. Reduction of false positives

6.5.1   DETECTION OF LUNG NODULES

In this chapter, some of the newly proposed nodule detection systems with CT images are presented.

In 2015, Kai-Lung Hua et al. [1] proposed two architectures: deep belief network (DBN) and convolutional neural network (CNN) for diagnosis of the malignant cells from CT images. The computation of texture features and morphology is not required in DBN and CNN architectures. To classify benign and malignant cells, a blend of unsupervised learning algorithm and consecutive supervised fine-tuning is used on the Lung Image Database Consortium (LIDC) data set. The outstanding results shown by experimental studies confirm that the deep learning architecture proposed by Kai-Lung Hua et al. outperformed the explicit feature computing CAD frameworks. In 2017, Shuo Wang et al. [2] implemented central focused convolutional neural networks (CF-CNN) in a system for segmentation of nodules in various 2-D and 3-D volumetric CT scans. After comparing the results of the proposed model with a number of generally used lung nodule segmentation models, their performance is found optimistic in segmentation and achieved accuracy of DSC = 82.15% in LIDC and DSC = 80.02% in GDGH for two data sets. In 2018, Xinzhuo Zhao et al. [3] constructed a Novel Agile CNN to classify cancerous and noncancerous nodules from biomedical images. They have enhanced accuracy and malfunctioning of the projected CNN system by using the characteristics of weight initialization, rate of learning, size of training batch, dropout, and kernel size. With this agile structure, their proposed system has achieved higher accurateness of 0.822 and an area under the curve (AUC) of 0.877. Chance of overfitting is less. This CNN architecture can classify lung nodules for small data sets. In 2019, Goran Jakimovski and Danco Davcev [4] implemented a system for classification with convolutional deep neural network (CDNN). From the results obtained, the Double CDNN algorithm is compared with that of regular CDNN, and it is found that it has higher accuracy of 99.6% with a 0.76 threshold rate and sensitivity of 99.9%, respectively. The uniqueness of this system based on deep neural networks with CT images is that Double CDNN is able to identify lung cancer from early stages, like 2, 3, and 4, but regular CDNN cannot detect lung cancer at stage 4.

Anum Masood et al. [5] implemented a system with deep fully convolutional neural network (FCNN) in 2018, which is IoT based. After recognition of pulmonary nodule and categorization of benign and malignant nodules, this system can classify the lung cancer in four stages. Their system has achieved accuracy of 96.33% and sensitivity of 83.67% with DFCNet.

All the CAD systems mentioned in the preceding discussion are compared in Table 6.1.

TABLE 6.1

Comparison of CAD Systems for Nodule Detection

Study	Year	Sample Size	Database	Techniques	Sensitivity (%)	Specificity (%)	Accuracy (%)
Kai-Lung Hua et al. [1]	2015	1,010	LIDC	CNN, DBN	73.4	82.2	
Shuo Wang et al. [2]	2017	2,610 + 74	LIDC, CT database from GDGH	CF-CNN			(DSC = 82.15%, LIDC) (DSC = 80.02%, GDGH) respectively
Xinzhuo Zhao et al. [3]	2018	1,018	LIDC-IDRI	Hybrid CNN of LeNet and AlexNet			82.23
Goran Jakimovski et al. [4]	2019	6,080	LONI database	Double convolution neural network (Double CDNN)	0.99912	0.8769	0.9962
Anum Masood et al. [5]	2018	2,101	LIDC-IDRI, RIDER, SPIE challenge, LUNA, database from Shanghai Hospital No. 6	CNN- deep fully convolutional neural network (DFC-Net)	75.35	80.59	77.61
					80.91	83.22	86.02
					75.23	86.46	89.67
					83.67	96.17	96.33

6.5.2   CAD System for False Positive Reduction

For enhancement of performance of the automated system, reduction of false positives is necessary. Several systems with false positive reductions are discussed here.

Hongsheng Jin et al. [6] have implemented a method in 2018, with a deep 3-D residual convolution network for reduction of false positives. This system is compared with others, and it is found that with the SPC layer, lung nodules can be detected more appropriately. They have performed the online selection of hard sample and multitest approaches, for improvement of performance and efficiency of this approach. In 2018, Hongyang Jiang et al. [7] constructed a well-organized automated recognition model enhanced by a Frangi filter based on multigroup patches on biomedical images. They have united images from two categories. A four-channel CNN system is used to help radiologists. This model can classify lung cancer into four stages and 4.7 false positives per scan with sensitivity of 80.06%, and 15.1 false positives per scan with sensitivity of 94% is achieved. From the outcome, it was found that performance of recognition of pulmonary nodules is enhanced, and the false positive cases are reduced with the multigroup patch-based learning. In 2019, Genlang Chen et al. [8] implemented a model to efficiently outline the nodules within a sensible response time. They have integrated segmentation of lung nodules and removal of false positives to achieve higher precision and low cost of time by tuning the network structures. Sensitivity rate for segmentation is 97.78% in this system along with an accuracy rate of 90.1%. In 2017, Qi Dou et al. [9] constructed 3-D CNNs for detection of pulmonary nodules. For the verification of this system, they have used the LUNA16 challenge, which was held in collaboration with ISBN 2016. This competent system has scored 82.7% as a false positive reduction rate. Different nodule detection methods are compared with respect to sensitivity and false positive per scan in Table 6.2.

TABLE 6.2

Comparison between Different Nodule Detection Methods

Study	Year	Database	Sample Size	Key Techniques	Sensitivity (%)	False Positive per Scan
Hongsheng Jin et al. [6]	2018	LUNA-16	888	3-D CNN, residual learning, special pooling and cropping (SPC) layer, online hard sample selection (OHSS), multitest	98.3	7
Hongyang Jiang et al. [7]	2018	LIDC-IDRI		CNN	80.06 / 94	4.7f / 15.1
Genlang Chen et al. [8]	2019	LIDC-IDRI	1018	2-D fully convolutional network (2-D FCN), 3-D filtration	97.8	Accuracy = 90.1 with 6% false positive rate
Qi Dou et al. [9]	2017	LIDC data set	888	2-D CNN, 3-D CNN	90	8

6.6 RECENT APPLICATIONS OF DEEP LEARNING FOR DETECTION OF LUNG CANCER

From our study, we have found that deep learning can be used on various types of data along with biomedical images for recognition of pulmonary cancer. We have compared and analyzed the applications of deep learning for recognition of pulmonary cancer.

Recently, deep learning has established amazing accuracy in lung cancer detection tasks by analyzing images. Therefore, CAD systems are suitable for performing as a clinical tool. Both in public and private domains of research, works involving deep learning have grown and have a wide range of applications. The implementation of deep learning algorithms to Big Data in the healthcare region is a branch of this development. Several implementations of deep learning for recognition of pulmonary cancer are listed here in this section.

In 2019, Yiwen Xu et al. [10] assessed deep learning frameworks to predict clinical outputs by scrutinizing time series CT images with local advanced NSCLC. The manner in which deep learning helps in tracking of the phenotype of the tumor and the condition of the lung cancer patient with respect to radiation therapy and CT scan follow-ups is revealed in this research work. Presentation of survival and prediction of prognosis has increased after the inclusion of timepoints with neural networks CNN and RNN. In 2021, Xinrong Lu et al. [11] proposed the finest system to perceive pulmonary cancer in early phases using preprocessing of biomedical images and deep learning from CT images. They have designed CNN architecture for cancer diagnosis. They have also used a metaheuristic known as the marine predators method to enhance the CNN. Results obtained from their comparison table show that the precision of this system is greater than other systems as pre-trained neural networks, which include CNN ResNet-18, GoogLeNet, AlexNet, and VGG-19. Precision, sensitivity, and specificity achieved by this system are 93.4%, 98.4%, and 97.1%, respectively. In 2020, Mark Kriegsmann et al. [12] utilized the CNN framework to categorize the three classes of pulmonary cancer viz. pulmonary adenocarcinoma (ADC), pulmonary squamous cell carcinoma (SqCC), and SCLC. They have established a quality control (QC) channel to impartially identify cases of mixed tumors that require additional immunohistochemistry (IHC) justification of trustworthy entity classification. Outcomes of the implemented system emphasize advantages and disadvantages of the CNN framework to classify morphology-based tumors. In 2016, in their study, Wenqing Sun et al. [13] have applied and compared three deep learning algorithms with conventional CAD techniques. The highest accuracy after using DBNs is 0.8119, better than the 0.7940 calculated with conventional CADx methods. After comparison of the results of the established system, the immense potential of deep learning and computer learned characteristics used in research involving biomedical images is confirmed.

In 2022, during the COVID-19 pandemic Gopi Kasinathan et al. [14] proposed a cloud-based lung tumor detector that segmented CT images, detected tumors, and classified the severity level of the tumor using M-CNN model. They have generated e-records with patient name, details of the tumor, and severity level. The authors have transferred e-records over cloud to radiologists, so that the records can be virtually monitored and e-diagnosed involuntarily. They have compared their results with existing techniques and found that for tested segmented images the proposed smart lung tumor detection model has achieved 97% accuracy in stage classification of tumor. In 2016, Ryota Shimizu et al. [15] constructed a system for analysis of pulmonary cancer with input data produced by human urine from a gas chromatography mass spectrometer (GC-MS). They also combined multiple sensors for detection of gases with low concentration. The authors have normalized the input data and used a neural network structure stacked autoencoder to check whether the patient is suffering from pulmonary cancer. They have evaluated their proposed method by comparing specificity, accuracy, and sensitivity and found that their system has achieved 90% accuracy and worked well. In 2020, Asuntha et al. [16] projected a framework to detect cancerous nodules from medical images of lung and classify lung cancer to predict its severity. They have used best feature extraction techniques viz. histogram of oriented gradients (HoG), scale-invariant feature transform (SIFT), wavelet transform-based characteristics, local binary pattern (LBP), and Zernike Moments. The authors have extracted characteristics like texture, geometry, volume, and intensity, then they have applied the fuzzy particle swarm optimization (FPSO) method to choose the finest characteristic and reduce the computational complexity of CNN. They have evaluated their proposed model on both online data set LIDC and an offline data set from Arthi Scan Hospital. From the results obtained, it is observed their model has achieved 94.97% accuracy, which is better than other existing systems. In 2021, Hadi Hashemzadeh et al. [17] implemented a dependable system for classification between cancerous and noncancerous cells. They grew well-liked NSCLC lines in a microfluidic chip and stained with phalloidin and obtained images from an IX-81 inverted Olympus fluorescence microscope. The authors have created an image analysis workflow based on deep learning that can classify images from pulmonary cancer cell-lines into six categories, viz. five cancer cell lines (P-C9, SK-LU-1, H-1975, A-427, and A-549) and one normal cell line (16-HBE). In order to pick the top model, they have evaluated five important CNN architectures – GoogLeNet, ResNet, AlexNet, SqueezeNet, and Inceptionvon – from their database with lung cancer cell lines. Results obtained from the system confirmed that ResNet18 is a competent and hopeful process for classification of lung cancer cell lines. Their system has achieved accuracy in classification of 98.37% and an F1-Score of 97.29%. In 2021, Aydın et al. [18] introduced a system based on the CNN model for tumor detection and classification of cancer as small and nonsmall cell carcinoma, as well as adenocarcinoma-squamous cell lung carcinoma. They have used CT images of the thorax for this system. The proposed CNN system has achieved F1 and Score values of 0.95, 0.81, and 0.87. In 2021, Kaimei Huang et al. [19] presented a system to predict target-drug therapy from a group of available drug therapies. They have applied deep convolution Gaussian mixture model for normalization of images. This system identifies the gene mutations in lung cancer from a stained pathological slice using CNN and Res-Net. This system has better precision of 86.3%.

Coudray et al. [20] presented a system using deep learning to classify and predict mutation from nonsmall lung cancer. They have predicted six categories of mutated genes in lung adenocarcinoma (LUAD) from pathology images.

6.7   RECENT APPLICATIONS OF EXPLAINABLE AI-BASED DEEP LEARNING FOR DETECTION OF CANCER

There is a substantial problem with deep learning techniques in that these models are black box algorithms and hence are basically indescribable. In medical applications, these black boxes may be biased in some way, and this can lead to consequences. Therefore, we need approaches to understand black boxes in a better way. Such approaches are known as explainable artificial intelligence or interpretable deep learning.

In 2019, Manu Siddhartha et al. [21] used the random forest to predict the survival status of lung cancer patients in postoperative life expectancy. Then they interpreted the random forest ensemble machine learning model to find out the reasons for particular predictions also known as explanatory artificial intelligence (XAI). They used a thoracic surgery patient's data, which was collected all together from Wroclaw Thoracic Surgery Centre in the years 2007 and 2011.

6.8   METHODS AND MATERIAL

The database used in our study is IQ-OTH/NCCD and the Kaggle open database, which contains 2,056 images representing CT scans of Dicom format. We have not used any preprocessing in our model. The number of these slices range from 80 to 200 slices, each of them representing an image of the human chest with different sides and angles. These cases can be grouped into three categories: normal, benign, and malignant. Out of these images, 1,425 images are of benign and malignant tumorous lungs, and 631 images are of normal lungs. In our study, we have worked on the Integrated Development Environment (IDE) PyCharm Community Edition 2021.3.1 and implemented a simple CNN model and the InceptionV3 CNN Model. These cases can be grouped into three categories: normal, benign, and malignant. Out of these images, 1425 images are of benign and malignant tumorous lungs and 631 images are of normal lungs. Before training the model, the image data set is split into training and testing sets. In our model, 80% of the database images are chosen for training the model, and 20% of them are used for testing. The selection of the images is random. Once the model is trained, the tumor is classified as either cancerous or noncancerous.

6.9   RESULTS

6.9.1   Simple CNN Model's Results

The configuration used for the aforementioned output was GPU: Nvidia GTX 1650Ti; GPU memory: 4 GB; RAM: 8 GB DDR4; and a Train–Test ratio 4:1. This device is mentioned in Table 6.3 as "proposed device." Figure 6.9 shows the confusion matrix of the simple model.

6.9.1.1   Graphical Analysis of the Results

From the results produced by the simple CNN model, we can analyze the model's training and testing accuracy, as well as its training and testing loss, and we can also

TABLE 6.3

Performance Difference of the Simple CNN Model in Different Devices

Device	Accuracy (%)	Precision (%)	Specificity (%)	Sensitivity (%)	Epochs (N)	Train–Test Ratio (T:V)	Time Taken (mm:ss.ms)
Proposed device	98.05	99.30	98.31	95.12	50	4:1	02:08.65
Proposed device	93.44	93.18	82.35	94.23	10	4:1	01:16.66
Proposed device	97.73	98.61	96.70	95.65	50	7:3	01:59.57
Proposed device	88.97	87.67	67.03	93.84	10	7:3	01:09.15
Local device	96.35	96.95	92.43	94.82	10	4:1	01:11.46
Google colab	97.08	97.62	94.11	95.72	50	4:1	01:14.61
Google colab	97.24	98.15	95.60	95.08	50	7:3	01:11.18
Kaggle	98.54	98.64	96.63	98.29	50	4:1	01:16.83
Kaggle	93.51	91.93	79.12	98.63	50	7:3	00:48.92

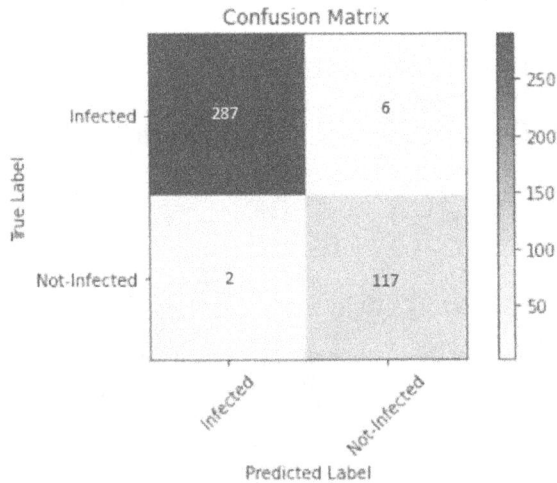

FIGURE 6.9 Confusion matrix of the simple CNN model.

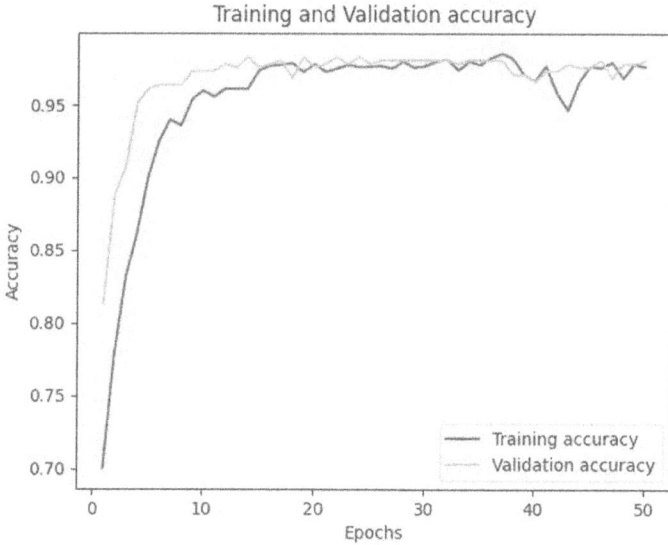

FIGURE 6.10   Graph for training and validation accuracy of the simple CNN model.

compare the model's accuracy and loss at the same time for both the training and testing data. The training accuracy and loss graph (Figure 6.10) is on the lower side because of the initial heavy loss while training. The graphs generated by the analysis are shown in Figures 6.10–6.13.

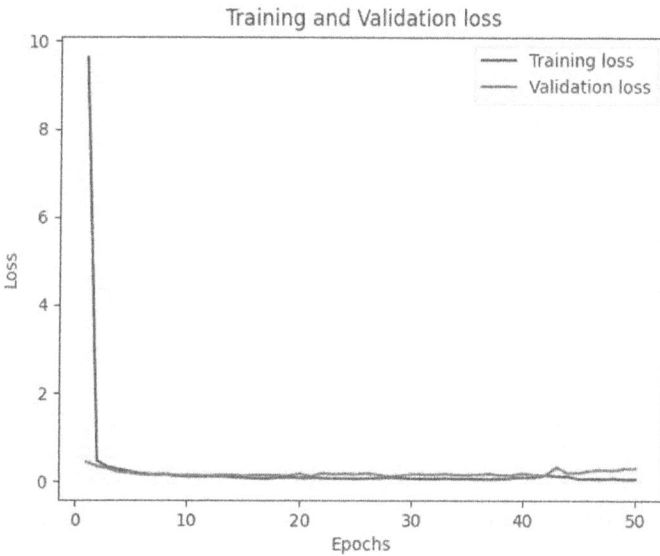

FIGURE 6.11   Graph for training and validation loss of the simple CNN model.

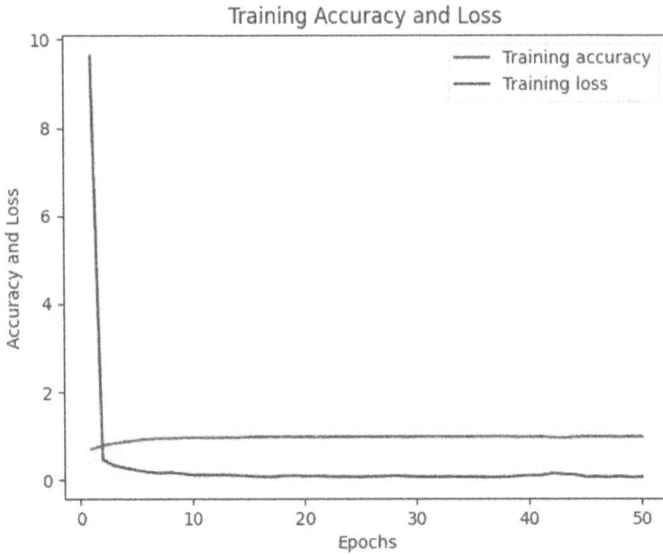

FIGURE 6.12   Graph for training accuracy and loss of the simple CNN model.

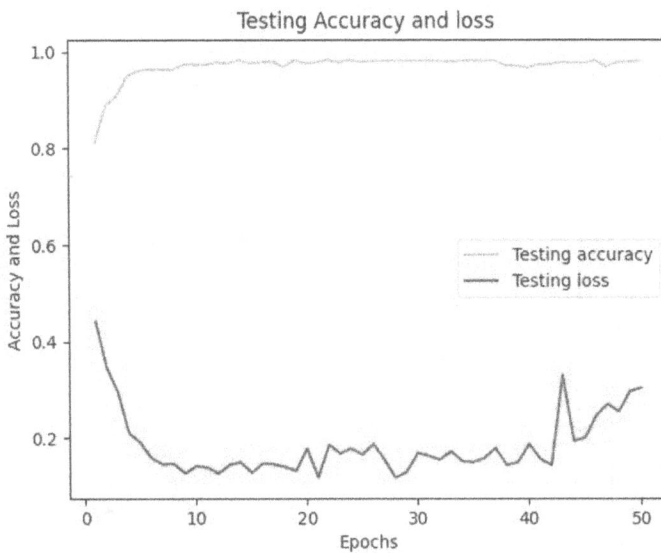

FIGURE 6.13   Graph for validation and loss of the accuracy and loss of the simple CNN model.

6.9.1.2 Difference in Performance in Different Configurations

The model was run on a local device with the configuration GPU: Nvidia GTX 1050; GPU memory: 4 GB and RAM: 8 GB DDR4, Google Collab with GPU: Nvidia Tesla K80; GPU memory: 12 GB and RAM: 16 GB DDR4 and Kaggle; with GPU: Nvidia Tesla P100, GPU memory: 16 GB and RAM: 16 GB DDR4. The results are shown in a tabulated fashion in Table 6.3.

6.9.2 INCEPTIONV3 CNN MODEL'S RESULTS

The complete output of the InceptionV3 CNN Model in our personal computer was as shown in Figure 6.14.

The configuration used for the above output was GPU: Nvidia GTX 1650Ti; GPU memory: 4 GB, RAM: 8 GB DDR4; and Train-Test ratio 4:1. This device is mentioned in the table below as "proposed device." Figure 6.14 shows the confusion matrix of InceptionV3.

6.9.2.1 Graphical Analysis of the Results

From the results produced by the InceptionV3 model, we can analyze the model's training and testing accuracy, as well as its training and testing, loss and we can also compare the model's accuracy and loss at the same time for both the training and testing data. The graphs generated by the analysis are shown in Figures 6.15–6.18.

Comparison between the different models based on GPU: Nvidia GTX 1650Ti, GPU Memory: 4 GB, RAM: 8 GB DDR4 and Train-Test ratio 4:1 for 10 epochs is given in Table 6.4.

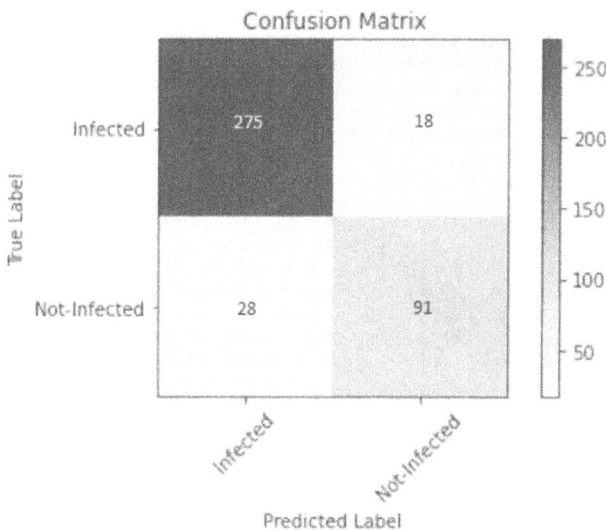

FIGURE 6.14 Confusion matrix of InceptionV3.

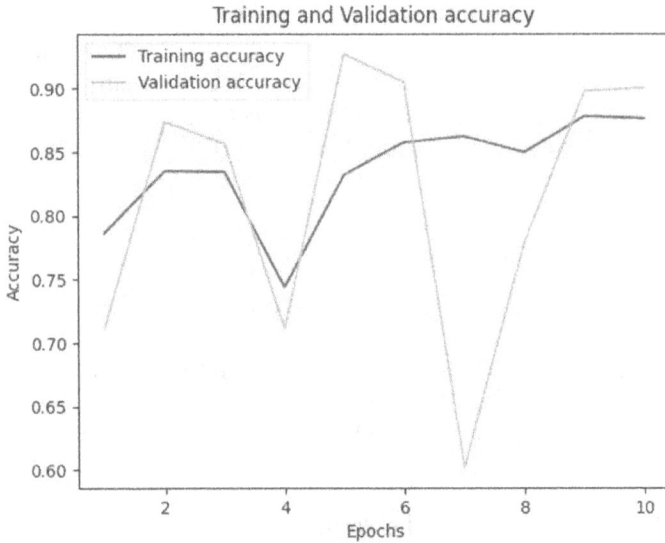

FIGURE 6.15 Graph for training and validation accuracy of the InceptionV3 CNN model.

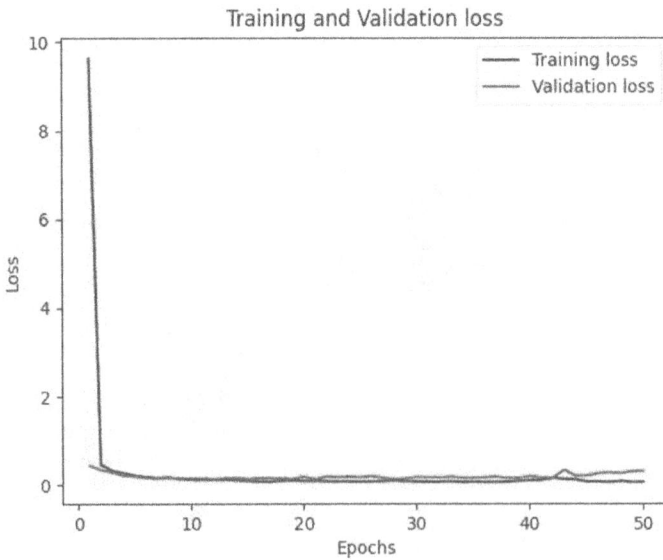

FIGURE 6.16 Graph for training and validation loss of the InceptionV3 CNN model.

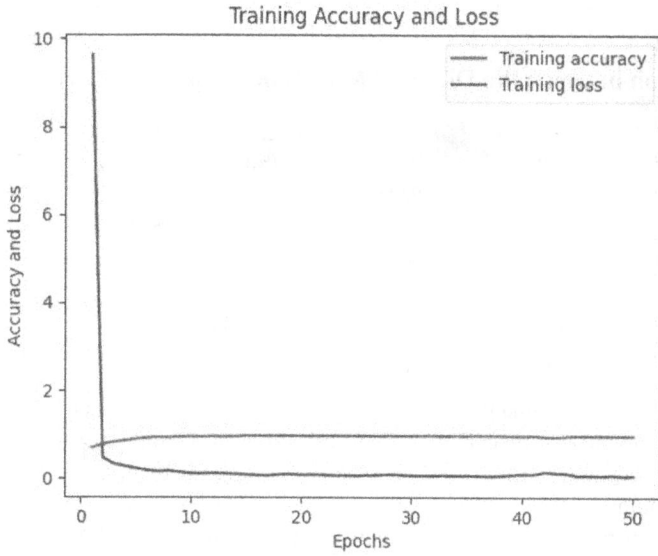

FIGURE 6.17   Graph for training accuracy and loss of the InceptionV3 CNN model.

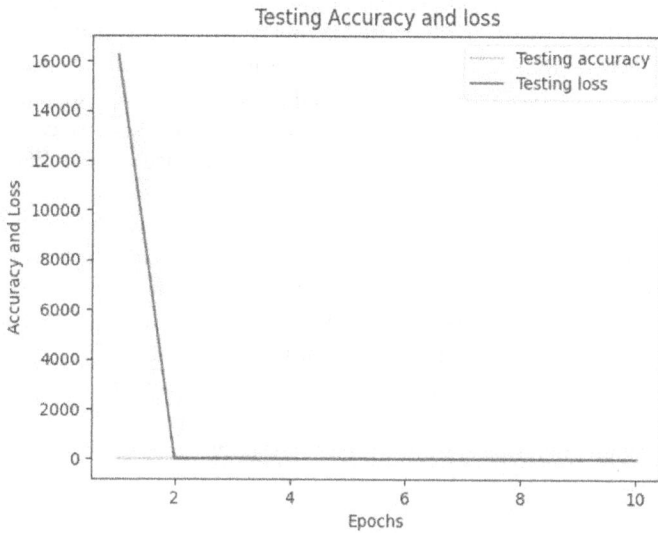

FIGURE 6.18   Graph for testing accuracy and loss of the InceptionV3 CNN model.

TABLE 6.4
Comparison between the Different Models on Proposed Device

CNN Architecture	Accuracy (%)	Precision (%)	Specificity (%)	Sensitivity (%)	Run Time (mm:ss.ms)
Simple CNN	93.44	93.18	82.35	94.23	01:16.66
InceptionV3	88.83	90.75	76.47	83.48	11:42.65

6.10 METHODS OF DETECTION OF LUNG CANCER SPECIFICALLY FOR SMOKERS

Several studies have found that 90% of cases of pulmonary cancer in men and 70–80% of cases in women are because of smoking cigarettes. Despite a smaller number of patients in nonsmokers in comparison to smokers, recently there has also been a notable rise in number of cases of lung cancer in nonsmokers. Therefore, evaluation of lung cancer in nonsmokers has become an interesting research topic. We will explore the techniques used for detection of pulmonary cancer both for smokers and nonsmokers. There exist quite a few risk factors of pulmonary cancer in nonsmokers, too, viz. passive smoking, cooking fumes in villages, radon, exposures to environmental pollution, genetic factors, underlying lung disease, oncogenic viruses, and estrogens.

Methods of detecting lung cancer in smokers include the following:

1. **Screening with low-dose chest CT:** Low-dose spiral CT scan is a sort of screening test that is used for recognition of pulmonary cancer at the initial phase in heavy smokers. This test does not help in detection of cardiovascular diseases like cancer in light smokers or nonsmokers.

    In 2018, Nikolas Lessmann et al. [22] presented an automatic method for recognition of coronary artery, thoracic aorta and cardiac valve calcification in low-dose chest CT. They have used CNN in two stages for identification of potential calcification inside the complete image, without segmentation and localization of anatomical structures. For coronary artery, thoracic aorta, aortic valve, and mitral valve calcifications, this method has acquired F1-Scores of 0.89, 0.89, 0.67, and 0.55. The results show the system can reliably perform cardiovascular risk assessment from low-dose chest CT images from screening of pulmonary cancer. In 2020, Sanne G. M. van Velzen [23] implemented a deep learning calcium scoring method for quantification of coronary and thoracic calcium. This system development is strong, in spite of considerable dissimilarity in CT protocol. To improve the performance, this algorithm was augmented with CT protocol–specific images.

2. **Pulmonary function tests:** PFTs are important study for the supervision of cases with suspected or formerly diagnosed respiratory disease. Smoking is considered one of the major reasons equally for cancer and chronic obstructive pulmonary disease (COPD). This study found close correlation amid smoking, obstructive lung diseases, and pulmonary cancer.

    In 1987, Melvyn S. Tockman et al. [24] tested the hypothesis that in cases of male smokers, if a patient has airways obstruction, then there is higher probability that he has pulmonary cancer too. They discovered, using the log-linear technique, that there is significant association between airways obstruction and lung cancer, while investigators found only a weak association between initial forced expiratory values (FEVj) and lung cancer mortality.

In 2010, E. Calabro et al. [25] stated in their research work that in lung cancer screening trials, baseline pulmonary function tests are important. They have shown that a modest decrease in $FEV_1\%$ indicates risk of pulmonary cancer in smokers not having COPD, as FEV_1 is considered the surrogate marker.

In 2009, R. P. Young et al. [26] found in their study that obstructive pulmonary function raises the risk of pulmonary cancer by sixfold; and pulmonary cancer and COPD are strongly associated, because both of them result from shared pathogenic mechanisms. From this close association, the authors clinically implied that spirometry can be widely used for early detection of patients with risk of lung cancer.

3. **Chest X-ray:** The common test suggested by doctors to check abnormalities in lung is a chest X-ray.

In 2019, Yu Gordienko et al. [27] developed a preprocessing system to segment lung images and exclude bone shadow from chest X-rays. This approach can assist doctors to detect suspicious lesions and nodules in patients. The results showed higher precision and loss results in analysis of lung cancer.

Different research works based on methods of detection of lung cancer are analyzed in Table 6.5.

TABLE 6.5
Comparison of Methods for Detection Pulmonary Cancer in Smokers

Study	Year	Database	Sample Size	Techniques Used	Score
Nikolas Lessmann et al. [22]	2018	National Lung Screening Trial database of CT images (NLST)	1,744	CNN	F1-Scores of 0.89, 0.89, 0.67, and 0.55
Sanne G. M. van Velzen [23]	2020	National Lung Screening Trial database of CT images (NLST)	7,240	CNN	0.92 (95% CI: 0.91, 0.93)
Melvyn S. Tockman [24]	1987	Database from IPPB trial and Johns Hopkins Lung Project	667 + 3,728	Spirometry	
E. Calabro et al. [25]	2010	Database from Multicentric Italian Lung Detection (MILD) project	3,806	Spirometry	
R. P. Young et al. [26]	2009			Spirometry	
Yu. Gordienko et al. [27]	2019	JSRT data set, BSE-JSRT data sets	247 + 247	U-Net-based CNN	

6.11   FUTURE RESEARCH DIRECTIONS

In the future work, we plan to perform PFT-based analysis of normal or abnormal lungs and study about research works based on correlation amid obstructive lung diseases and pulmonary cancer. We will study utilization of detection of COPD for timely recognition of pulmonary cancer among smokers and nonsmokers. Our work will apply deep learning techniques in detection of pulmonary cancer in smokers and nonsmokers both in online data sets and real-time data sets to be obtained from ABV Regional Cancer Centre, Agartala, Tripura.

6.12   CONCLUSION

In this chapter, we have presented a general idea of implementation of neural networks for recognition of lung cancer using CT images of the lung. We discussed the categories of lung cancer in our world and presented a brief discussion of architectures of deep neural networks to detect pulmonary cancer and classify lung cancer into four stages. With our study, we have found that CAD systems based on deep learning are more convenient to use compared to conventional CAD because it reduces the load of image preprocessing and feature extraction from images. Methods used for identification of lung cancer in smokers have been discussed in this chapter. In our study, we have found several applications of deep learning with various data types viz. lung CT images, cell lines of lung, and urine for recognition of pulmonary cancer. These applications can be viewed as a promising tool to assist radiologists for second opinions. In this study, we implemented a simple CNN model and InceptionV3 CNN Model and found accuracy of 93.44% and 88.83% respectively. In our future research works, we would like to implement XAI for predicting the cancerous images.

BIBLIOGRAPHY

1. Hua Kai-Lung, Hsu Che-Hao, Hidayati, Shintami Chusnul, Cheng Wen-Huang, and Chen Yu-Jen. "Computer-aided classification of lung nodules on computed tomography images via deep learning technique." *Onco Targets and Therapy* 8 (2015): 2015–2022. doi: 10.2147/OTT.S80733. eCollection 2015.
2. Wang Shuo, Zhou Mu, Liu Zaiyi, Liu Zhenyu, Gu Dongsheng, Zang Yali, Dong Di, Olivier, Gevaert, and Tian Jie. "Central focused convolutional neural networks: Developing a data-driven model for lung nodule segmentation." *Medical Image Analysis* 40 (2017): 172–183. doi: 10.1016/j.media.2017.06.014.
3. Zhao Xinzhuo, Liu Liyao, Qi Shouliang, Teng Yueyang, Li Jianhua, and Qian Wei. "Agile convolutional neural network for pulmonary nodule classification using CT images." *International Journal of Computer Assisted Radiology and Surgery* 13(4) (2018): 585–595. doi: 10.1007/s11548-017-1696-0.
4. Jakimovski, Goran, and Davcev, Danco. "Using double convolution neural network for lung cancer stage detection." *Applied Sciences* 9 (2019): 427. doi: 10.3390/app9030427.
5. Anum, Masood, Sheng Bin, Li Ping, Hou Xuhong, Wei Xiaoer, Qin Jing, and Feng Dagan. "Computer-assisted decision support system in pulmonary cancer detection and stage classification on CT images." *Journal of Biomedical Informatics* 79 (2018): 117–128. doi: 10.1016/j.jbi.2018.01.005.

6. Hongsheng, Jin, Zongyao, Li, Ruofeng, Tong, and Lanfen, Lin. "A deep 3D residual CNN for false positive reduction in pulmonary nodule detection." *Medical Physics* 45(5) (2018): 2097–2107. doi: 10.1002/mp.12846. Epub 2018 Mar 25.

7. Jiang Hongyang, Ma He, Qian Wei, Gao Mengdi, and Li Yan. "An automatic detection system of lung nodule based on multi-group patch-based deep learning network." *IEEE Journal of Biomedical and Health Informatics* 22(4) (2018): 1227–1237. doi: 10.1109/JBHI.2017.2725903.

8. Chen Genlang, Zhang Jiajian, Zhuo Deyun, Pan Yuning, and Pang Chaoyi. "Identification of pulmonary nodules via CT images with hierarchical fully convolutional networks." *Medical & Biological Engineering & Computing* 57 (2019): 1567. doi: 10.1007/s11517-019-01976-1.

9. Dou Qi, Chen Hao, Yu Lequan, Qin Jing, and Heng Pheng-Ann. "Multi-level contextual 3D CNNs for false positive reduction in pulmonary nodule detection." *IEEE Transactions on Biomedical Engineering* 64(7) (2017): 1558–1567. doi: 10.1109/TBME.2016.2613502.

10. Xu Yiwen, Hosny, Ahmed, Zeleznik, Roman, Parmar, Chintan, Coroller, Thibaud, Franco, Idalid, Mak, Raymond H., and Aerts, Hugo J. W. L. "Deep learning predicts lung cancer treatment response from serial medical imaging." *Clinical Cancer Research* 25(11) (2019): 3266–3275. doi: 10.1158/1078-0432.CCR-18-2495.

11. Lu Xinrong, Nanehkaran, Y. A., and Fard, Maryam Karimi. "A method for optimal detection of lung cancer based on deep learning optimized by marine predators algorithm." *Computational Intelligence and Neuroscience* (2021): 3694723. doi: 10.1155/2021/3694723.

12. Kriegsmann, M., Haag, C., Weis, C. A., Steinbuss, G., Warth, A., Zgorzelski, C., Muley, T., Winter, H., Eichhorn, M. E., Eichhorn, F., Kriegsmann, J., Christopoulos, P., Thomas, M., Witzens-Harig, M., Sinn, P., von Winterfeld, M., Heussel, C. P., Herth, F. J. F., Klauschen, F., Stenzinger, A., and Kriegsmann, K. "Deep learning for the classification of small-cell and non-small-cell lung cancer." *Cancers (Basel)* 12(6) (2020): 1604. doi: 10.3390/cancers12061604. PMID: 32560475; PMCID: PMC7352768.

13. Sun Wenqing, Zheng Bin, and Qian Wei, "Computer aided lung cancer diagnosis with deep learning algorithms." *Proceedings of SPIE 9785, Medical Imaging 2016: Computer-Aided Diagnosis*, 97850Z (24 March 2016). doi: 10.1117/12.2216307.

14. Kasinathan, G., and Jayakumar, S. "Cloud-based lung tumor detection and stage classification using deep learning techniques." *BioMed Research International* (2022): 4185835. doi: 10.1155/2022/4185835. PMID: 35047635; PMCID: PMC8763490.

15. Shimizu R., et al. "Deep learning application trial to lung cancer diagnosis for medical sensor systems." *2016 International SoC Design Conference (ISOCC)* (2016), pp. 191–192. IEEE. Jeju, South Korea. doi: 10.1109/ISOCC.2016.7799852.

16. Asuntha, A., and Srinivasan, A. "Deep learning for lung cancer detection and classification." *Multimedia Tools and Applications* 79 (2020): 7731–7762. doi: 10.1007/s11042-019-08394-3.

17. Hashemzadeh, H., Shojaeilangari, S., Allahverdi, A., et al. "A combined microfluidic deep learning approach for lung cancer cell high throughput screening toward automatic cancer screening applications." *Scientific Reports* 11 (2021): 9804. doi: 10.1038/s41598-021-89352-8.

18. Aydın, Nevin, Celik, Ozer, Aslan, Ahmet Faruk, Odabas, Alper, Dundar, Emine, and Sahin, Meryem Cansu. "Detection of lung cancer on computed tomography using artificial intelligence applications developed by deep learning methods and the contribution of deep learning to the classification of lung carcinoma." *Current Medical Imaging* 17(9) (2021): 1137–1141. doi: 10.2174/1573405617666210204210500.

19. Huang, K., Mo, Z., Zhu, W., Liao, B., Yang, Y., Wu, F-X. "Prediction of target–drug therapy by identifying gene mutations in lung cancer with histopathological stained image and deep learning techniques." *Frontiers in Oncology* 11 (2021): 642945. doi: 10.3389/fonc.2021.642945.

20. Coudray, Nicolas, et al. "Classification and mutation prediction from non-small cell lung cancer histopathology images using deep learning." *Nature Medicine* 24 (2018): 1559–1567. doi: 10.1038/s41591-018-0177-5.

21. Siddhartha, Manu, Maity, Paramita, and Nath, Rajendra. "Explanatory artificial intelligence (XAI) in the prediction of post-operative life expectancy in lung cancer patients." *International Journal of Scientific Research* 8(12) (2019): 23–28. doi: 10.36106/ijsr.

22. Lessmann, Nikolas, van Ginneken, Bram, Zreik, Majd, de Jong, Pim A., de Vos, Bob D., Viergever, Max A., and Išgum, Ivana. "Automatic calcium scoring in low-dose chest CT using deep neural networks with dilated convolutions." *IEEE Transactions on Medical Imaging* 37(2) (2018): 615–625. doi: 10.1109/TMI.2017.2769839.

23. van Velzen, Sanne G. M., Lessmann, Nikolas, Velthuis, Birgitta K., Bank, Ingrid E. M., van den Bongard, Desiree H. J. G., Leiner Tim, de Jong Pim A., Veldhuis Wouter B., Correa Adolfo, Terry, James G., Carr, John Jeffrey, Viergever, Max A., Verkooijen, Helena M., and Išgum, Ivana. "Deep learning for automatic calcium scoring in CT: Validation using multiple cardiac CT and chest CT protocols." *Radiology* 295 (2020): 66–79. doi: 10.1148/radiol.2020191621.

24. Tockman, Melvyn S., Anthonisen, Nicholas R., Wright, Elizabeth C., and Donithan, Michele G. "Airways obstruction and the risk for lung cancer." *Annals of Internal Medicine* 106 (1987): 512–518. doi: 10.7326/0003-4819-106-4-512.

25. Calabro, E., Randi, G., La Vecchia, C., Sverzellati, N., Marchiano, A., Villanie, M., Zompatori, M., Cassandro, R., Harari, S., and Pastorino, U. "Lung function predicts lung cancer risk in smokers: A tool for targeting screening programmes." *European Respiratory Journal* 35 (2010): 146–151. doi: 10.1183/09031936.00049909.

26. Young, R. P., Hopkins, R. J., Christmas, T., Black, P. N., Metcalf, P., Gamble, G. D., "COPD prevalence is increased in lung cancer, independent of age, sex and smoking history." *European Respiratory Journal* 34(2) (2009): 380–386. doi: 10.1183/09031936.00144208. Epub 2009 Feb 5. PMID: 19196816.

27. Gordienko, Yu., Gang Peng, Hui Jiang, Zeng Wei, Kochura, Yu., Alienin, O., Rokovyi, O., and Stirenko, S. "Deep learning with lung segmentation and bone shadow exclusion techniques for chest X-ray analysis of lung cancer." Hu, Z., et al. (eds.), Springer International Publishing AG, part of Springer Nature (2019): ICCSEEA 2018, AISC 754, pp. 638–647. "Advances in Computer Science for Engineering and Education. ICCSEEA 2018. Advances in Intelligent Systems and Computing." doi: 10.1007/978-3-319-91008-6_63.

28. Das, S., and Majumder, S. "Lung cancer detection using deep learning network: A comparative analysis." *2020 Fifth International Conference on Research in Computational Intelligence and Communication Networks (ICRCICN)*, 2020, pp. 30–35. IEEE. Bangalore, India. doi: 10.1109/ICRCICN50933.2020.9296197.

29. Faridoddin, Shariaty, and Mojtaba, Mousavi. "Application of CAD systems for the automatic detection of lung nodules." *Informatics in Medicine Unlocked* 15 (2019): 100173. doi: 10.1016/j.imu.2019.100173.

30. Han Guanghui, Liu Xiabi, Zheng Guangyuan, Wang Murong, and Huang Shan. "Automatic recognition of 3D GGO CT imaging signs through the fusion of hybrid resampling and layer-wise fine-tuning CNNs." *Medical & Biological Engineering & Computing* 56 (2018): 2201–2212. doi: 10.1007/s11517-018-1850-z.

31. Kumar, D., Wong, A., and Clausi, D. A. "Lung nodule classification using deep features in CT images." *2015 12th Conference on Computer and Robot Vision*, 2015, pp. 133–138. IEEE. Halifax, NS, Canada. doi: 10.1109/CRV.2015.25.

32. Makaju, Suren, Prasad, P. W. C., Alsadoona, Abeer, Singh, A. K., and Elchouemi, A. "Lung cancer detection using CT scan images." *Procedia Computer Science* 125 (2018): 107–114.

33. Mets, Onno M., et al. "Identification of chronic obstructive pulmonary disease in lung cancer screening computed tomographic scans." *Journal of the American Medical Association* 306(16) (2011): 1775.

34. Terdale, Shamala B., and Kulhalli K. V. "CAD system for lung cancer detection using ANN." *IOSR Journal of Electronics & Communication Engineering (IOSR-JECE)*, 11–15. ISSN: 2278–2834, ISBN: 2278–8735.
35. Tran, Giang Son, Nghiem, Thi Phuong, Nguyen, Van Thi, Luong, Chi Mai, Burie, Jean-Christophe. "Improving accuracy of lung nodule classification using deep learning with focal loss." *Hindawi Journal of Healthcare Engineering* (2019): 1–9. Article ID 5156416. doi: 10.1155/2019/5156416.
36. van der Velden Bas, H. M., Kuijf, Hugo J., Gilhuijs, Kenneth G. A., Viergever, and Max A. "Explainable artificial intelligence (XAI) in deep learning-based medical image analysis." *Medical Image Analysis* 79 (2022): 102470. doi: 10.1016/j.media.2022.102470.

7 Cervical Cancer Screening Approach Using AI

D. Santhi[1], M. Carmel Sobia[2], and M. Jayalakshmi[3]
[1]Department of Biomedical Engineering, Mepco Schlenk Engineering College, Virudhunagar, Tamil Nadu, India
[2]Department of Electrical and Electronics Engineering, PSR Engineering College, Virudhunagar, Tamil Nadu, India
[3]Department of Computer Science, Kalasalingam University, Srivilliputhur, Tamil Nadu, India

CONTENTS

7.1 INTRODUCTION

Based on a World Health Organization (WHO) document, cervical malignancy distresses more than 300,000 individuals over a period of 12 months, and 85% of such deaths take place in much less advanced nations [1]. The uncommon growth of abnormal cells in the body is cancer. These are termed malignant cells, which start from one abnormal cell, then multiply out of control into malignant tumors. Cervical cancer (CC) is one of the most common cancers that affect women, ranked after breast cancers. According to a statistical report, one woman dies every minute from this disease. CC is a communal women's destroyer in emerging and established countries [2].

The definition of human papillomavirus (HPV)-related conditions was published on February 26, 2016, and provides vital information for the population of India on cervical cancer. CC mainly affects women over 15 years of age, and the aforementioned statistical report found that around 453.02 million are affected by CC, and the annual number of cases are 122,844. Further, CC causes the death of 67,477 persons.

DOI: 10.1201/9781003324430-9

CC is cancer arising from the cervix, part of the female reproductive system. It is present in between the uterus and vagina. The cervix is about two to three centimeters long, in the lower and narrower part of the uterus. The cancer cells originate from the cervix.

First, the regular cells of the cervix develop into precancerous cells and then grow to be cancerous cells. Infection of cervical epithelium via HPV is considered the cause of cancer. Potentially precancerous cells inside the cervix can be detected by way of cervical screening, the usage of a pap smear (also referred to as a cervical smear), wherein epithelial cells are scraped from the surface of the cervix and examined beneath a microscope. Cervical screening diagnoses the disorder at an early precancerous stage. Cervical cancer is preventable if precancerous lesions are detected with adequate screening and are adequately treated. The cancerous transformation of cervical cells is associated with improved nucleus length and decreased cytoplasm length.

On the pap smear slide, cancerous cells display a substantially better nucleus-to-cytoplasm (NC) ratio than normal cells [3], and abnormal cells typically benefit from a darker shade after the fixation technique and pap staining. This color depth difference can discriminate among normal and cancerous cells [4, 5]. Take a look at what has to be accomplished on various ordinary cells to distinguish normal and abnormal cells. There are three forms of everyday cells: superficial, intermediate, and parabasal cells. The superficial cells are the giant cells, which are polygonal in form and very flat. Intermediate cells are comparable in appearance but small in length, and have large and round nuclei.

The parabasal cells are smaller in size and have large nuclei. These normal cells can easily be misclassified as abnormal in an automatic screening system. Studying and identifying the normal cells is necessary for the cancer screening system to avoid misclassification. It is beneficial to reduce the misclassification of abnormal cancerous cells and improve the diagnosis. We proposed a technique to distinguish numerous types of normal cells that could be later useful to hit upon abnormal cells from the pap smear cell images.

This chapter proceeds as follows. Literature reviews are given in Section 7.2. The techniques and algorithms are in Sections 7.3 and 7.4. Section 7.8 demonstrates the practical consequences. Conclusions are given in Section 7.9.

7.2   LITERATURE REVIEW

Published literature about cervical cancer screening is done carefully, and the essence of the findings is presented in this section. Meng-Husiun Tsai et al. [6] expand a cytoplast and nucleus contour (CNC) detector from cervical smear images. They confirmed the biorganization enhancer to make a simple separation for the pixels among two objects and the maximal color difference (MCD) method to draw the exact nucleus contour. Wang Xiaoning et al. [7] proposed classifying the segmented single cervical cell nuclei using a backpropagation neural network.

Sun Y. Park et al. [8] presented a domain-specific automated image analysis framework to detect the starting stage of the cancerous and abnormal stage of the uterine cervix. They focused on a window-built execution estimate system for 2-D image analysis, focusing on image realignment's inherent difficulty. Ajala Funmilola et al. [9] presented a fuzzy-k means algorithm combining fuzzy c-means and k-means for MRI brain images. Yang-Mao et al. [10] proposed a trim-meaning filter that can effectively remove impulse and Gaussian noises but still preserves the sharpness of object boundaries. Santhi et al. [11] proposed a novel K-means nearest neighbor algorithm, combining K-means with morphology and Fuzzy to segment exudates in retinal images. Genctava et al. [12] proposed an unsupervised approach for the segmentation and classification of cervical cells. The segmentation process involved automatic thresholding to separate the cell regions from the background, Lin et al. [13] proposed a fuzzy logic CBIR (content-based image retrieval) system for finding textures. In CBIR system, a user can submit textual descriptions and/or visual examples to find the desired textures. After the initial search, the user can give relevant and/or irrelevant examples to refine the query and improve the retrieval efficiency. Chen et al. [14] developed a semiautomatic system to discriminate the cervical cells from original cells. A software application incorporating characteristics, inclusive of photographs reviewing and standardized denomination of report names, was also designed to facilitate and standardize the workflow of mobile analyses.

In 2019, Araújo et al. [15] developed CNN's method to segment the cervical cell image size (1,392 × 1,040 pixels) through an electron microscope, and Lin et al. [16] developed convolutional neural networks to categorize irregular cells using a single CC image with an average dimension of (110 × 110 pixels), sensibly arranged through physical localization and abstracting electron microscope images. The recognition of low-grade squamous intraepithelial lesions (LSIL) leads to shorter continuation intervals. The methods [15] and [16] require physical involvement to find and get single image or images of region of interest (ROI). The preceding scenarios are not enough for wholly programmed whole slide imaging (WSI) investigation in cervical high-grade squamous intraepithelial lesions (HSILs) inspection. This survey suggests a deep learning algorithm on cervical HSILs analysis and action using Papanicolaou staining, spotting, and determination of HSILs for advanced therapy recommendation.

7.3 MATERIALS AND METHODS

The cervical cell image contains the nucleus and cytoplasm, and their characteristics are most important to identify the normal and abnormal cells. Segmentation of these regions from the cervical cell images is necessary to differentiate the cancerous cells from the normal ones. So, we mainly focused on the cell nucleus and cytoplasmic region because the abnormal characteristics are most predominant there. The segmentation of cytoplasm and nucleus from the cervical cell images is carried out in various stages and presented step by step. In the preprocessing location, cervical images are resized to 120 × 120 for further processing. Resized images are converted to gray images with the different intensity values varying from 0 to 255. It is well suited to apply Otsu's thresholding to segment the cytoplasm, and this is discussed later in this chapter. In this work, images from the Herlev dataset are used for analysis. It contains 194 normal cells found in pap smear images. This includes 72 superficial cells in the image, 72 intermediate cells in the pap smear, and 50 parabasal epithelial cells, as shown in Table 7.1.

TABLE 7.1
Data Set

Herlev Data Set (Pap Smear Cells)	
Number of normal cells	194
Number of superficial cells	74
Number of intermediate cells	70
Number of para basal cells	50

7.4   CYTOPLASM SEGMENTATION

Segmentation is partitioning the image into various segments for further analysis. Thresholding is an effective technique for segmenting images having nimble objects at the dark historical past. Here, Otsu's threshold method segments the cytoplasm region from the cervical cell. There were 60 images (20 superficial cells, 20 intermediate cells, and 20 parabasal cells) from the dataset from Herlev. Preprocessed images are for Otsu's thresholding techniques to segment the cytoplasm. A single threshold value acts as a cutoff value for the entire image. Figure 7.1 illustrates the cytoplasm region obtained from Otsu's process from its original appearance. This method segments the cell's cytoplasm, but it is not suited for images having a blurred boundary. Morphological operations can overcome this problem for segmenting the cytoplasm.

When extracting the cytoplasmic region, basic morphological operations include erosion, reconstruction, and dilation. The erosion operation shrinks an image according to the shape of the structuring element. It removes objects that are smaller than the shape. The reconstruction operation restores the original forms of the objects that remain after erosion. After performing reconstruction, dilation is done. The dilation step regrows the remaining things left by the erosion operation, by the same shape. The result obtained is converted into a binary image. This method is done for another dataset containing 75 images (25 superficial cells, 25 intermediate cells, and 25 parabasal cells) chosen from the Herlev dataset. Figure 7.2 illustrates the individual steps.

The extracted features from the segmented results differentiate the normal cells from the abnormal ones. The technique adopted in this method was a neural network.

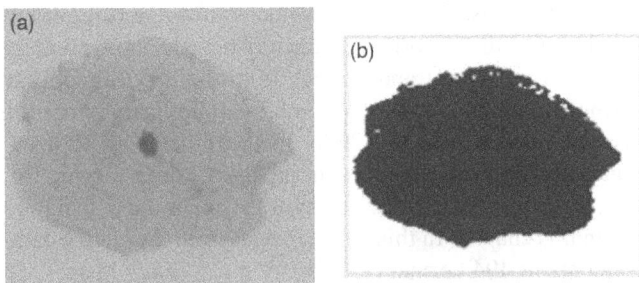

FIGURE 7.1   (a) Original image; (b) cytoplasm region obtained from threshold.

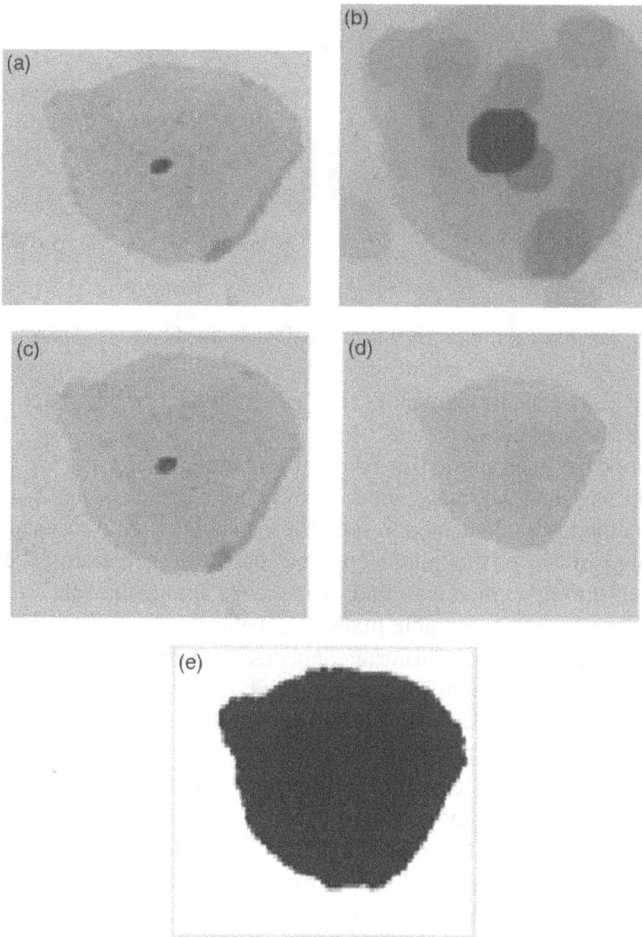

FIGURE 7.2 (a) Original image; (b) eroded image; (c) reconstructed image; (d) dilated image; (e) cytoplasm region after binarization.

The experimental analysis and static characteristics were calculated using the NPR tool in MATLAB. The nucleus of the cervical cells is segmented using color thresholding and k-means clustering for the single cells collected from the Herlev dataset.

7.5 SEGMENTATION OF THE NUCLEUS

The nucleus is the smallest region in the cell image, and it is essential to segment the nucleus because cells variation is mainly based on nucleus characteristics. The method used to segment the nucleus is described in this section. In this chapter, the threshold color method is used to segment the nucleus of the cervical cell. The size of the nucleus image is tiny compared to the size for the normal one. The global threshold technique will not give an improved departure of the nucleus. Therefore, color

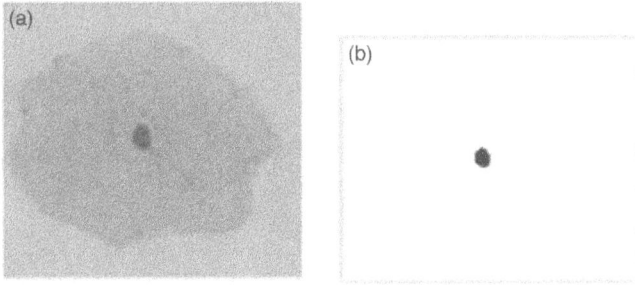

FIGURE 7.3   (a) Original image; (b) nucleus region obtained by color thresholding.

thresholding [3] is done to segment the nucleus from the cytoplasm and background based on the intensity measurement.

This method has been applied on a dataset containing 60 images. Figure 7.3 shows the original image and the image obtained from color thresholding. A segmentation clustering method is implemented to segment the nucleus in the cervical cell.

Clustering is a way of grouping techniques based on their features. The concept behind the clustering method is to find their groups among the data. A cluster typically contains a set of comparable pixels that belong to a particular place and are distinct from different areas. Clustering depends upon characteristics of pixels such as shape and texture. K-means logic and fuzzy c-means methods are the two main types of clustering. Here, k-means clustering is used to segment the nucleus from the cytoplasm. K-means is a type of clustering that splits the data into clusters. The k-means clustering method clusters the groups based on the intensity and color of the image. Here, the intensity is chosen as the main criterion to segment the three groups, namely background, cytoplasm, and the nucleus.

Figure 7.4a shows the original RGB image, and Figure 7.4b–d shows the three clusters, namely background, nucleus, and cytoplasm, respectively. From Figure 7.4, it is observed that the three clusters, namely cluster 1 (background), cluster 2 (nucleus), and cluster 3 (cytoplasm), obtained from the k-means clustering for the

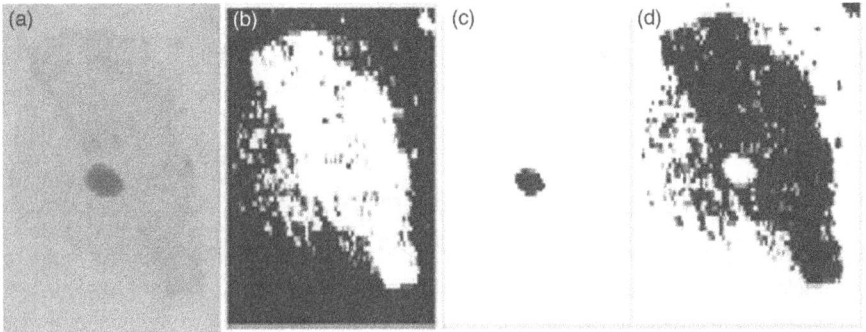

FIGURE 7.4   (a) Original image; (b) cluster 1 (background); (c) cluster 2 (nucleus); (d) cluster 3 (cytoplasm).

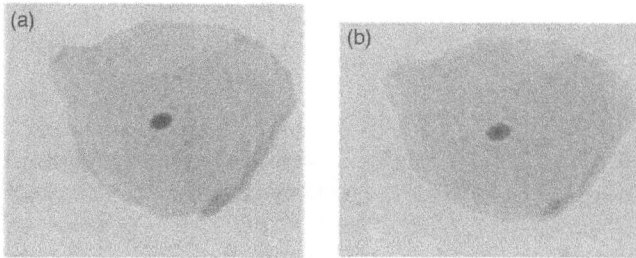

FIGURE 7.5 (a) Original image; (b) image with the final edge detected.

intensity values of background (0.7), nucleus (0.25), and cytoplasm (0.45), segments the nucleus aptly from the cytoplasm and background. This algorithm is not suitable for segmenting the background and cytoplasm. So the k-means algorithm is adapted to segment the nucleus from the cell images.

The detection of a contour of cytoplasm is done through an edge detection algorithm. Many edge detection techniques are available; from these, Canny's localization algorithm [5, 17, 18] was selected as the best. Then, the morphological operation is performed to eliminate the lesser area in and around the cytoplasm. Finally, identified edges overlapped on the grayscale images through object analysis. Figure 7.5 shows the edge detection image obtained from the binary image.

7.6 FEATURE EXTRACTION

Types of cervical cells can be differentiated by cell characteristics such as size, shape, color, and texture. Herlev University has provided a table of characteristics, shown in Table 7.2, for different types of cervical cells. Based on these findings, 17 features were removed in the cytoplasm and nucleus through the global threshold and color threshold method. Haralick features suggested by Haralick [19], entropy, energy, contrast, homogeneity, and linearity, were extracted from the images. Three Tamura features proposed by Tamura et al. [20], coarseness, roughness, and contrast of the image, were measured. Moreover, the entropy and the contrast of the co-occurrence matrix are also used to analyze textures in the cell. Thirty-one features have been extracted for the cytoplasm and nucleus obtained by image processing methods, such as morphological operation and the k-means clustering method. This

TABLE 7.2
Characteristics for Pap Smear Cells

Cell	Area	Nucleus-to-Cytoplasm Ratio	Nucleus Color	Cytoplasm Color
Superficial cells	Small	Small	Dark	Light
Intermediate cells	Small	Medium	Dark	Light
Parabasal cells	Small	Medium	Dark	Dark

TABLE 7.3
Extracted Features

S. No.	Features	S. No.	Features	S. No.	Features
1	Nucleus area	11	Nucleus width	21	Cytoplasm contrast
2	Cytoplasm area	12	Cytoplasm width	22	Cytoplasm correlation
3	N/C ratio	13	Nucleus length	23	Cytoplasm energy
4	Cytoplasm perimeter	14	Cytoplasm length	24	Cytoplasm homogeneity
5	Nucleus perimeter	15	Nucleus elongation	25	Cytoplasm equivdiameter
6	Maximum gross perimeter	16	Cytoplasm elongation	26	Nucleus equivdiameter
7	Average gross perimeter	17	Nucleus contrast	27	Cytoplasm eccentricity
8	Nucleus entropy	18	Nucleus correlation	28	Nucleus eccentricity
9	Cytoplasm entropy	19	Nucleus energy	29	Cytoplasm centroid (x)
10	Nucleus roundness	20	Nucleus homogeneity	30	Cytoplasm centroid (y)
				31	Cytoplasm roundness

software coding is developed using the image processing toolbox of MATLAB and extracted the 31 features shown in Table 7.3.

Feature selection is carried out to minimize the error rate and attain perfection in classification using a neural network. An analysis of variance (ANOVA) test is performed for selection. After statistical analysis, only the morphometric variables that show significant difference are chosen for classification purpose. On performing an ANOVA test on 31 features, only three features show the most significant deviation ($p < 1$) among three groups (group 1, superficial and parabasal cells; group 2, intermediate cells and parabasal cells; and group 3, superficial and intermediate cells). The three features with their probability are shown in Table 7.4.

7.7 CLASSIFICATION

A neural network is used to train the evaluated feature values to differentiate the abnormal cells from the original. Here, a feed-forward backpropagation method is used to distinguish the normal from original cells. To organize the three types of normal cervical cells, three features from the ANOVA test are selected, with high

TABLE 7.4
Selected Features and Their Probability Determined by an ANOVA Test

	P Value		
Features	Superficial with Parabasal Cells	Intermediate and Parabasal Cells	Superficial with Intermediate Cells
Cytoplasm contrast	0.013	0.0079	0.0087
Cytoplasm homogeneity	−0.0029	−0.0003	−0.0007
Nucleus correlation	−0.1227	−0.0657	−0.0364

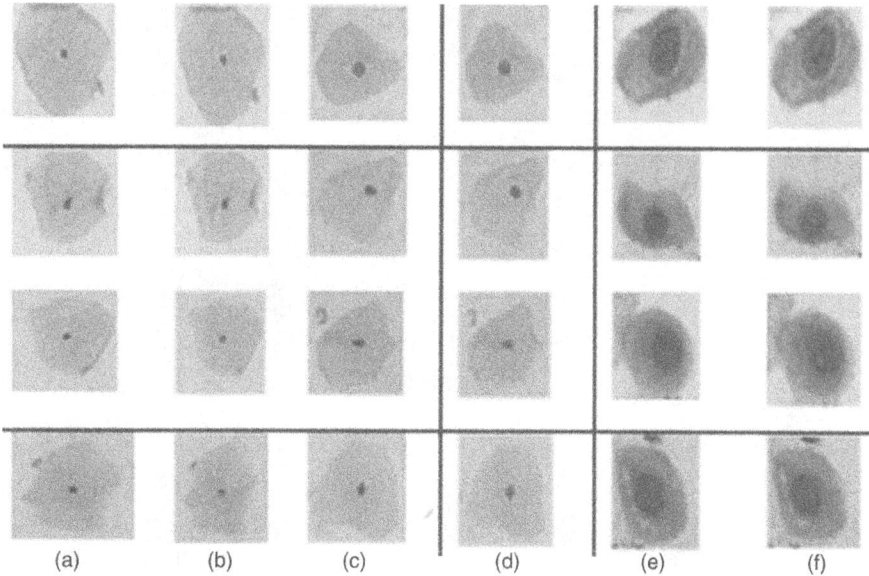

(a)   (b)   (c)   (d)   (e)   (f)

FIGURE 7.6 (a) Superficial input images (column 1); (b) contour detected superficial resultant images (column 2); (c) intermediate input images (column 3); (d) contour detected intermediate resultant images (column 4); (e) parabasal cell input images (column 5); (f) contour detected parabasal cell in resultant images (column 6).

variance among the three groups. For every kind of normal cell, the 25–75 samples were divided into 60% training samples and 40% test samples. A backpropagation training algorithm does the classification for the network. The transfer function for the hidden and output layers is chosen as a sigmoid and linear transfer function. Forty-five samples containing 15 for each type of normal cervical cells are used for training the network. Thirty samples were selected as 10 of each kind of normal cervical cells and used for testing. The target vector for the normal superficial cells, normal intermediate cells, and the normal parabasal cells is taken as [1 0 0] T, [0 1 0] T, and [0 0 1] T, respectively. Four different images from superficial, intermediate and parabasal category and its contour-detected resultant images are shown in Figure 7.6.

7.8 EXPERIMENTAL RESULTS

The neural network trains the evaluated feature values to differentiate the abnormal cells from the original ones. Here, a feed-forward backpropagation method categorizes the normal from original cells. To organize the three types of normal cervical cells, three features from the ANOVA test are selected, with high variance among the three groups. The 25–75 samples were divided into 60% training samples and 40% test samples for every type of normal cell. A backpropagation training algorithm does the classification used for the network. The transfer function for the hidden and output layers is chosen as a sigmoid and linear transfer function. Forty-five samples contained 15 for each type of normal cervical cells to train the network.

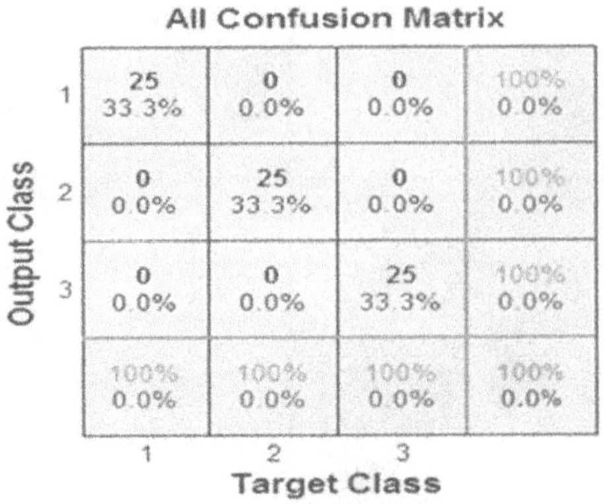

All Confusion Matrix

	1	2	3	
1	25 33.3%	0 0.0%	0 0.0%	100% 0.0%
2	0 0.0%	25 33.3%	0 0.0%	100% 0.0%
3	0 0.0%	0 0.0%	25 33.3%	100% 0.0%
	100% 0.0%	100% 0.0%	100% 0.0%	100% 0.0%

Output Class (vertical) — Target Class: 1 2 3

FIGURE 7.7 Confusion matrix.

Thirty samples were selected as 10 of each normal cervical cells were used for testing. The target vector for the normal superficial cells, normal intermediate cells, and the normal parabasal cells are taken as [1 0 0] T, [0 1 0] T, and [0 0 1] T, respectively.

In this study, three nominated features are for training and testing the data for neural networks that classify the superficial, parabasal, and intermediate cells. Based on the backpropagation neural network, we can obtain the confusion matrix to identify the designed network's training, validation, and testing accuracy. Figure 7.7 illustrates the confusion matrix for the designed backpropagation neural network.

Then all confusion matrices will give the overall network behavior for the training, validation, and testing. For the whole, 75 samples were used for the testing and validation of the designed backpropagation neural network, and the network obtained 100% accuracy. In this work, the three features, namely, contrast and homogeneity of cytoplasm and nucleus correlation, are enough to classify the standard cell in the cervical images. Jeremey Jordan proposed [21, 22] that ResNet50 in CNN. The ResNet50 model has taken less time to train the models than other machine learning algorithms. Many algorithms are in CNN, but residual neural networks gave good accuracy. This net also solves the overlapping blocks and upgrades the features.

7.9 CONCLUSION

The images used in this study are from Herlev. For implementation of detection and analysis, the morphological operation is used. The k-means clustering algorithm is used to segment the nucleus region from the cell. This algorithm is specifically designed for 75 normal CCs, 25 images are normal superficial cells, 25 images are normal intermediate cells and 25 of them are normal parabasal cells, respectively. Classification accuracy of 100% is attained. A limitation of this algorithm is prediction of the image. The prediction of carcinoma is a tedious issue. According to a researchers' survey, ResNet50 gives precise results in prediction and classification of cells, whereas CNN gives a lower percentage (44%) in prediction of classes. ResNet50 gives good results by identifying the correct classification of the cells. The literature survey states that the proposed method can be used for advanced image dataset.

REFERENCES

1. Shimizu, Y. Elimination of cervical cancer as a global health problem is within reach. World Health Organization. 2020. https://www.who.int/reproductivehealth/topics/cancers/en/.
2. Noorani, Hussein Z. Assessment of techniques for cervical cancer screening project director, Ottawa Canadian Coordinating Office for Health Technology Assessment 1997, monograph, CCOHTA report 1997: 2E, p. 33.
3. Das, A., Kar, A., and Bhattacharyya, D. (2011). "Preprocessing for Automating Early Detection of Cervical Cancer." *15th International Conference on Information Visualisation*, 597–600. https://doi.org/10.1109/IV.2011.89.
4. Al-amri, Salem Saleh, Kalyankar, N. V., and Khamitkar, S. D. "Image segmentation by using threshold techniques." *Journal of Computing* 2 (2010), ISSN.
5. Sharma, Nikita, Mishra, Mahendra, and Shrivastava, Manish. "Colour image segmentation techniques and issues: An approach." *International Journal of Scientific & Technology Research* 1(4) (2012): 9–12.
6. Tsai, Meng-Husiun, Chan, Yung-Kuan, Lin, Zhe-Zheng, Yang-Mao, Shys-Fan, and Huang, Po-Chi. "Nucleus and cytoplast contour detector of cervical smear image." *Pattern Recognition Letters* 29 (2008): 1441–1453.
7. Xiaoning, Wang, Jianwei, Zhang, Yue, Xin, Wanpeng, Wang, and Minchao, Lian. "LCT image recognition for cervical cells based on BP neural network." *IEEE International Conference on Computer Science and Network Technology*, Changchun, China, pp. 1479–1483, 2012. DOI:10.1109/ICCSNT.2012.6526200.
8. Park, Sun Y., Sargent, Dustin, and Lieberman, Richard. "Domain-specific image analysis for cervical neoplasia detection based on conditional random fields." *IEEE Transactions on Medical Imaging* 30(3) (2011): 867–868.
9. Funmilola, A. Ajala, Oke, O. A., Adedeji, T. O., Alade, O. M., and Adewusi, E. A. "Fuzzy k-c-means clustering algorithm for medical image segmentation." *Journal of Information Engineering and Applications* 2(6) (2012): 21–32. ISSN 2224–5782.
10. Yang-Mao, S.-F., Chan, Y.-K., and Chu, Y.-P. "Edge enhancement nucleus and cytoplast contour detector of cervical smear images." *IEEE Transactions on Systems, Man, and Cybernetics, Part B (Cybernetics)* 38(2) (2008): 353–366. doi: 10.1109/TSMCB.2007.912940.
11. Santhi, D., Manimegalai, D., and Karkuzhali, S. "Diagnosis of diabetic retinopathy by exudates detection using clustering techniques." *Biomedical Engineering: Applications, Basis and Communications* 26(6) (2014): 1450077-1–13.
12. Genctava, Aslı, Aksoya, Selim, and Onder, Sevgen. "Unsupervised segmentation and classification of cervical cell images." *Pattern Recognition* 45 (2012): 4151–4168.
13. Lin, H. C., Chiu, C. Y., and Yang, S. N. "Finding textures by textual descriptions, visual examples, and relevance feedbacks." *Pattern Recognition Letters* 24 (2003): 2255–2267.
14. Yung-Fu Chen. "Semi-automatic segmentation and classification of pap smear cells." *IEEE Journal of Biomedical and Health Informatics* 18 (2014): 94–108.
15. Araújo, F. H., et al. "Deep learning for cell image segmentation and ranking." *Computerized Medical Imaging and Graphics* 72 (2019): 13–21.

16. Lin, H., Hu, Y., Chen, S., Yao, J., and Zhang, L. "Fine-grained classification of cervical cells using morphological and appearance based convolutional neural networks." *IEEE Access* 7 (2019): 71541–71549.

17. Frei, W., and Chen, C. "Fast boundary detection: A generalization and new algorithm." *IEEE Transactions on Computers* C-26(10) (1977): 988–998.

18. Canny, J. "A computational approach to edge detection." *IEEE Transactions Pattern Analysis and Machine Intelligence* 8(6) (1986): 679–698.

19. Haralick, R. M., Shanmugam, K., and Dinstein, I. H. "Textural features for image classification." *IEEE Transactions of Systems, Man, and Cybernetics* SMC-3(6) (1973): 610–621.

20. Tamura, H., Mori, S., and Yamawaki, T. "Texture features corresponding to visual perception." *IEEE Transactions of Systems, Man, and Cybernetics* 8(6) (1978): 460–473.

21. Jordan, Jeremy. Common architectures in convolutional neural networks. https://www.jeremyjordan.me/convnet-architectures/. 2021.

22. Sobia, M. Carmel, and Abudhahir, A. "An efficient adaptive network-based fuzzy inference system with mosquito host-seeking for facial expression recognition." *Autosoft* 24(4): 1–15.

8 Progression Detection of Multiple Sclerosis in Brain MRI Images

Santosh Chede[1] and Surekha Washimkar[2]
[1]D. Y. Patil College of Engineering and Technology, Kolhapur, Maharashtra, India
[2]Priyadarshini College of Engineering, Nagpur, Maharashtra, India

CONTENTS

8.1 INTRODUCTION

Multiple sclerosis (MS) is also known as the disseminated sclerosis or encephalomyelitis disseminate. It is a demyelinating disease that degrades the protecting covers of nerve cells in the spinal cord and brain. The ability of parts of the nervous system to communicate is distrusted by this damage, resulting in various indication and symptoms. It is quite possible that between attacks symptoms may disappear totally as if affected; conversely, long-lasting neurological problems and damage may occur, especially as the disease advances. Understanding of the cause of the disease is not up to the mark. It is assumed that the underlying mechanism of the nerves gets destroyed because of the resistant system or failure of the myelin-generating cells.

DOI: 10.1201/9781003324430-10

133

Suggested causes for this include hereditary and ecological factors such as infections. MS is generally diagnosed on the presenting marks, indications, and the outcomes supporting medical tests.

This disease usually affects humans aged 20–50 years and is more common in women than men. MS is coined after the numerous scars (sclera, better known as plaques or lesions) that live on the white matter present in the brain and spinal cord in particular [1]. There are a number of new treatments and diagnostic methods that are under development.

MRI is used to capture correct information of the disease diagnosis. This also allows monitoring lesions, as shown in Figure 8.1. With appropriate data for each patient, a processing system developed for image analysis of pathology must be adaptable to practical breaches like changing camera settings and acquisition enough to change the quality of images. There are numerous identified approaches that are used to distinguish T1 brain tissue's white matter (WM), gray matter (GM), cerebrospinal fluid (CSF), and T2 modality that shows the lesions and cerebrospinal fluid (CSF). For detection of lesions, the segmentation of brain tissue plays a crucial role. The accurate detection of lesions is a challenging assignment. Manual segmentation

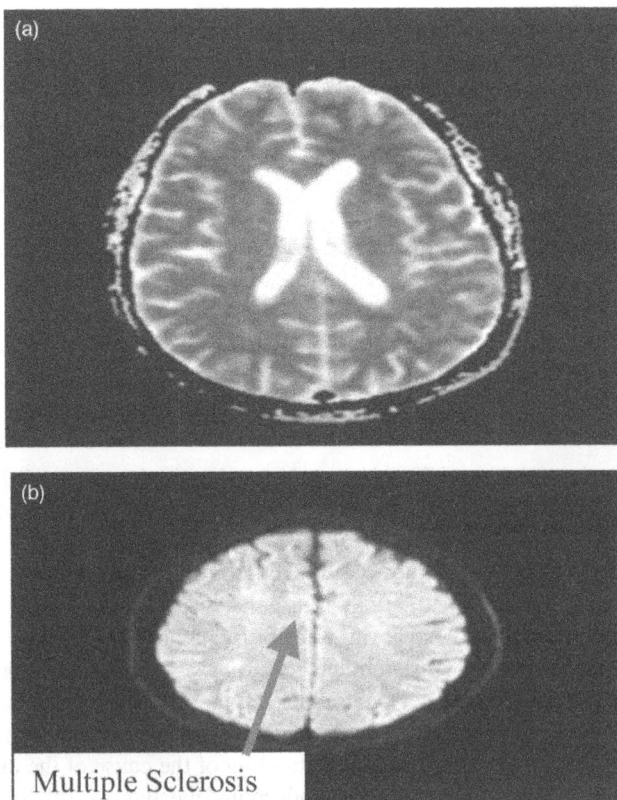

FIGURE 8.1   (a) Normal brain MRI image; (b) MS brain MRI image.

is done by a neurologist to extract the region of interest. A number of semiautomatic and automatic segmentation methods are available for identifying or segmenting MS lesions based on 2D MRI images. Extraction of quantitative information from an image is based on mathematical analysis called texture analysis [2]. An image is a mixture of pixels characterized by spatial location and gray-level intensity variation. This method proposes amplitude modulation (AM) frequency modulation (FM) for segmentation of brain MRI images [3]. A multimethod segmentation like one that applies saliency map, fuzzy C-means (FCM), and an adaptive iterative threshold-based algorithm is used with AM-FM to extract the region of interest. Various features like morphological, local binary pattern, and Gabor features are extracted. To record the real-time progressive detection of the disease, the same developed work is simulated in Very High Speed Integrated Circuit Hardware Description Language (VHDL) simulation and implemented on field-programmable gate array (FPGA) to show classification results [4].

8.2 MATERIAL AND DATA ACQUISITION

Lesion size varies from patient to patient. Some have small lesions, some have medium, and some have large lesions. Data of 20 real patients in the form of MR images have been collected from different reputable hospitals of the city for both males and females. The images are of T1-weighted, T2-weighted sagittal, and coronal with all angles. The lesion can be seen at least at two angles. A 1.5 Tesla MRI machine is used for capturing brain images. Out of the total disease images, some are of initial stages and rest are of progressive weeks. Normal brain images of 25 healthy subjects are acquired from MRI laboratories. As there is variation in image brightness between follow-up and baseline images, a normalization algorithm has been used. To get all gray image levels, the original histogram is stretched and shifted [5].

8.3 LITERATURE REVIEW

MRI is used to show MS lesions throughout the central nervous system (CNS) and for diagnostic purposes to solve the problem of complexity in a patient's examination. To indicate diagnostic weight of findings and their incorporations into the clinical analysis, MRI classes of evidence for MS are used [6]. There is also the semiautomatic method of image segmentation, which presents t-mixture-based medical image segmentation. The parameter of this model is first estimated, and posterior probabilities of the pixels of images are computed. The image was further segmented using Bays decision rule for minimum error [7]. Texture analysis can be performed in three different MRI units on T1- and T2-weighted MR images. This approach uses quantitative methodology for depiction of pathologic and healthy brain tissues like white matter, gray matter, cerebrospinal fluid, edema, and tumors. Each selected brain region of interest was characterized with both several texture parameters and its mean gray-level values. MR brain images contain texture features that can reveal discriminant factors for tissue classification and image segmentation [8]. To detect spatial deviations in gray-level values within an image and to provide useful information on the structures observed, texture analysis techniques are used. Application of various protocols to intra- and interscanner variations in the case of MRI are sensitive to acquisition conditions [9]. The classical texture analysis features are extracted with the help of texture analysis on MR images. To differentiate between normal-appearing white matter (NAWM), normal white matter (NWM) and MS, a set of texture attributes has been used. Texture analysis is performed on brain MRIs of patients. Texture features from gray-level cooccurrence matrices (GLCM) has been selected and classified for tissue discrimination. Three statistical analysis methods – redundancy analysis (RDA), principal components analysis (PCA), and linear discriminant analysis (LDA) – and two classifications – K-NN and ANN – are applied to seek high classification accuracy [10]. A solution to use MRI to carry early diagnosis of MS stems from the subtle pathological changes in the CNS. Texture analysis is performed on MR images of MS patients. Normal control and a combined set of texture features are explored in order to better discriminate tissues between MS lesions, NAWM, and NWM. Features are extracted from gradient matrix, run length (RL) matrix, gray level co-occurrence matrix (GLCM), autoregressive (AR) model and wavelet analysis [11]. The use multi-scale AM-FM texture analysis of MS using magnetic resonance (MR) images from brain is advantageous and also proves association between disease development and lesion texture. AM-FM physiognomies are responsible in differentiating between NWM and NAWM, NAWM and lesions, and NWM and lesions. AM-FM provides complementary information to classical texture analysis features like the gray scale, median, and contrast [3]. Such an approach can be realized using FPGA implementation [12]. FPGA using Xilink System Generator (XSG) can be applied to execute various image augmentation algorithms like thresholding, contrast stretching, and negative transformation [13]. Different enhancement methods using frequency domain and spatial domain to improve the visual eminence can be realized using FPGA [14]. Image enhancement techniques using Verilog Hardware Descriptive Language focus on image augmentation in a spatial domain to process contrast stretching threshold algorithms for hardware implementation [11]. Numerous image processing operations can be implemented using FPGA [11]. MATLAB Simulink blocks and XSG are utilized for FPGA implementation [15]. The FPGA Cyclon III Altera system is used to implement various image-processing algorithms in the spatial domain such as contrast stretching, median filter, and histogram equalization. In literature review, survey of various papers on texture analysis of the AM-FM method and on FPGA implementation has been conducted. Researchers have proposed numerous methods for disease detection in brain MRI images. These methods mainly include atrophy analysis of brain white matter, changes in the pathological parameter of brain as the disease progresses, and its correlation with expanded detectability status scale. Several segmentation and feature extraction techniques have been proposed by researchers to help to find features of the lesion in the region of interest and to detect the disease and its progression. To see the progression of the disease, MRI scans at different time points are required. Hence there is a possibility of intensity variation between scans. To solve this, intensity normalization methods were suggested by the researcher. A texture analysis method was given by the researcher for segmentation and extracting the features of medical images. One of the texture analysis methods, called AM-FM, was used by researcher in various medical applications for detection of disease. AM-FM demodulation is a basic module. With improvement in segmentation and feature extraction techniques, an effective AM-FM demodulation and image reconstruction technique is developed.

8.4   PROPOSED SYSTEM

The system proposed has four important steps to find and segment MS from brain images. These main stages are image preprocessing, target segmentation, feature attribute, and categorization. The proposed methodology clearly is shown in Figure 8.4.

8.4.1   STEP 1: PREPROCESSING

The initial stage in projected method is preprocessing of the brain MRI image. To lower the noise by a 3×3 median filter and to prepare the brain MRI image for further processing, the preprocessing of an image is done. These steps give improved image appearance and image eminence for more indemnity and ease in MS detection.

8.4.2   STEP 2: TARGET SEGMENTATION

The next step after refining the MRI image of the brain is to segment the MS MRI image. An image foreground is separated from its background by segmentation. The processing period for further operations is saved by segmenting an image that must be applied to the image. Some of the techniques are explained as follows:

1. **Fuzzy C-means algorithm**

   Constrained soft clustering algorithm is the best clustering algorithm [16]. This algorithm is useful to find a soft partition of a given data set by which an element in the data set partially belongs to multiple clusters. Let us consider an example $X = \{x_1, x_2, x_3 \ldots x_n\}$ and $P = \{c_1, c_2, c_3 \ldots c_k\}$, where X is a set of n number of data points and P is a set of k number of clusters. Each of the points here belongs to one or more clusters depending on its degree of membership. Point x_i belongs to cluster c_j as long as its degree of membership to c_j, produced by membership function $\mu c_j(x_i)$, is more than zero. The center of each cluster and the decision of to which cluster points these clusters belong are computed for clustering a data set [17]. To find the center of a cluster, the sum of the distance between points in the cluster and its center is used as the criterion in FCM to use an objective function J. The function needs to be minimized with respect to P. It is depicted as follows:

$$J_{m(P,V)} = \sum_{j=1}^{k} \sum_{i=1}^{n} (\mu_j(x_k))^m \|x_i - v_j\|^2 \qquad (8.1)$$

   This formula incorporates the fuzzy membership degree μ_c and surplus parameter "m," a weighted exponent of fuzzy membership that determines the value of the measure to which partial members of the cluster affect the result. Where x_i is the value of the data point under consideration, and v_j is the center of cluster c_j. V is initiated with some prototype value at the beginning of the process. For updating the membership degrees, the function J is minimized by using the following equation and V iteratively until $|V_i - V_{i-1}| < e$.

$$\mu_{cj}(x_i) = \frac{1}{\sum_{j=1}^{k}\left(\frac{\|x_i - v_j\|^2}{\|x_i - v_j\|^2}\right)^{\frac{1}{m-1}}} \tag{8.2}$$

Here $1 \leq j \leq k$ and $1 \leq i \leq n$.

$$vj = \frac{\sum_{i=1}^{n}\left(\mu_{cj}(x_i)\right)^m x_i}{\left(\mu_{cj}(x_i)\right)^m} \tag{8.3}$$

This not only speeds up the process but ensures computation in the main memory, thereby reducing disk access during the process [18].

2. **AM-FM image segmentation**

According to the AM-FM model, an image can be modeled by way of the superposition of sinusoidal components, which is represented by following equation [19]:

$$I(x,y) = \sum_{k=1}^{k} a_k(x,y)\cos(\emptyset_k(x,y)), w_k(x,y)\nabla\emptyset_k(x,y) \tag{8.4}$$

Here each of the k components is a movable AM-FM signal with instantaneous amplitude $a_k(x,y)$ and instantaneous frequency w_k. The decomposition of an image in terms of the aforementioned problem is ill posed due to computation of an infinity of AM and FM signals yielding the same image. The separation of an idle AM-FM component can be achieved by using filtering with a multiband Gabor filter bank, where the output of each filter can then be denoted as a mono-component that lends itself to an effective demodulation algorithm and is instinctively interpretable [20].

If $f(x, y)$ is a mono-component, in a 2D AM-FM signal its spatially varying amplitude $a(x, y)$ can be interpreted as modeling a local image contrast, while the instantaneous frequency vector $\omega(x, y) = \nabla\varphi(x, y)$ describes locally emergent spatial frequencies:

$$f(x,y) = a(x,y)\cos[(\phi(x,y))] \tag{8.5}$$

Efficient estimation of the modulation component of the AM-FM signals can be accompanied via the energy separation algorithm. Let $f(x,y)$ be a

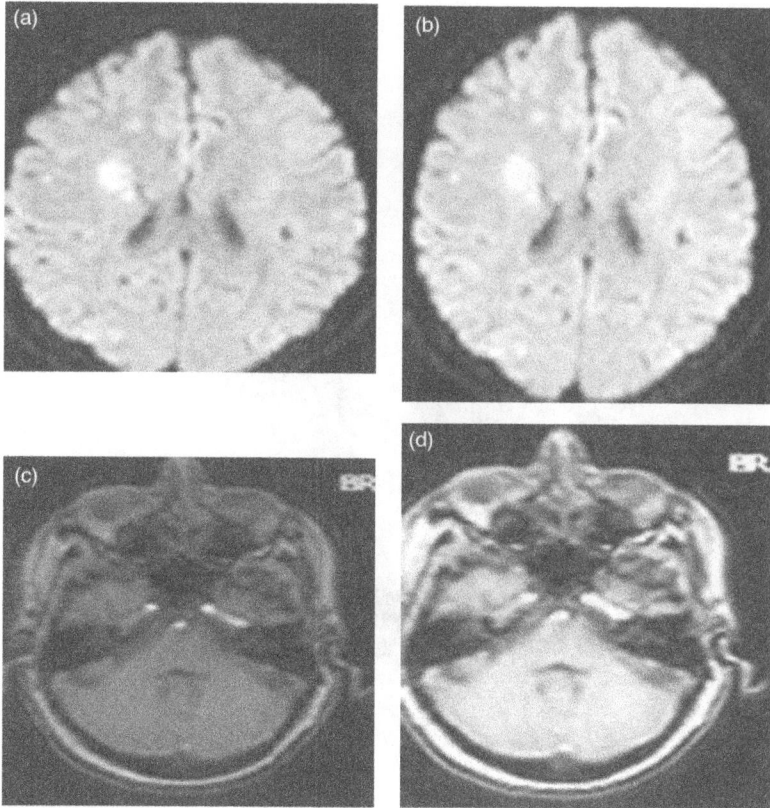

FIGURE 8.2   (a and b) AM-FM segmented images; (c and d) Brain MRI input images.

double-differentiable continuous-space real-valued input function, and then the operator is defined as

$$\varnothing(f)(x,y) \triangleq \|\nabla f(x,y)\|^2 - f(x,y)\nabla^{2*} f(x,y) \qquad (8.6)$$

Figure 8.2(a) shows the input brain MRI image, and Figure 8.2(b) shows images after AM-FM segmentation in different amplitudes and angles

3. **The saliency map detection model**

This model is used to get the area of interest by reducing the unwanted region from the image. Calculation of the salient map is accomplished with features like intensity, color, and orientation. To get the salient region of the image, Gaussian filter and hypercomplex algorithms are used. Binary and Gaussian filters have been applied to get the smooth image, which further removes the noise from the image [19].

For an explicit illustration of an image objects, the saliency map is used. To detect image objects in a saliency, simple threshold segmentation is used. The object map $R(x)$ is obtained with $I(x)$ of an image [21].

$$R(x) = \{\blacksquare \left(1 \text{ if } I(x) > \text{threshold}, 0 \text{ otherwise}\right)$$

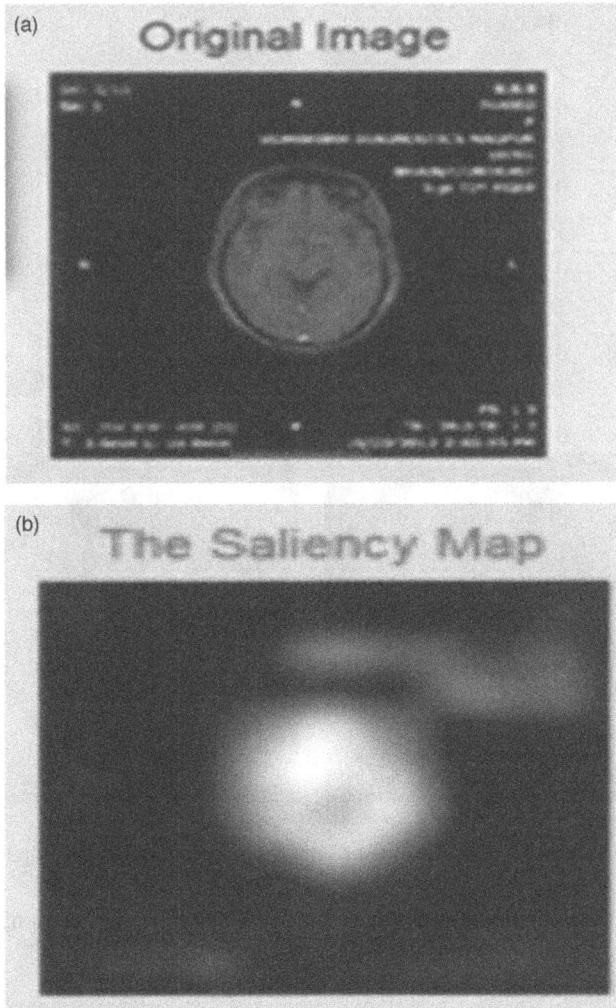

FIGURE 8.3 (a) Cognitive normal; (b) saliency map brain.

Empirically, threshold set $= m\ (I(x)) \times 3$ and $m\ (P(x))$ is the mean intensity of the saliency map. The threshold assortment is a trade-off difficulty between disregard of objects and false alarm. The image objects can be easily obtained from their respective positions in the input image when object map $R(x)$ is generated. Various targets are extracted consecutively. Figure 8.3 (a and b) shows normal brain and saliency map images respectively.

8.4.3 STEP 3: FEATURE EXTRACTION

In this stage, the input image helps to analyze the objects, to extricate the most important attributes that represent various object classes. Classifiers use attributes as inputs and assign the class that they represent. The original data are reduced through feature extraction by measuring certain properties and attributes that distinguish one input pattern from another. The classifier gets the characteristics of the input type by the extracted feature by considering the description of the relevant properties of the image into feature vectors. The following attributes are extracted in this proposed system: (i) shape attributes – circularity, irregularity, area, perimeter, shape index; (ii) intensity attributes – mean, variance, standard variance, median intensity, skewness, and kurtosis; and (iii) texture attributes – contrast, correlation, entropy, energy, homogeneity, cluster shade, and sum of square variance. The efficacy of texture-based MS detection, segmentation, and categorization helps to describe the MS surface variation. It is expected to be different from the non-MS region, which leads to increase the certainty of fine extraction. To classify the images into different categories to observe the progression of disease, a linear classifier like the multifeature K-NN classifier is used. Work flow of methodology is mentioned in Figure 8.4.

A. **Training phase**

The proposed system is trained by an image database of different classes. The brain MRI image is given as input to the system, and the input image is processed by AM-FM segmentation. To find the region of interest and the important area of an image, a saliency map detection technique is used. The output image created has only a salience image, and to extract features from the image, an output image created by AM-FM segmentation is used.

B. **Evaluation phase**

For evaluation, the features are stored in the database with the disease name. The progress pattern of the patient is estimated initially and compared with pattern stored in trained database. Hence the future state of the patient is predicted with the pattern matching patient history. For further segmentation, an adaptive iterative threshold-based algorithm is used. Threshold is calculated for each iteration. The results are obtained for an iteration value from 1 to 5. In each iteration, brighter components are selected, while the darker components are removed. Iteration value must be kept optimum for optimized results, and iteration 2 gives the best output results for disease progression.

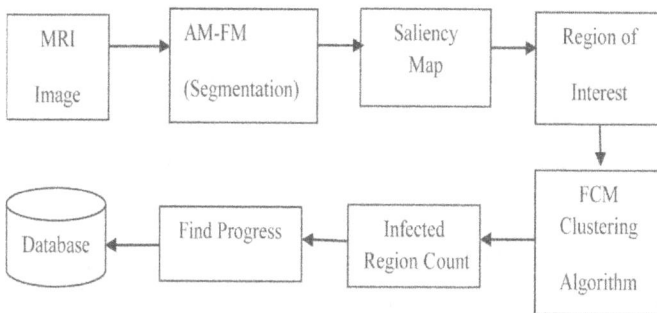

FIGURE 8.4 Workflow diagram.

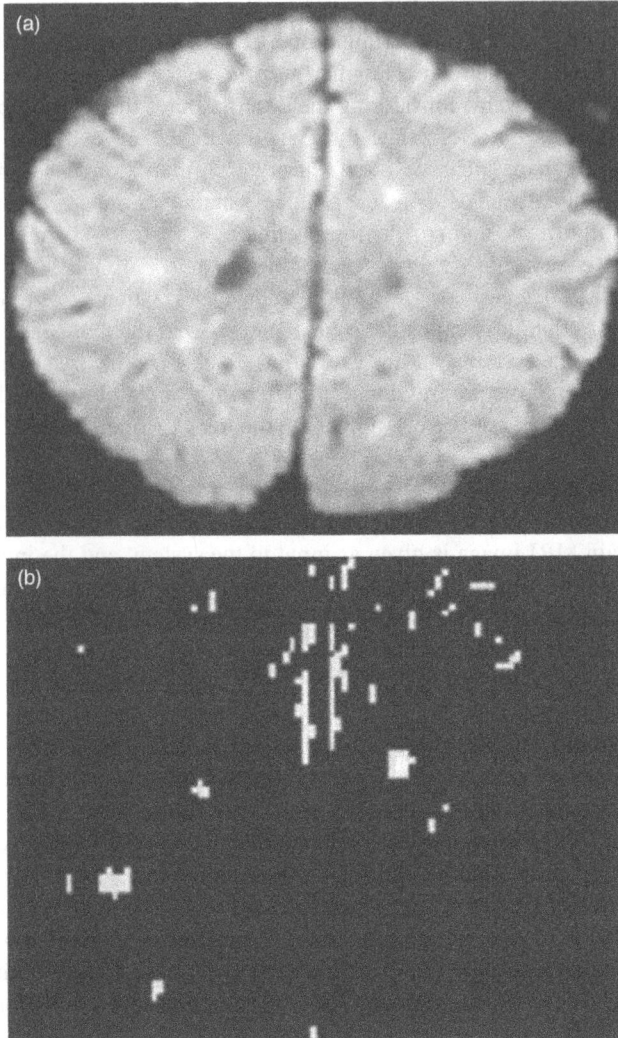

FIGURE 8.5   (a) Normal brain MRI image; (b) segmented image.

Figure 8.5(a) shows the normal brain MRI image, and Figure 8.5(b) shows the image after multimethod segmentation. The same developed work in MATLAB is simulated in the VHSIC Hardware Description Language (VHDL) environment for implementation in real time. Accordingly, sclerosis state evaluation is shown in Figure 8.6.

8.5   VHDL SIMULATION

The test image for verification of class is input to MATLAB. After applying automatic (saliency map) and semiautomatic AM-FM segmentation maximum a posteriori (MAP) segmentation and maximal region features (MRF), the features are

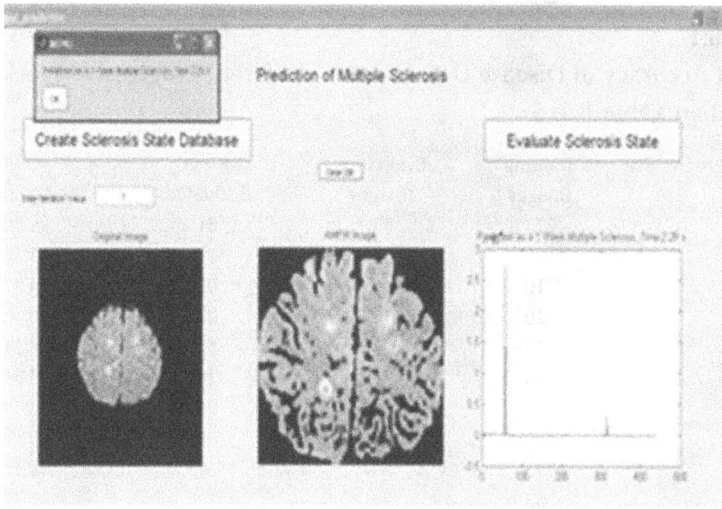

FIGURE 8.6   Sclerosis state evaluation.

extracted. The extracted features from MATLAB are exported in a .do file (TCL file), shown in Figure 8.7. The .do file is in a matrix form that contains the pixel value of the images. This .do file is input for VHDL processing. Tables 8.1 and 8.2 show the different classes of disease through the simulation software Modelsim. Figure 8.8 represents one of output classes of disease progression. The same developed work in MATLAB is simulated in the VHDL environment for implementation in real time.

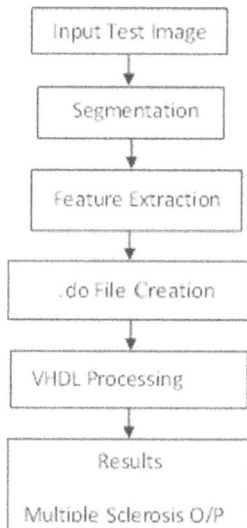

FIGURE 8.7   Flowchart of MATLAB to VHDL processing.

TABLE 8.1

Percent Accuracy of Disease Detection for Different Progressive Weeks of Iteration Value 1 to 5

Disease Progressive Weeks	Training Images	Evaluated Images	Correctly Evaluated	% Accuracy
1	273	53	51	96.66
24	53	29	19	65.51
96	10	06	02	33.33
144	20	10	03	30
1	273	53	52	98.11
24	53	29	22	75.86
96	10	06	05	83.33
144	20	10	08	80
1	273	53	52	98.11
24	53	29	12	41.37
96	10	06	04	66.66
144	20	10	08	80
1	273	53	40	75.47
24	53	29	20	68.96
96	10	06	04	80
144	20	10	06	60
1	273	53	40	75.47
24	53	29	16	55.17
96	10	06	03	50
144	20	10	06	60

TABLE 8.2

Accuracy of Progression Detection of MS in Brain MRI Images by VHDL Simulation

Disease Progressive Weeks	Training Images	Evaluated Images	Correctly Evaluated	% Accuracy
1	85	73	69	69/73 = 94.25
24	35	29	28	28/29 = 96.55
96	10	6	3	3/6 = 50
144	20	10	8	8/10 = 80
Normal Subject	20	10	9	9/10 = 90

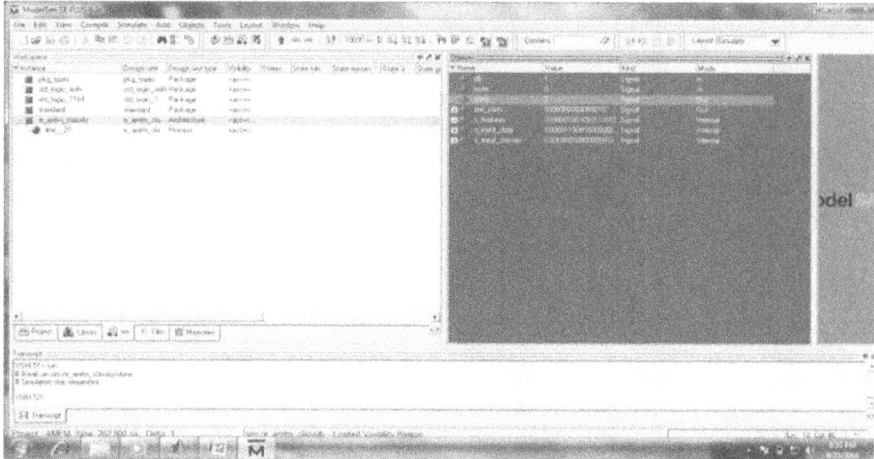

FIGURE 8.8   Output class indication.

8.6   SYSTEM ARCHITECTURE

The system architecture shown in Figure 8.9 consists of the classifier model along with additional digital blocks to test the complete system on FPGA. The input clock to the system is the 50 MHz oscillator on DE2 board. The output is connected to a seven segment display.

8.7   DESIGN FLOW

Figure 8.10 shows the design flow for FPGA. The extracted features from MATLAB are exported in a .do file. The contents of the .do file are stored in memory. The memory inside the FPGA has been distributed between block RAM and distributed RAM to make it faster. The extracted features are written in a package in VHDL.

8.7.1   POWER OPTIMIZATION

Load-enabled registers are group of flip-flops to share the same clock and synchronous control signals that are inferred from the same HDL variable. Clock gating is applied to synchronous load-enabled registers. Synchronous load-enabled, synchronous set, synchronous reset, and synchronous toggle are the functions of synchronous control signals. The registers are implemented by Design Compiler, which is used to implement registers with the help of feedback loops. These registers maintain the same logic value through multiple cycles with the penalty of power. Clock gating saves power by eliminating the unnecessary activity associated with reloading register banks. This is carried for reduced power consumption. Designs that benefit most from clock gating are those with low-throughput data paths.

8.7.2   RTL VIEW OF THE CLASSIFIER FOR ALL CLASSES

See Figure 8.11.

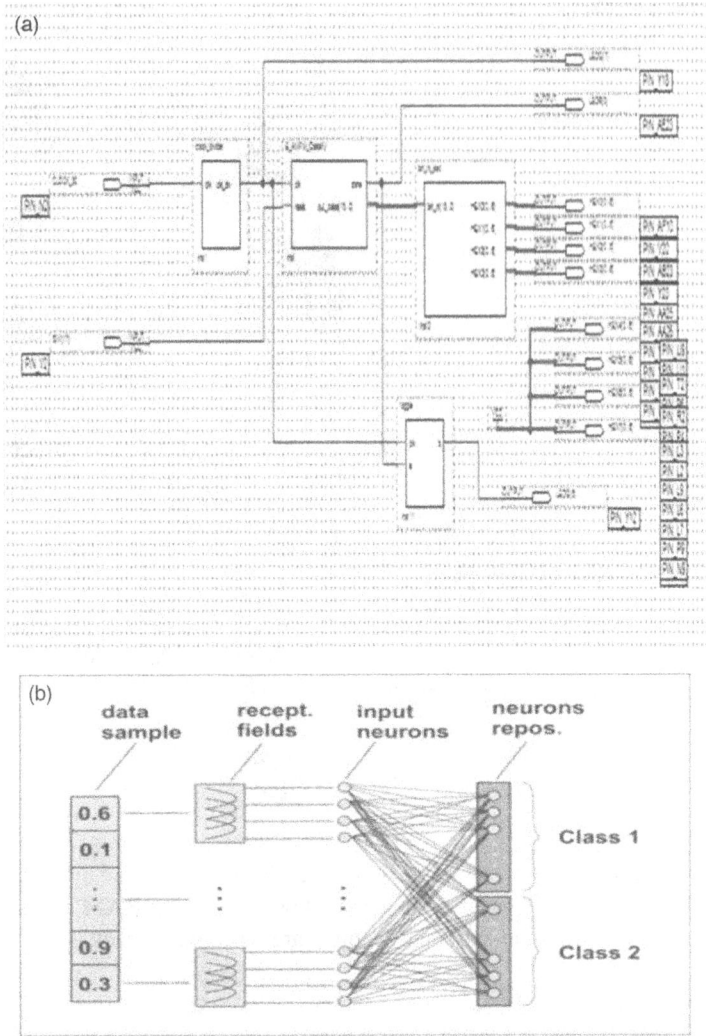

FIGURE 8.9 System architecture.

8.7.3 MAXIMUM FREQUENCY FOR COMPLETED SYSTEM

Figure 8.12 describes the maximum frequency of design. The design achieved a maximum frequency of 225 MHz on FPGA, making it highly efficient for medical science.

8.8 RESULT OF FPGA IMPLEMENTATION

Table 8.3 and Figure 8.13 present results of FPGA implementation. Table 8.3 displays results for progression of MS, and Figure 8.13 shows the output classes.

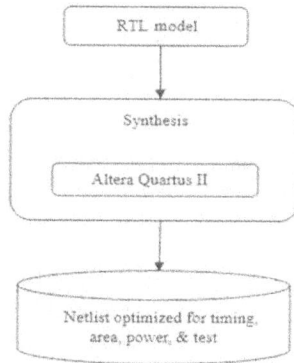

FIGURE 8.10   FPGA design flow.

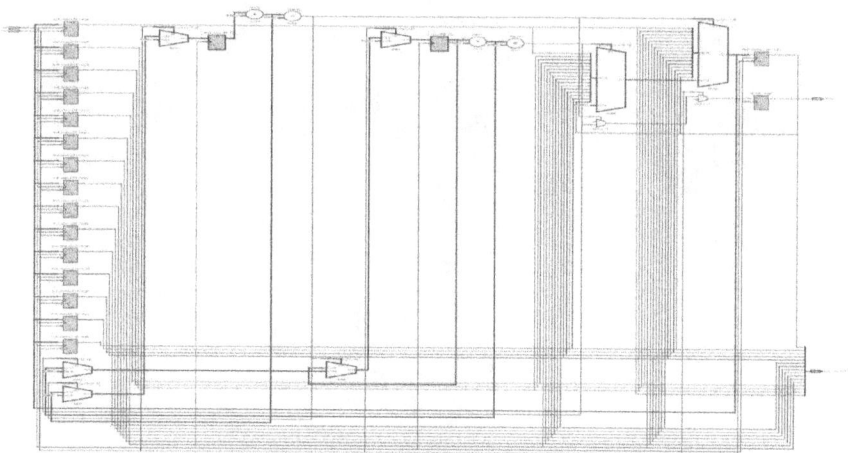

FIGURE 8.11   RTL view of the classifier for all classes.

	Value	
From	E_AMFM_Classify:inst|v_feat_count[0]	
To	E_AMFM_Classify:inst|v_count[0]	
Clock period	4.309 ns	
Frequency	232.07 MHz	

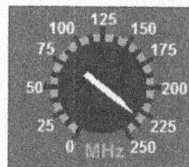

FIGURE 8.12   Maximum frequency for complete system.

TABLE 8.3
Results Obtained for Progression of Disease on FPGA

Diseased Progressive Weeks	Name of the Class	Test Image Input Class	FPGA Output Class
1 week	Class 1	0000000000000001	0001
24 week	Class 2	0000000000000010	0010
96 week	Class 3	0000000000000011	0011
144 week	Class 4	0000000000000100	0100
Normal subject	Class 5	0000000000000101	0101

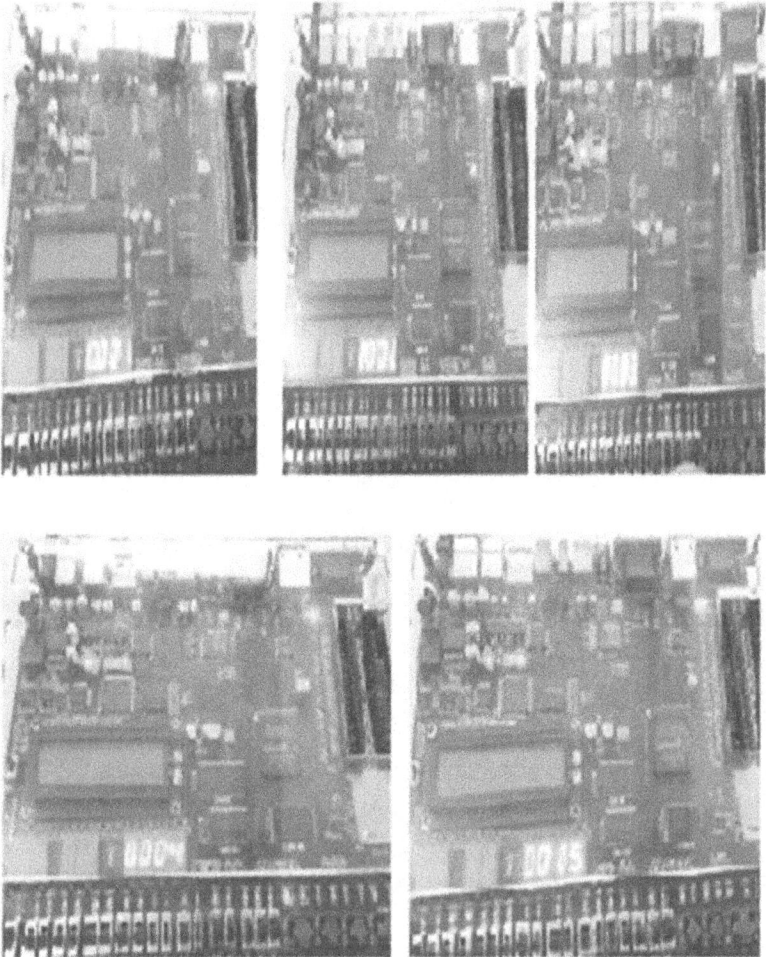

FIGURE 8.13   Results of FPGA showing output classes.

8.9 CONCLUSION

Texture-based segmentation techniques like AM-FM (semiautomatic) and saliency maps (automatic) applied on the real patient images give excellent classification results when the extracted feature file (the .do file) is simulated in the VHDL environment. The results in the table show that the accuracy is 94% and is best for the initial week of the disease diagnosis of the patient, which helps in predicting the disease in its earlier stages. The same work is implemented on FPGA by storing the value of the .do file in memory to give the classification result of the disease progression. Figure 8.13 and Table 8.3 show results of FPGA showing output classes. The hardware implementation of proposed work helps in the future for real-time processing of the disease that may speed up the process of disease verification.

REFERENCES

1. J. Sastre-Garriga, et al., Gray and white matter volume changes in early primary progressive multiple sclerosis: A longitudinal study, Brain, vol. 128, pp. 1454–1460, 2005.
2. J. Zhang, L. Tong, L. Wang, and N. Li, Texture analysis of multiple sclerosis: A comparative study, Magnetic Resonance Imaging, vol. 26, no. 8, pp. 1160–1166, 2008.
3. C.P. Loizou, V. Murray, M.S. Pattichis, I. Seimenis, M. Pantziaris, and C.S. Pattichis, Multiscale amplitude-modulation frequency modulation (AM-FM) texture analysis of multiple sclerosis in brain MRI mages, IEEE Transactions on Information Technology in Biomedicine, vol. 15, no. 1, pp. 119–129, January 2011.
4. Tarek M. Bittibssi, Gouda I. Salama, Yehia Z. Mehaseb, and Adel E. Henawy, Image enhancement algorithms using FPGA, International Journal of Computer Science & Communication Networks, vol. 2, no. 4, pp. 536–542, 2015.
5. C.P. Loizou, I. Siemens, M. Pantziaris, and C.S. Pattichis, "Brain MR image normalization in texture analysis of multiple sclerosis," Proceedings of the 9th International Conference on Information Technology and Application in Biomedicine, ITAB 2009, Larnaca, Cyprus, pp. 5–7, November 2009.
6. Fazekas (Graz), "The contribution of magnetic resonance imaging to the diagnosis of multiple sclerosis," 43rd International Neuropsychiatric PULA Symposium.
7. C.A. Plagan, and T. Leena, "Brain structure segmentation of Magnetic Resonance imaging using t-mixture algorithm," 3rd International Conference on Electronics Computer Technology, vol. 3, pp. 446–450, 2011.
8. S. Heridou-Meme, MRI texture analysis on texture test objects, normal brain and intracranial tumors, Magnetic Resonance Imaging, vol. 21, pp. 989–993, 2003.
9. G. Collewet, M. Strzelecki, and F. Marriette, Influence of MRI acquisition protocols and image intensity normalization methods on texture classification, Magnetic Resonance Imaging, vol. 22, pp. 81–91, 2004.
10. Jing Zhang, Lei Wang, and Longzheng Tong, "Feature reduction and texture classification in MRI texture analysis of multiple sclerosis," IEEE International Conference on Complex Medical Engineering, pp. 752–756(36), 2007.
11. Iuliana Chiuchisan, Marius Cerlinca, Alin-Dan Potorac, and Adrian Graur, "Image enhancement methods approach using Verilog Hardware Descriptive Language," 11th International Conference on Development and Application Systems, pp. 144–148, May 17–19, 2012.
12. K. Anil Kumar, and M. Vijay Kumar, Implementation of image processing lab using xilinx system generator, Advances in Image and Video Processing, vol. 2, no. 5, pp. 27–35, September 25, 2014.

13. Kalyani A. Dakre, and P.N. Pusdekar, Review on image enhancement using hardware co-simulation for biomedical operations, International Journal of Advanced Research in Computer Engineering & Technology, vol. 3, no. 12, pp. 4438–4441, December 2014.

14. S.O. Nirmala, T.D. Dongale, and R.K. Kamat, Review on image enhancement techniques: FPGA implementation perspective, International Journal of Electronics Communication and Computer Technology, vol. 2, no. 6, pp. 270–274.

15. Mohammed Yusuf Khan, Masarath Nayeem Tayyaba, M.A. Raheem, Ayesha Siddiqua, and Syed Sameena, Image enhancement and hardware implementation of edge detected vascular images using Simulink model, International Journal of Advanced Research in Computer and Communication Engineering, vol. 3, no. 4, pp. 6385–6388, 2014.

16. Y. Yong, Z. Chongxun, and L. Pan, A novel fuzzy c-means clustering algorithm for image thresholding, Measurement Science Review, vol. 4, no. 1, pp. 11–19, 2004.

17. A. Rui, and J.M.C. Sousa, "Comparison of fuzzy clustering algorithms for classification," International Symposium on Evolving Fuzzy Systems, pp. 112–117, 2006.

18. S. Chen, and D. Zhang, Robust image segmentation using FCM with spatial constraints based on new kernel-induced distance measure, IEEE Transactions on Systems, Man and Cybernetics, vol. 34, pp. 1907–1916, 1998.

19. T. Liu, J. Sun, N. Zheng, X. Tang, and H.Y. Shum, "Learning to detect a salient object," Proceeding IEEE International Conference on Computer Vision and Pattern Recognition, pp. 1–8, July 2007.

20. Victor Murray, Paul Rodríguez, and Marios S. Pattichis, Multiscale AM-FM demodulation and image reconstruction methods with improved accuracy, IEEE Transactions on Image Processing, vol. 19, no. 5, pp. 1138–1152, May 2010.

21. X. Hou, and L. Zhang, "Saliency detection: A spectral residual approach," Proceeding IEEE Conference on Computer Vision and Pattern Recognition.

9 Artificial Intelligence Clustering Techniques on Dermoscopic Skin Lesion Images

V. Saravana Kumar[1], M. Kavitha[2], S. Anantha Sivaprakasam[3], E. R. Naganathan[4], Sunil Bhutada[1], K. G. Suma[5], Lakshmi Priya[4], and M. Sakthivel[6]
[1]Sreenidhi Institute of Science and Technology, Hyderabad, Telangana, India
[2]S A Engineering College, Chennai, Tamil Nadu, India
[3]Rajalakshmi Engineering College, Chennai, Tamil Nadu, India
[4]GITAM University, Bengaluru, Karnataka, India
[5]Lovely Professional University, Punjab, India
[6]Mohan Babu University, Tirupati, Andhra Pradesh, India

CONTENTS

9.1 INTRODUCTION

Dermoscopy is an inconspicuous diagnostic system for the observation of pigmented skin injuries and one of the greatest momentous imaging procedures for melanoma analysis [1]. At the same time, its indicative exactitude overall relies upon the familiarity of the dermatologists, the optical illumination and evaluation of this type of picture is monotonous, and a few computer-based hold up verdict systems of computerized dermoscopic pictures [2–4] have been obtainable. Besides, a faithful ground truth database of bodily segregated pictures [5, 6] is imperative for the progression and appreciation of planned division and grouping techniques. Even supposing the masters among dermatologists keep up the ground truth database, there is a prerequisite for the perfection of description devices that can boost up the manual division of dermoscopic pictures [7], and by the side of these lines makes this task simpler and, in addition, realistic for dermatologists.

Image processing [8] plays a vital role in systematic processing for image analysis [9] in MATLAB. This image analysis operates for uplifting purposes for early analysis of any infection [10]. At present, skin malignancy is a typical sickness, and its preliminary identification [11] and fix is noteworthy. It spectacularly helping by exploiting the emphasis on data mining and segmentation [12–14] techniques. This strategy requires fiscal know-how as it uses many exorbitant gadgets and afterward operates by each person. At the moment, unbelievable deception is possible in the automatic image processing [15] modus operandi. It provides the useful information about the lesion with the help of clinical gadgets. It is perceived as premature and dealing with skin malignant growth might diminish the instability and fear of patients. The things to see should offer a known quantitative process to subsequently examine the disease. The most noteworthy test is the structure evaluation [16, 17] prior to the obligation of conclusion. In consequence of the embarrassing measure of available information, there is perhaps myriad leaning if the structure appraisal doesn't led properly. This chapter provides a review of the means necessary to clearly analyze skin malignant growth [18] by using dissimilar pictures of a range of dangers.

9.2   K-MEANS CLUSTERING ALGORITHM

Machine learning algorithms are put forward by unsupervised [19] learning by a clustering process, namely the K-Means clustering algorithm. It is an iterative approach, simple and interesting to implement. The algorithm provides a smooth, classical unsupervised clustering method. Most researchers start their research career using this method. Its aim is to segregate the given data into k clusters. It starts from certain (K) initial values called seed points, where each cluster is defined, such as an adaptively varying centroid. It computes the squared distance of inputs and centroids besides doled-out inputs to the adjoining centroid.

For clustering issues, let us deliberate a set of n items $I = \{1,....n\}$ make as K-clusters. For every object $i \in I$, present a cluster of m features $\{x_{ij}: j \in J\}$, where x_{ij} denotes the jth features of the item i quantifiable. Let $x_i = (x_{ij},....x_{im})^T$ refer to the feature vector of the item i and $X = (x_1,....x_n)$ refer to the data set.

The clustering mission can be restructuring as an optimization problem that diminishes the subsequent clustering objective role:

$$\min J(U,V) = \sum_{k=1}^{K} \cdot \sum_{i \in I} u_{ik} \|x_i - v_k\|_p^p$$

below the succeeding restraints:

$$\sum_{k=1}^{K} u_{ik} = 1, u_{ik} \epsilon \{0,1\}, \forall i \epsilon I, k = 1,....K,$$

where $p = 1,2$. For $k = 1,....K$, $v_k \epsilon R^m$ is the kth cluster archetype and for any $i \epsilon I$, u_{ik} sign posts that the item $i \epsilon k$th cluster. K-Means is an effective algorithm to work out the clustering problem for $p = 1$ and $p = 2$.

For the accompanying, let the cluster archetype matrix $V = [v_1, v_2, ...v_k] \epsilon R^{m \times K}$ besides the membership matrix $U = [u_1,....u_n] \epsilon R^{K \times n}$, such as $v_i = (v_{i1},....v_{im})^T$ and $u_i = (u_{i1},....u_{iK})^T$.

This algorithm works out the clustering problem repeatedly as follows.

Step 1: Assign repetition index $t = 0$ and arbitrarily pick out K diverse items as the preliminary cluster archetypes $\{v_k^t: k = 1,...K\}$.

Step 2: Assign $t = t + 1$ and upgrade the membership matrix U^t by setting the cluster archetype matrix V^{t-1}.

For any $i \epsilon I$, arbitrarily pick out $k^* \epsilon \arg\min\{||x_i - v_k^{t-1}||_p: k = 1,....k\}$, and set $u_{ik^*}^t = 1$ and for any $k \neq k^*$, set $u_{ik}^t = 0$.

Step 3: Upgrade the cluster archetype matrix V^t by setting the membership matrix U^t. Once $p = 1$ for any $k = 1,...K$ and $j \epsilon J$ fixed v_{kj}^t as the median of the jth feature values of these items in cluster k. Once $p = 2$, for any $k = 1,...K$, set v_k^t as the centroid of these items in cluster k; that is,

$$v_k^t = \left(1/\sum_{i \epsilon I} u_{ik}\right) \sum_{i \epsilon I} u_{ik} x_i$$

Step 4: If, for any $i \epsilon I$ and $k = 1,...K$, w.k.t $u_{ik}^t = u_{ik}^{t-1}$, then discontinue and return to U and V; or else, go to Step 2.

The algorithm of this method could be written as

1. Arbitrarily choose "c" cluster centers.
2. Estimate the distance of entire data points and each center.
3. With the least distance, the data are assigned to a cluster.
4. Recompute the center positions using (Step 2).
5. Recompute the distance of every data point and every center.
6. If no data were reallocated, then stop, or else reiterate from Step 3.

9.3   ROBUST K-MEANS (RKM) CLUSTERING METHOD

The clustering issue might be expressed as a mini-max robust optimization problematic by dint of interval data. The Robust K-Means clustering process could cluster the inadequate data deprived of claim for the loss features of data and afford robust clustering outcomes that are insensitive to estimate error. In 2008, Professor Karsin introduced an augmentation of the K-Means algorithm that removes the outlier entitled as RKM [20]. It utilizes the information bottleneck scheme as an establishment for its solution to classical clustering issues. In the information theory point of view, clustering is for lossy compression in view of the ratio of datum to clusters. The objective is to keep hold of large amounts of pertinent information regarding the locality of the data points, although compressing the data, it would seem, is eager for as few clusters as possible.

This compression by means of the Lagrange parameter λ, the clustering decisive factor of RKM [21], is therefore

$$\max\left[I(x,c) - \lambda I(c,i)\right]$$

$$p(c\,|\,1)$$

where i, c, and x are the data index, cluster index, and locations of the datum, respectively. The objective is to engage a tremendous amount of pertinent information, prearranged by the compression parameter λ. The temperature λ assumes a part in which the algorithm carries on. For any value λ < 1, the routine converges to a "hard" K-Means elucidation, however, contingent upon its precise value, incline to reveal fewer affectability to initial centroid placement. For a λ value of 1, the subsequent equations are precisely that of the soft K-Means approach. In this manner, the RKM approach can act like previously defined algorithms; nonetheless, the algorithm can be tuned through the λ parameter to fabricate an effective and precise supplementary solution.

The algorithm of this method could be written as

1. Arbitrarily choose "c" cluster centers.
2. Estimate the distance of entire data points and each center.
3. Assign the data to the closest cluster.
4. If any outlier occurs, then remove it.
5. Recompute the center positions using Step 2.
6. Recompute the distance of every data point and every center.
7. If no data were reallocated, then stop or else reiterate from Step 3.

9.4   SEGMENTATION USING K-MEANS

Theoretically, it is a classic approach. Now that it is elementary and prompt, it is desirable in practice. It segregates the input data set keen on K-Clusters. Every cluster is delineated by an adaptively shifting centroid, starting from a few initial values that are intended as seed points. K-Means reckons the squared distances between the inputs and centroids and designates inputs to the nearest centroid. Evidently, the overall performance of the K-Means algorithm [22] relies upon preliminary cluster centers, while the final partition depends on the initial configuration. The flow of the K-Means technique for segmentation of Skin Cancer Image is demonstrated in Figure 9.1.

This work is carried out with the K-Means clustering procedure. Skin lesion images have been given as input. Convert these dermoscopic image into L*a*b* [19]. Assign the number of clusters as three, then three centroids are selected randomly.

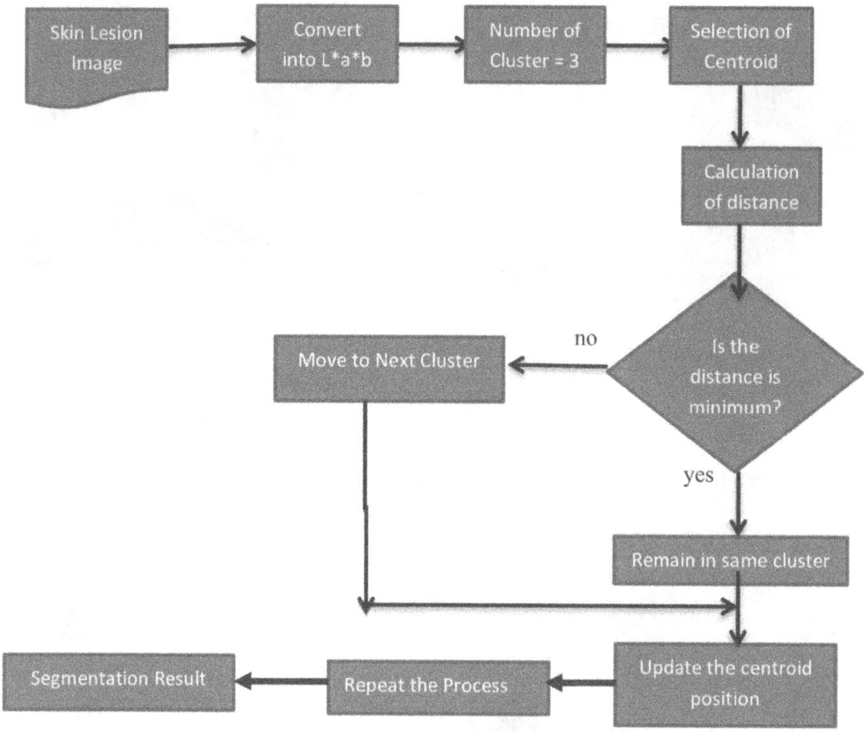

FIGURE 9.1   Flow chart for K-Means technique for segmentation of skin cancer image.

The Euclidean distance measure has been used for clusters, i.e., if this distance is less than average, remain in that cluster, otherwise expel into another cluster. Repeat the same process till the result converges.

9.5   SEGMENTATION USING RKM

This work is put forward with the RKM. Since it is worked based on centroid points, there is a need to define the number of clusters. Consistent with the reference of the ground truth image, define the number of clusters as three. This initial centroid is placed randomly in the given image, and the clustering process is started. For grouping the cluster, a Euclidean distance measure is used. If the distance is average, the centroid remains in that cluster; otherwise, it is expelled into the next cluster, as with K-Means. The prime difference is that if any outlier [23] occurs, it is removed during grouping. Repeat the same process until you reach the final results. The flow of RKM technique for segmentation of Skin Cancer Image is demonstrated in Figure 9.2.

The K-Means algorithm has been analyzed and experimented with. Its performance is always good if the centroid is taken correctly. Generally, K-Means results are unreliable, because the algorithm segments the object based on the centroid; however, the centroid could be selected randomly.

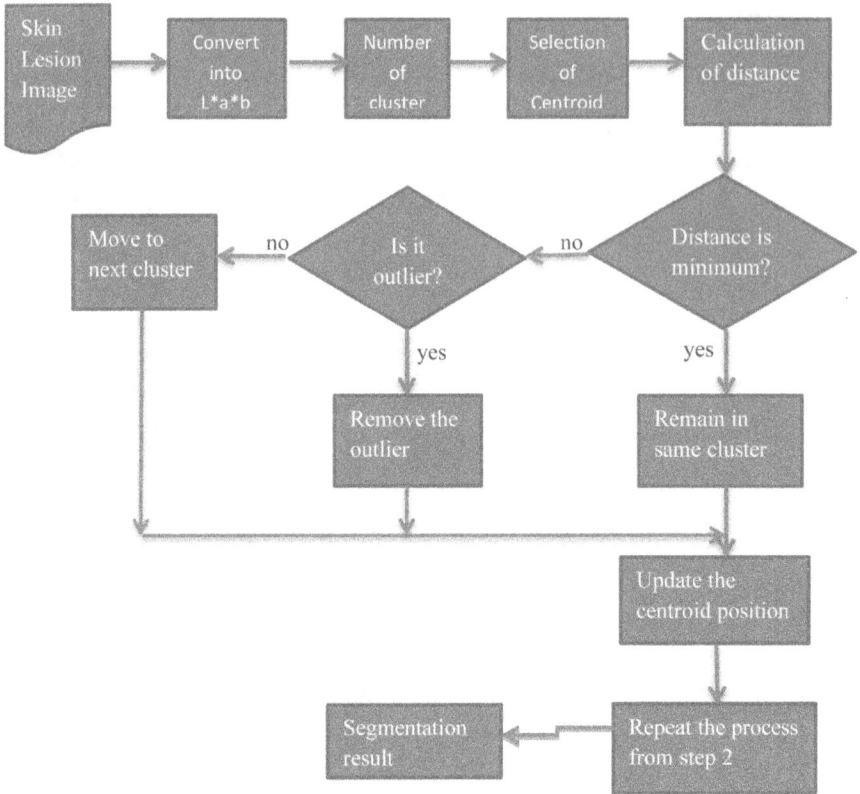

FIGURE 9.2 Flow chart of robust K-Means technique for segmentation on dermoscopic image.

RKM has been analyzed and implemented on skin lesion data sets, and it is considered highly accurate.

9.6   RESULT ANALYSIS

The outcomes are analyzed in various scenarios. Initially the analysis was carried out with pixel wise cluster, i.e., pixels were cluster for this method. Besides, the analysis is carried out in terms of means, standard deviation, variance, and, in addition, time complexity. Figures 9.3.1–9.3.5 portray the results using K-Means and RKM for various skin lesion images.

9.6.1   PERFORMANCE BASED ON PIXELS

In keeping with the guidance of the ground truth image, these skin lesion images are segmented with three clusters. The total number of pixels, say 270,000 of an image, has been grouped into these three clusters.

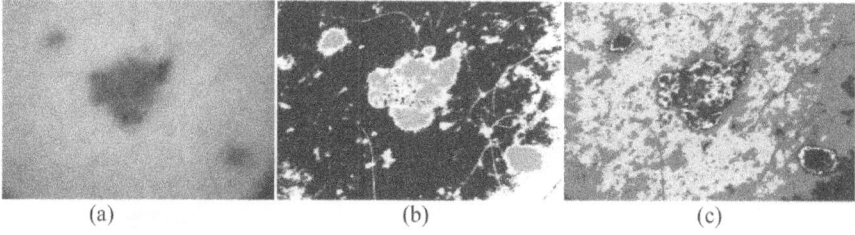

FIGURE 9.3.1 (a) Input, (b) K-Means, (c) RKM.

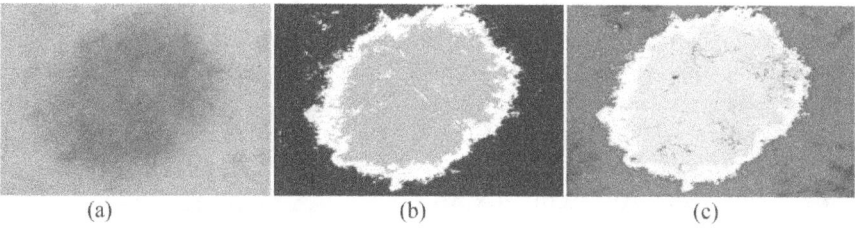

FIGURE 9.3.2 (a) Input, (b) K-Means, (c) RKM.

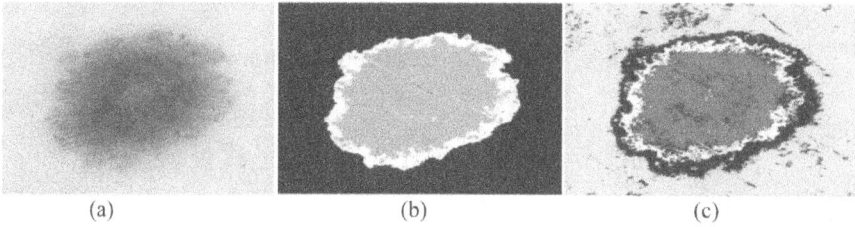

FIGURE 9.3.3 (a) Input, (b) K-Means, (c) RKM.

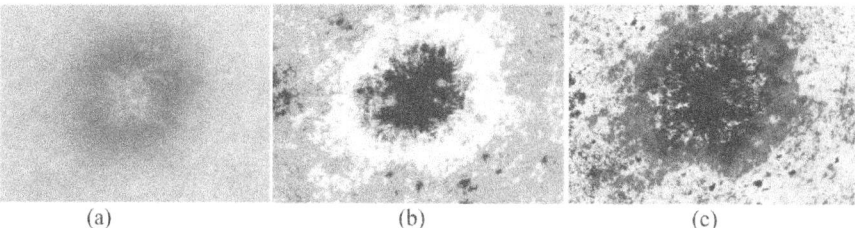

FIGURE 9.3.4 (a) Input, (b) K-Means, (c) RKM.

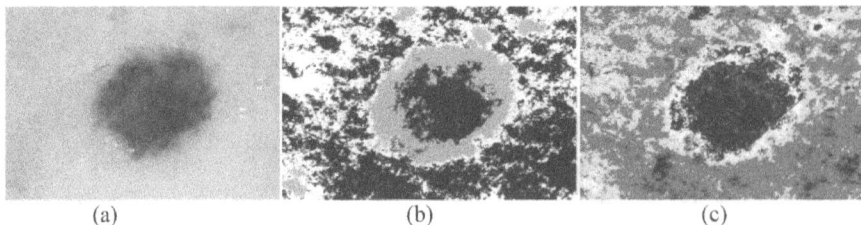

(a)   (b)   (c)

FIGURE 9.3.5   (a) Input, (b) K-Means, (c) RKM.

Tables 9.1–9.5 portray the number of pixels that are clustered as a result. The number of clusters is outlined in advance in keeping with its ground truth. The K-Means segregate into three clusters, and the total number of pixels is clustered into these parts. The Robust K-Means produces the result of a loss of pixels for all cases. It is a trimmed process, so few pixels were lost. Figures 9.4–9.8 portray its corresponding charts.

9.6.2   TIME TAKEN TO EXECUTE FOR RKM

Table 9.6 portrays the time taken to execute. For various skin lesion images on dermoscopic image analysis, RKM takes a number of seconds for segmentations. Figure 9.9 portrays the time taken in chart form.

TABLE 9.1
Performance Based on Pixels for Skin-Image_1

Cluster	K-Means	RKM
1	194,193	104,216
2	15,607	117,811
3	60,200	7,886
Total	270,000	**229,913***

* The result we received is loss of some pixels, because RKM is remove the outlier if occurs. That is the difference of K-Means and RKM.

TABLE 9.2
Performance Based on Pixels for Skin-Image_2

Cluster	K-Means	RKM
1	141,380	131,242
2	84,124	81,809
3	44,496	42,694
Total	270,000	**255,745**

TABLE 9.3
Performance Based on Pixels for Skin-Image_3

Cluster	K-Means	RKM
1	172,306	47,983
2	70,052	152,217
3	27,642	20,026
Total	270,000	**220,226**

TABLE 9.4
Performance Based on Pixels for Skin-Image_4

Cluster	K-Means	RKM
1	31,361	55,527
2	148,323	95,785
3	90,316	38,287
Total	270,000	**189,599**

TABLE 9.5
Performance Based on Pixels for Skin-Image_5

Cluster	K-Means	RKM
1	60,536	115,633
2	27,908	73,903
3	151,556	22,829
Total	270,000	**212,365**

Pixel Clustered for Image_1

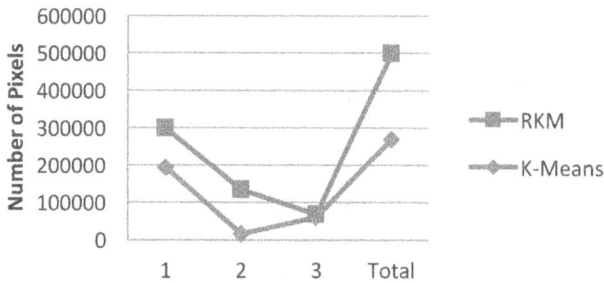

FIGURE 9.4 Chart of pixels clustered for Image_1.

Pixel Clustered for Image_2

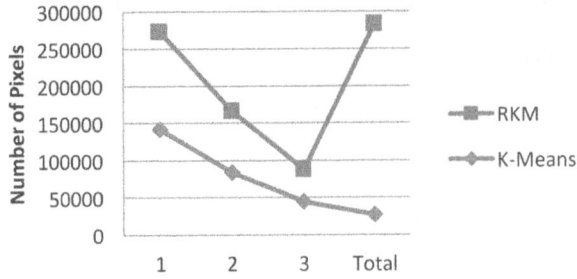

FIGURE 9.5   Chart of pixels clustered for Image_2.

Pixel Clustered for Image_3

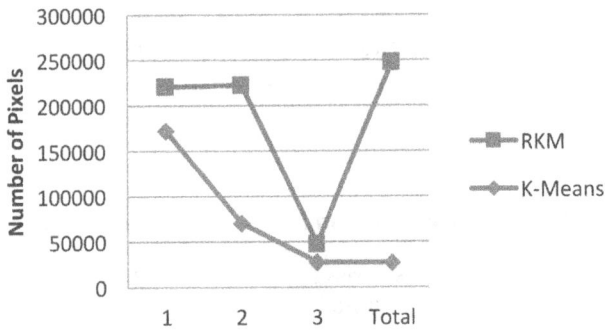

FIGURE 9.6   Chart of pixels clustered for Image_3.

Pixel clustered for image_4

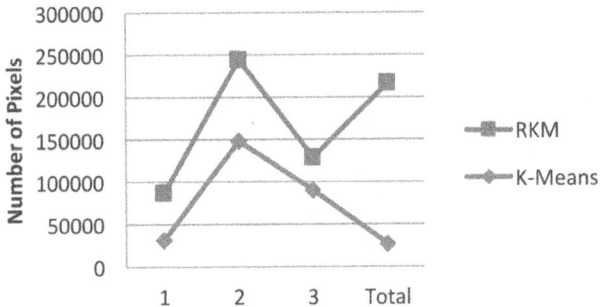

FIGURE 9.7   Chart of pixels clustered for Image_4.

Pixels Clustered for Image_5

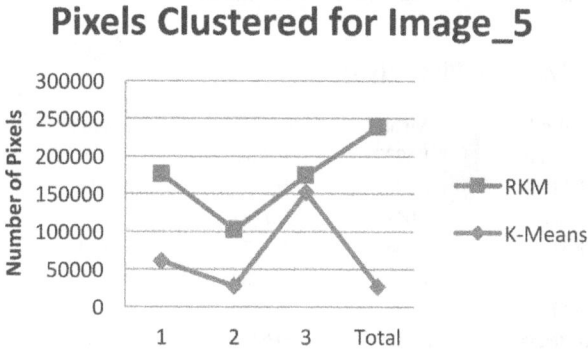

FIGURE 9.8 Chart of pixels clustered for Image_5.

TABLE 9.6
Time Taken for Execution

Image	Time Taken (Seconds)	
	K-Means	**RKM**
Image_1	1.9188	24.0022
Image_2	2.0280	42.6805
Image_3	1.7628	24.5824
Image_4	2.1528	38.0552
Image_5	2.0904	38.9657

Time Taken Chart

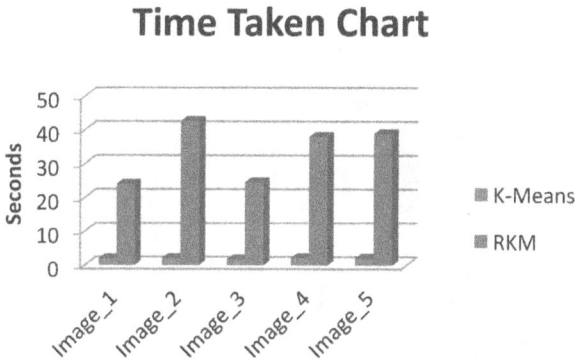

FIGURE 9.9 Chart of time taken for RKM.

TABLE 9.7
Statistical Analysis and Pixel Idx List

Image	Method	Mean	Std. Dev	Variance	Pixel Idx List
Image_1	K-Means	1.5037	0.8342	0.6959	345,807
	RKM	1.3463	0.7627	0.5817	475,871
Image_2	K-Means	1.6412	0.7481	0.5597	398,620
	RKM	1.5665	0.8170	0.6674	423,013
Image_3	K-Means	1.4642	0.6734	0.4535	367,694
	RKM	1.5278	0.8754	0.7663	541,791
Image_4	K-Means	2.2184	0.6348	0.4030	508,639
	RKM	1.3406	1.0506	1.1038	564,874
Image_5	K-Means	2.2260	0.9195	0.8456	449,464
	RKM	1.2294	0.8791	0.7728	482,002

9.6.3 STATISTICAL ANALYSIS REPORT FOR RKM

Table 9.7 depicts the results of statistical terms, namely Means, Std Dev, and Variance for various dermoscopic skin lesion images. Figure 9.10 portrays the table's corresponding chart. This table will help to perform the classification by mapping with corresponding ground truth images.

9.7 CHAPTER CONCLUSION

This chapter puts forward the segmentation of dermoscopy skin lesion images. For the segmentation process, unsupervised clustering methods, namely K-Means and the enhanced clustering method RKM, have been carried out. The results produced

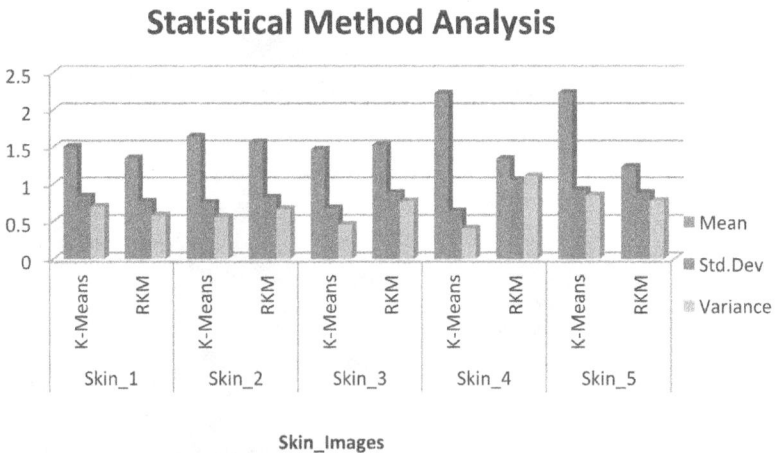

FIGURE 9.10 Chart for statistical method analysis using RKM.

by RKM are analyzed in different scenarios. RKM takes nominal time to segment the skin lesion properly. Despite segregating properly, RKM produces(leads) over segmentation results for most of the images. Moreover, this method produces a result with certain loss of pixels because it is a trimmed process.

REFERENCES

1. Remero Lopez Adria et al. "Skin Lesion Classification from Dermoscopic Images Using Deep Learning Techniques," IEEE, 13th IASTED International Conference on BioMedical Engineering, Austria, (2017). https://doi.org/10.2316/P.2017.852-053.
2. Adjed Faouzi et al. "Segmentation of Skin Cancer Images Using an Extension of Chan and Vese Model," 7th International Conference on Information Technology and Electrical Engineering (ICITEE), Chiang Mai, Thailand, (2015). https://doi.org/10.1109/ICITEED.2015.7408987.
3. Ferreira P.M., Mendonca T., Rozeira J. and Rocha P. "An Annotation Tool for Dermoscopic Image Segmentation," 1st International Workshop on Visual Interfaces for Ground Truth Collect Ion in Computer Vision Applications, (2012). https://doi.org/10.1145/2304496.2304501.
4. Schaefer Gerald et al. "Colour and Contrast Enhancement for Improved Skin Lesion Segmentation," In Computerized Medical Imaging and Graphics, vol. 35-2, pp. 99–104 (2011). https://doi.org/10.1016/j.compmedimag.2010.08.004.
5. Wang Ning et al. "Skin Lesion Image Segmentation Based on Adversarial Networks," In KSII Transaction on Internet & Information Systems, vol. 12, no. 6 (2018). http://doi.org/10.3837/tiis.2018.06.021 ISSN: 1976–7277.
6. Oludayo O. et al. "Segmentation of Melanoma Skin Lesion Using Perceptual Colour Difference Saliency with Morphological Analysis," In Hindawi – Mathematical Problems in Engineering Feb (2018). https://doi.org/10.1155/2018/1524286.
7. Barata C., Celebi M.E. and Marques J.S. "A Survey of Feature Extraction in Dermoscopy Image Analysis of Skin Cancer," In IEEE Journal of BioMedical and Health Informatics, vol. 23, pp. 1096–1109 (2015). https://doi.org/10.1109/JBHI.2018.2845939.
8. Sivaprakasam Ananth and Kumar V. Saravana et al. "Wavelet Based Cervical Image Segmentation Using Morphological and Statistical Operations," In Journal of Advanced Research in Dynamical & Control Systems, vol. 10, no. 3 (2018). http://www.jardcs.org/abstract.php?archiveid=3838.
9. Sivaprakasam S. Anantha and Naganathan E.R. "Segmentation and Classification of Cervical Cytology Images Using Morphological and Statistical Operation," In ICTACT Journal on Image and Video Processing, vol. 7, no. 3 (2017). https://doi.org/10.21917/ijivp.2017.0208.
10. Cham Aruba and Cham Bill. "Treatment of Skin Cancer with a Selective Apoptotic-Inducing Curaderm^{BEC5} Topical Cream Containing Solasodine Rhamnosides," In International Journal of Clinical Medicine, vol. 6, pp. 326–333 (2015). http://dx.doi.org/10.4236/ijcm.2015.65042.
11. Unver Halil Murar and Ayan Enes. "Skin Lesion Segmentation in Dermoscopic Images with Combination of Yolo and Grabcut Algorithm," In Diagnostics – MDPI Publications, vol. 9, no. 3, pp. 1–21. https://doi.org/10.3390/diagnostics9030072.
12. Kumar V. Saravana and Naganathan E.R. "Segmentation of Hyperspectral Image Using JSEG Based on Unsupervised Clustering Algorithms," In ICTACT Journal on Image and Video Processing, vol. 06-02 (2015). https://doi.org/10.21917/ijivp.2015.0168.
13. Kumar V. Saravana and Naganathan E.R. "Hyperspectral Image Segmentation Based on Particle Swarm Optimization with Classical Clustering Methods," In Advances in Natural and Applied Sciences, vol. 9, no. 12, pp. 45–53 Aug (2015). http://www.aensiweb.net/AENSIWEB/anas/anas/2015/August/45-53.pdf.

14. Kumar V. Saravana and Naganathan E.R. et al. "Multiband Image Segmentation by Using Enhanced Estimation of Centroid (EEOC)," In Information – An International Interdisciplinary – Journal, Tokyo, Japan July, vol. 17-A, pp. 1965–1980 (2014). http://www.informationiii.org/abs_e2.html#No7(A)-2014.
15. Okuboyejo Damilola A. et al. "Automatic Skin Disease Diagnosis Using Image Classification," In The World Congress on Engineering & Computer Science, vol. 2 (2013), USA. http://www.iaeng.org/publication/WCECS2013/WCECS2013_pp850-854.pdf.
16. Kavitha M. and Hong Tzung-Pei et al. "Fuzzy Clustering Technique for Segmentation on Skin Cancer Dermoscopic Images," In Fuzzy Mathematical Analysis and Advances in Computational Mathematics, Part of the Studies in Fuzziness and Soft Computing, vol. 419, pp. 81–89 (2022). https://link.springer.com/chapter/10.1007/978-981-19-0471-4_6.
17. Kavitha M. and Kumar V. Saravana et al. "An Empirical Study on Image Segmentation Techniques for Detection of Skin Cancer," In Journal of Pharmaceutical Research International, vol. 33, no. 10, pp. 71–81 (2021). https://doi.org/10.9734/jpri/2021/v33i1031235.
18. Zortea Maciel et al. "Automatic Segmentation of Dermoscopic Images by Iterative Classification," In Hindawi – International Journal of Biomedical Imaging, vol. 2011, July (2011). https://doi.org/10.1155/2011/972648.
19. Kavitha M. and Kumar V. Saravana et al. "Dermoscopic Skin Lesions Images Segmentation Using Enhanced Clustering Technique," In Journal of Theoretical and Applied Information Technology, vol. 100, no. 3 (2022). http://www.jatit.org/volumes/Vol100No3/12Vol100No3.pdf.
20. Li Jinhua et al. "Robust K-Median and K-Means Clustering Algorithms for Incomplete Data," In Mathematical Problems in Engineering (2016). http://dx.doi.org/10.1155/2016/4321928.
21. Garcia-Escudero Luis Angel and Gordaliza Alfonso. "Robustness Properties of K-Means and Trimmed K-Means," In Journal of the American Statistical Association, vol. 94, no. 447, pp. 956–969 Sep (1999). https://doi.org/10.1080/01621459.1999.10474200.
22. Kavitha M. et al. "Classical Clustering Technique for Segmentation of Skin Cancer Image," In TEST Engineering and Management, Trade Journal – Mattingley Publishing Co, Inc, pp. 5753–5758 June (2020). http://testmagzine.biz/index.php/testmagzine/article/view/8412.
23. Kavitha M. et al. "Enhanced Clustering Technique for Segmentation on Dermoscopic Images," IEEE - 4th International Conference on Intelligent Computing and Control Systems (ICICCS 2020), Madurai, TN, May (2020), pp. 956–961. https://doi.org/10.1109/ICICCS48265.2020.9121102.

10 Automated Alzheimer's Disease Detection with Optimized Fuzzy Neural Network

Preeti Topannavar[1], D. M. Yadav[2], and Varsha Bendre[3]
[1]Department of Electronics & Telecommunication Engineering, GHRCEM, Savitribai Phule Pune University, Pune, Maharashtra, India
[2]Department of Electronics & Telecommunication Engineering, SND College of Engineering and Research Centre, Yeola, Savitribai Phule Pune University, Pune, Maharashtra, India
[3]Department of Electronics & Telecommunication Engineering, Pimpri Chinchwad College of Engineering, Pune, Maharashtra, India

CONTENTS

10.1 INTRODUCTION

The Alzheimer's disease (AD) is a very common neurological disorder observed in older people. There is a considerable delay between the onset of AD and its diagnosis, which can be confirmed by autopsy only. Thus the early detection of AD is very difficult and there is a need of intelligent means to support the clinicians for

DOI: 10.1201/9781003324430-12

personalized, early, and accurate diagnosis of the disease. In brain-related diseases, structure, and MR image-based biomarkers identify structural differentiation in the white and gray matter cells and tissues. Mild cognitive impairment (MCI) samples have more deterioration than normal samples but less than AD samples. Especially, entorhinal and hippocampal cortical deterioration is significant in MCI due to AD patients. But it is very difficult for clinicians to detect the smaller changes just by visual assessment. Thus the use of a computational model for defining the biomarkers significantly for the prediction of MCI patients is needed.

For Alzheimer's disease detection using MR imaging techniques, various classical methods were suggested previously. Some researchers are also focusing on the use of wavelet decomposition methods in which actual image size reduction by extracting unique characteristic features is performed. On the other hand, discrete wavelet transform (DWT) still has a skipping property while extracting features compared to continuous wavelet transform (CWT). Also, applying CWT is the right choice for extracting lossless feature coefficients. The combinational discrete and CWT transforms offer the best approach for keeping complexity low and extracting lossless features. The 2D dual-tree complex wavelet transform (DTCWT) for feature extraction in medical image processing is explained in [1]. The method is modified to get extra angular features in terms of spatial characteristic coefficients, which when clubbed with an optimized fuzzy neural network classifier gives better performance. Though, the designing and analysis of this system is not so easy because of its complex structure. Few studies related to this can be found in the literature.

10.2   RELATED WORKS

Er [2] provided study of a computerized method with a deep learning approach for identification of MCI due to Alzheimer's disease. The method identifies different brain regions with the use of a three-dimensional Jacobian-based method. The track of difference between two consecutive brains is easily maintained using this strategy. The method shows accuracy of 87.2%. Pan [3] identified limitations in various methods involving neural network-based prediction of dementia from standard MRI (sMRI) images. The unique anatomical characteristic of each brain is ignored while identifying common features. Also, patch-based training focuses on limited regions of interest and hence global structural information about the brain is neglected. The authors provided use of an attention layer in a CNN-based approach for improving the performance in case of multiple combinations of the data sets. Du et al. [4] proposed analysis method using multitask sparse canonical correlation from multimodal quantitative traits (QT) brain images. The parameter decomposition and multitask learning advantage is the main outcome of using the method. The genetic image analysis with multiview using canonical correlation coefficients and weights is the main advantage of the method. Chan et al. [5] showed use of the wavelet method for identifying the brain connectivity parts. The identification of Alzheimer's disease is performed using the method. The motion artifact removal is the main target from fNIRS data. The signal processing approach is used for Alzheimer's disease detection. Authors considered topological constraints in filtering brain networks. Even with sparsity present in the network, it has shown the highest efficiency. Dada et al. [6] presented a fully automatic segmentation technique. The application considered is a brain MRI image in which the aging effect and AD are to be detected. The white matter hyperintensities are segmented using the linear segmentation method. The automatic segmentation shows almost 93% accuracy.

Mahanand et al. [7] presented a method for AD detection with the Integer Coded Genetic Algorithm along with the extreme learning machine (ELM) classifier. The morphometric analysis is used with a voxel-based approach in which respective best features are selected. The classifier shows 91.8% accuracy with 10 features compared to 86.84% accuracy using the support vector machine classifier for AD detection. Herrera et al. [8] have discussed two problems in AD detection using MRI images. The first one focuses on identification of AD and normal images from a data set of 1,000 images. The second problem focuses on identification of mild cognitive impairment patients, AD, and normal from MRI image data sets. The early diagnosis of dementia is possible using a solution to the second problem developed by authors. In the feature extraction stage, 2D discrete wavelet transform is used, and then principal component analysis (PCA) is applied for further feature reduction. Classification is done by a support vector machine (SVM)-based linear kernel classifier. The comparison using two methods of wavelet decomposition is done in which Daubechies and Haar wavelet is used. In both methods, performance is evaluated using PCA and without PCA in which Haar wavelet shows the highest performance of 96.23% accuracy and applying PCA improves the processing speed of classifier but reduces accuracy to 94.79%. Sweety et al. [9] used optimization technique for feature selection. The preprocessing with noise removal using the Markov random field method is done. The features are obtained using eigenvectors, mean, standard deviation, variance, area, perimeter, skewness, eccentricity, and kurtosis. The particle swarm optimization is used for feature selection and feature vector reduction, and classification is done using the decision tree.

Yang and Yang [1] showed use of DTCWT for feature extraction from MRI images. The results were evaluated using multilevel decomposition of DTCWT. Vector length, time, and wavelet coefficients were considered. The level 4 decomposition even maintains the uniqueness of the features from MRI images where AD disease is concerned. Udomhunsakul et al. [10] demonstrated spatial feature extraction and its application to MRI images. The 5×5-sized filters with 40 sets are used to extract the features, which maintains the scale and edge parameters as a characteristic feature. The preprocessing of an image is done using Gaussian 3×3 filters. Then the impact of noise removal is observed while using Gabor filter banks. Oleiwi [11] used texture-based segmentation method using k-means. The segmented image is further processed using a gray-level cooccurrence matrix for feature extraction. The features are then classified in AD and normal sets using a K-nearest neighbor classifier with 86.6% accuracy on the OASIS database. Alattas et al. [12] used simple and basic image processing methods such as thresholding, edge detection, and morphological operations to get brain dimensionality. The comparison of brain size is performed for AD patients' brain MRI images and normal brain MRI images in which dimensional difference study is shown. Zhang et al. [13] proposed a fuzzy min-max neural network-based classifier on the data core. The pattern classification is done with this classifier. It uses this overlapped neuron with novel membership function based on the data core, which differs from contraction processing.

Nandedkar et al. [14] proposed a classification approach, a min-max fuzzy neural network with compensatory neurons. In this classifier approach, pattern classes are represented as hyperbox fuzzy sets, and a novel compensatory neuron architecture gets activated whenever a test sample appears in the overlapped regions of different classes. Simpson et al. [15] suggested a fuzzy classifier that uses a fuzzy min-max learning system to obtain min-max points. In this, the nonlinear class boundaries in a single pass through the data are cultured easily to obtain the convergence faster. The degree of membership information obtained from the fuzzy set method for pattern classification has proven highly beneficial for high-level decision making. Kulkarni et al. [16] suggested FNN for pattern classification. The suggested method is an improvement over the radial basis function neural network (RBFNN). This method proposes obtaining the processing nodes in the hidden layers of the FNN supervised fuzzy clustering and pruning algorithm to get the precise number of clusters with the appropriate centroid and width. Mitra et al. [17] provided insightful understanding of fuzzy sets for pattern recognition and its combination procedure for combining with other methods of soft computing.

10.3 DESIGN METHODOLOGY

The stages involved in the detection of Alzheimer's disease are as shown in Figure 10.1. The feature extraction is an integral part of the system, which highlights and gathers all important features regarding AD from data sets of MR scans. The Kaggle [18] Alzheimer's data set consists of four stages of Alzheimer's disease, with standard images collected from different websites to test the accuracy of the model. It consists of T2 MR images. The T2 MR images are preferred since they represent maximum details as compared to T1 scans. The performance of the proposed method is evaluated using this database.

In earlier conventional tools, Fourier transform was popular for feature extraction. But the time and frequency feature extraction capability of wavelet transform is very good, so it has shown its impact in machine learning applications. The 2D discrete wavelet transform (2D-DWT) decomposes the image in four bands, which then reduces complexity of processing by using each band separately. The complex wavelet transform (CWT) is a complex valued extension of the standard discrete wavelet transform (DWT). The maximum characteristic features in terms of multiresolution and sparse representation of CWT, the more unique features can be obtained. The higher degree of shift invariance in its magnitude is main reason for obtaining important distinctive features in medical images. A drawback in simple

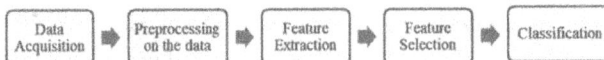

FIGURE 10.1   Block diagram of processing for the Alzheimer's detection method.

CWT is that it exhibits 2D redundancy in features as compared to a separable transform (DWT). On the other hand, for image features extraction, Kingsbury showed
use of dual tree CWT (DTCWT) in 1998. In DTCWT, two real DWTs are performed
while obtaining the subband features, and it also has imaginary part in secondary
DWT operations.

The features extracted by using coefficients extraction method should meet the
following conditions:

1. The decomposition should be perfectly reversible to get the original image
   back, which shows lossless decomposition and important features even for
   a small region of interest after decomposition.
2. The decomposed parts of the input vector must be a shift in half-sample of
   the other (h0 and g0).
3. The boundary condition in h0(1) and g0(1) must be by one and only one
   sample shift.

Orthogonal Q-shift filters were proposed by Kingsbury to meet these conditions
for 1D signal vectors. The idea can be extended for 2D by using equations (10.1) and
(10.2) which describe complex separable wavelet and scaling respectively with the
implementation of separable filters on first columns and then on rows in 2D DTCWT.

$$\psi 1 \ (x,y) = \varphi(x) \ (y),$$

$$\psi_2(x,y) = \psi(x)\varphi(y),$$

$$\psi 3 \ (x,y) = \psi(x)\psi(y) \tag{10.1}$$

$$\varphi(x,y) = \varphi(x)\varphi(y) \tag{10.2}$$

Here ψ ($\cdot$) and φ ($\cdot$) are complex wavelet and complex scaling functions, respectively. The proposed method combines four trees on columns and four trees on rows
to obtain 12 shift variant wavelets oriented at $\pm15°$, $\pm30°$, $\pm45°$, $\pm60°$, $\pm75°$, and $\pm90°$.
Two different sets of filters are used in two wavelet transforms to meet the first
condition mentioned earlier. Consider h0 (n), h1 (n), and g0 (n). g1 (n) represents
a low-pass and high-pass pair of filters for upper and lower separable filter banks,
respectively. Hence a complex wavelet can be denoted as

$$C(t) = h'(t) + jg'(t) \tag{10.3}$$

$$g'(t) = \text{Hilbert}\{h'(t)\} \tag{10.4}$$

Where $h'(t)$ and $g'(t)$ are real complex wavelet transforms of h(t) and g(t),
respectively.

Equation (10.4) denotes the relation such that the exact Hilbert transform of $h'(t)$
is $g'(t)$ for a lossless decomposition method. Another advantage of using DTCWT
is that there is no involvement of complex arithmetic during its implementation,
and also the input data rate is half that of the output data rate. In 2D DTCWT, the
coefficient extraction can be demonstrated, as shown in Figure 10.2. Respective 2D

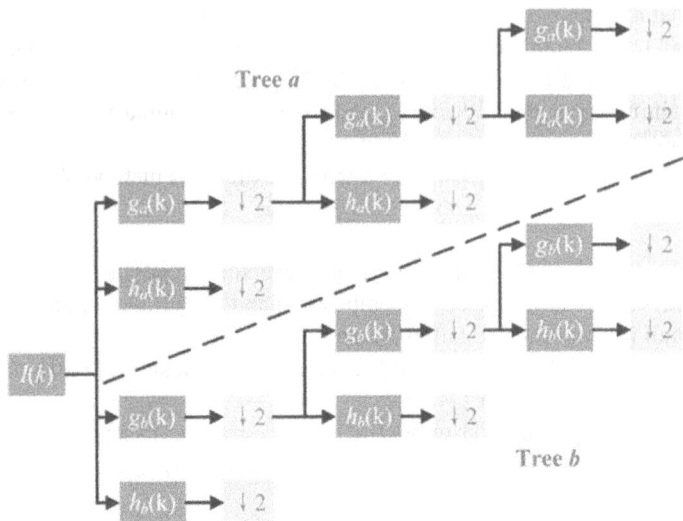

FIGURE 10.2 DTCWT decomposition.

DTCWT is applied for the decomposition of the input brain MRI image, and the resulting four-level decomposition is shown in Figure 10.3.

10.3.1 Design Requirements

Fuzzy neural network is a model fusion method that utilizes the neural network's learning capability with the noise handling ability of Fuzzy Learning. FNN is simply a three-layered feed-forward network consisting of the input layer, a hidden layer, and the output layer. Input and output layers are used for fuzzification and defuzzification, respectively. Hidden middle layer contains fuzzy directions. Generally, the connections between layers contain the fuzzy rule sets. Sometimes a fuzzy neural network is a five-layered network, in that fuzzy sets are contained in the second and fourth layers. The input fuzzy layer signifies the input connection functions for the fuzzy directions.

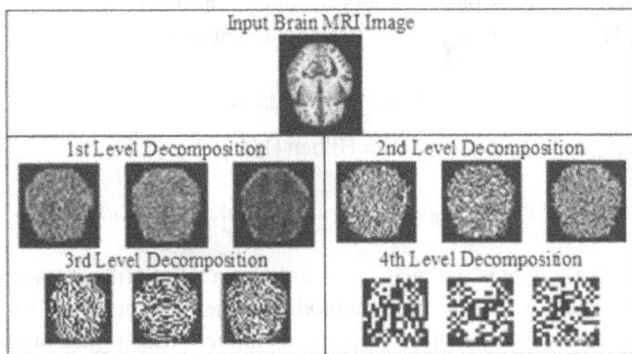

FIGURE 10.3 2D DTCWT four-level decomposition.

Enough input initiates the rules in the hidden middle layer to ignite. The weights among the fuzzy layers symbolize the fuzzy sets. The relative weights determine the relationship in each set, and that relationship can be varied using various training algorithms similar to the usual neural system. In FNN, the transfer functions are continuous in nature and used to pass the values to the output layer through the network. It is interpreted as degrees of membership in fuzzy sets. This is according to the fuzzy rules in the hidden middle layer. Fuzzy neural networks use the combination of strengths of neural networks and FL, making the FNN a very commanding hybrid model with the integration of expert knowledge. The use of fuzzy inference like a human makes the system easy to understand. The input from data set 1 [18] consists of four classes in which normal, very mild demented, mild demented, and moderate demented images are used. In data set 2 [19], seven classes of images are present: normal, meningioma, glioma, Pick's disease, Huntington's disease, sarcoma, and Alzheimer's disease. The features obtained from 2D DTCWT are very large in number, and hence to achieve convergence of FNN in a smaller number of epochs is the main requirement considered. To minimize the convergence iteration count and the system complexity, the feature reduction technique is applied. The feature reduction is possible by conventional methods such as linear discriminant analysis (LDA), principal component analysis (PCA) and independent component analysis (ICA). These methods again have limited capacity to reduce the features and are independent methods that provide output irrespective of the classifier requirement. The optimization algorithm can optimize the convergence during the training process, thereby achieving it faster. This approach is used for optimizing the classifier using GA for selecting the required features based on optimal solution and fitness, and hence the model converges earlier with maximum accuracy of classification.

10.3.2 FEATURE REDUCTION

The total number of features must be reduced to achieve faster convergence in the classifier. On the other hand, the accuracy should remain intact while selecting the features from a set of a large number of features. For the optimized processing requirement during classification, the GA can be used for selecting the features. Khehra et al. [20] have shown use of GA for selecting the features. Darwin's "survival of the fittest" principle is used in genetic algorithm. GA involves stages of selection, crossover, and mutation in which a new population is generated from old generation for a predefined number of iterations. Based on the fitness function, the optimum solution is obtained.

10.3.3 POPULATION ENCODING

In the proposed method, binary coded GA is used in which $2n$ possible feature sets are obtained for n number of total features. A binary set of n elements can be obtained by encoding, namely, $S = (k1, k2, ..., kn)$. The feature selection variable k_i can be given as

$$k_i = \begin{cases} 1, & feature\ is\ present\ in\ subset \\ 0, & otherwise \end{cases} \qquad (10.5)$$

In each defined string or chromosome, if a feature is selected, it is nominated as 1, else 0. Considering eight features for the classifier as the optimal feature set, S = (01001001) can be considered a feasible solution in which features at 2, 5, and 8 are selected.

10.3.4 FITNESS OF POPULATION

The fitness of the string is given by

$$F(Si) = CR(FNNSi) \qquad (10.6)$$

where CR is the classification rate of the classifier.

10.3.5 ALGORITHM

Step 1. Initialize GA parameters: population size = P (total number of features obtained from DTCWT); number of generations = Gmax (this number defines the maximum number of generations to be obtained, where the operation stops after getting Gmax, which is the optimal solution); probability of mutation = pm; probability of crossover = pc.

Step 2. Obtain P from the feature vector.

Step 3. Calculate fitness using equation (10.6).

Step 4. Apply the roulette wheel selection to select individuals.

Step 5. Apply crossover with respect to pc.

Step 6. Mutate based on pm.

Step 7. Get new offspring.

Step 8. If maximum iterations reached‖ G ≥ Gmax stop Else, go to Step 3.

10.4 RESULT AND ANALYSIS

The main disease to be detected is Alzheimer's disease from both the data sets. The performance of the proposed system is analyzed using twofold analysis in which the total data set is divided in two parts. The first part is used for training and second part for validation. The operation is applied on both the data sets and performance is evaluated. The performance of a simple system without optimization and with optimization is evaluated in which accuracy of classification is seen higher in optimization-based methods, and also time analysis is performed to evaluate the complexity level of the methods. Also, the results are compared with other classifiers having no optimization process. The classifiers used for comparison are probabilistic neural network (PNN) and artificial neural network (ANN). The training parameter configuration is as shown in Table 10.1 and represented in Figure 10.4.

In case of data set 2, the performance evaluation is done using confusion matrix in which true positive (TP) stands for input Alzheimer and detected as Alzheimer. True negative (TN) input is Alzheimer and detected as non-Alzheimer. Similarly, when input is non-Alzheimer, then false positive (FP) and false negative (FN) are

TABLE 10.1

Planning and Control Components

Parameter	Configuration Value
Epochs	1000
Learning rate	0.001
Number of hidden neurons	10
Gradient	$1e^{-25}$

detected as Alzheimer and non-Alzheimer, respectively. The formulae for accuracy, sensitivity, and specificity are given in Table 10.2. The performance values obtained for data set 1 for very mild, mild, and moderate demented images and data set 2 are given in Tables 10.3 and 10.4 and graphically represented in Figures 10.5 and 10.6, respectively. The performance values obtained for data set 1 for and data set 2 for feature reduction are given in Tables 10.5 and 10.6 and graphically represented in Figures 10.7 and 10.8, respectively.

In case of data set 1, there are three subsets of Alzheimer's with variation in stages from very mild to moderate, and hence each case has a different approach for considering confusion matrix parameters. The one against all for each Alzheimer's class is considered separately, and average performance is calculated to determine parameters accuracy, sensitivity, and specificity.

10.4.1 ANNOTATIONS

1. The accuracy of FNN is better over ANN and PNN. The addition of GA also further boosts accuracy due to its unique feature selection mechanism.
2. PCA, ICA, and LDA reduce feature dimensions up to certain limit, and hence fitness-oriented selection of features using GA improves the reduction performance with more convergence in the classifier.
3. The performance of the proposed method remains higher even in the case of inclusion of very mild Alzheimer's disease images and also when combined with other disease types.

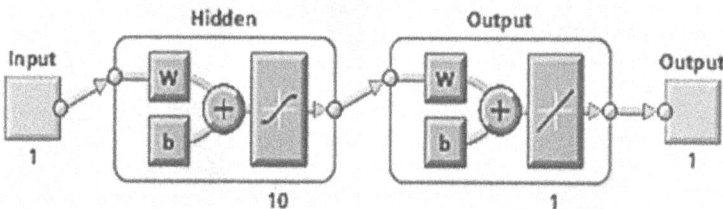

FIGURE 10.4 ANN architecture.

TABLE 10.2
Performance Parameters

Parameter	Formula
Sensitivity	$TPR = \dfrac{TP}{FN + TP}$
Specificity	$TNR = \dfrac{TN}{FP + TN}$
Accuracy	$ACC = \dfrac{TP + TN}{TP + TN + FP + FN}$

TABLE 10.3
Performance of Classifiers on Data Set 1

Method	Accuracy	Specificity	Sensitivity
FNN	0.94	0.875	0.878
FNN + GA	0.97	0.91	0.91
ANN	0.899	0.827	0.825
PNN	0.81	0.81	0.80

TABLE 10.4
Performance of Classifiers on Data Set 2

Method	Accuracy	Specificity	Sensitivity
FNN	0.96	0.88	0.90
FNN + GA	0.97	0.91	0.91
ANN	0.83	0.82	0.83
PNN	0.86	0.84	0.84

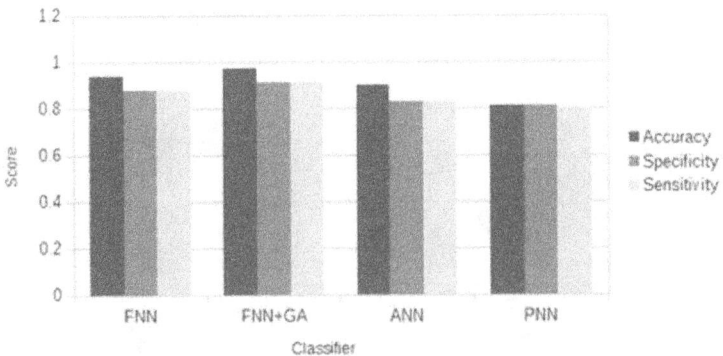

FIGURE 10.5　Performance of different classifiers on data set 1.

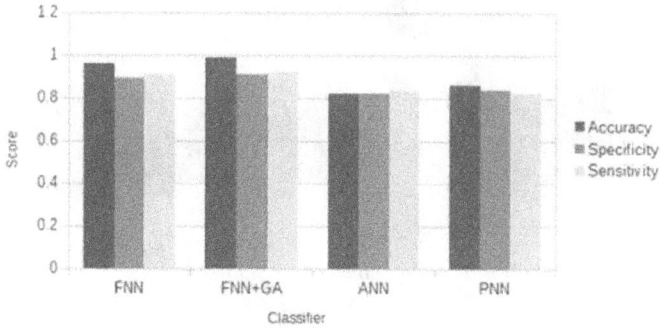

FIGURE 10.6 Performance of different classifiers on data set 2.

TABLE 10.5
Performance of Feature Reduction and Classifiers on Data Set 1

Method	Accuracy	Specificity	Sensitivity
FNN	0.96	0.89	0.91
FNN + GA	0.99	0.91	0.92
ANN	0.82	0.82	0.83
PNN	0.86	0.84	0.82

TABLE 10.6
Performance of Feature Reduction and Classifiers on Data Set 2

Method	Accuracy	Specificity	Sensitivity
FNN	0.95	0.85	0.90
FNN + GA	0.98	0.90	0.91
ANN	0.82	0.83	0.82
PNN	0.86	0.83	0.81

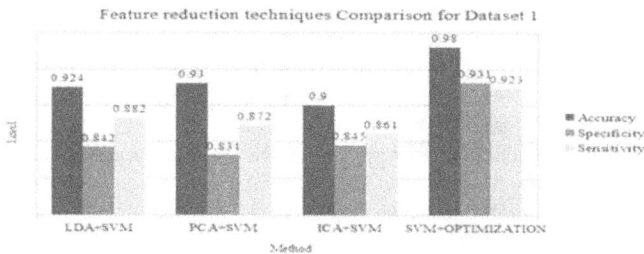

FIGURE 10.7 Different feature reduction techniques on data set 1.

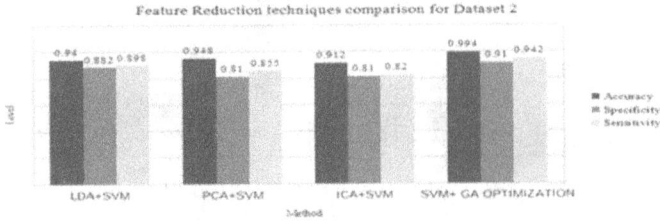

FIGURE 10.8   Different feature reduction techniques on data set 2.

10.5   CONCLUSION

This chapter presented the use of optimization algorithm over features extracted using 2D DTCWT method. The FNN classifier has shown better performance for application of four classes and seven classes while identifying Alzheimer's disease. The method shows no impact on performance even if very mild and mild cognitive impairment MRI images are included in the data set, which cause a performance-degrading problem in existing methods. The performance of GA-based feature selection and reduction is seen as satisfactory when compared to other feature reduction techniques in PCA, LDA, and ICA. The conventional feature reduction techniques have limited scope for feature size reduction while maintaining uniqueness of the features; on the other hand, GA shows better performance by reducing the overall complexity of the system. The overall results are outstanding when using the proposed method.

REFERENCES

1. P. Yang, and G. Yang, Image features extraction using the dual-tree complex wavelet transform & gray level co-occurrence matrix, Neurocomputing, vol. 197, 2016, pp. 212–220, doi: 10.1016/j.neucom.2016.02.061.
2. F. Er, and D. Goularas, Predicting the prognosis of MCI patients using longitudinal MRI data, IEEE/ACM Transactions on Computational Biology and Bioinformatics, p. 1, 2020, doi: 10.1109/TCBB.2020.3017872.
3. C. Lian, M. Liu, Y. Pan, and D. Shen, Attention-guided hybrid network for dementia diagnosis with structural MR images, IEEE Transactions on Cybernetics, vol. 52, no. 4, pp. 1–12, 2020, doi: 10.1109/TCYB.2020.3005859.
4. L. Du et al., Associating multi-modal brain imaging phenotypes and genetic risk factors via a dirty multi-task learning method, IEEE Transactions on Medical Imaging, vol. 39, no. 11, pp. 3416–3428, 2020, doi: 10.1109/TMI.2020.2995510.
5. Y. L. Chan, W. C. Ung, L. G. Lim, C.-K. Lu, M. Kiguchi, and T. B. Tang, Automated thresholding method for fNIRS-based functional connectivity analysis: Validation with a case study on Alzheimer's disease, IEEE Transactions on Neural Systems and Rehabilitation Engineering, vol. 28, no. 8, pp. 1691–1701, 2020, doi: 10.1109/TNSRE.2020.3007589.
6. M. Dadar et al., Validation of a regression technique for segmentation of white matter hyperintensities in Alzheimer's disease, IEEE Transactions on Medical Imaging, vol. 36, no. 8, pp. 1758–1768, 2017, doi: 10.1109/TMI.2017.2693978.
7. B. S. Mahanand, S. Suresh, N. Sundararajan, and M. A. Kumar, "ICGA-ELM Classifier for Alzheimer's Disease Detection."

8. L. J. Herrera, I. Rojas, H. Pomares, A. Guillén, O. Valenzuela, and O. Baños, Classification of MRI images for Alzheimer's disease detection, Proc. - Soc. 2013, pp. 846–851, 2013, doi: 10.1109/SocialCom.2013.127.

9. M. E. Sweety, and G. W. Jiji, Detection of Alzheimer disease in brain images using PSO and decision tree approach, Proc. 2014 IEEE Int. Conf. Adv. Commun. Control Comput. Technol. ICACCCT 2014, no. 978, pp. 1305–1309, 2015, doi: 10.1109/ICACCCT.2014.7019310.

10. S. Udomhunsakul, and P. Wongsita, Feature extraction in medical ultrasonic image, IFMBE Proc., vol. 15, pp. 267–270, 2007, doi: 10.1007/978-3-540-68017-8_69.

11. W. K. Oleiwi, Alzheimer disease diagnosis using the K-means, GLCM and K_NN, Journal of Babylon University/Pure and Applied Sciences, vol. 26, no. 2, pp. 57–65, 2017, doi: 10.29196/jub.v26i2.474.

12. R. Alattas, and B. D. Barkana, A comparative study of brain volume changes in Alzheimer's disease using MRI scans, 2015 IEEE Long Isl. Syst. Appl. Technol. Conf. LISAT 2015, vol. c, 2015, doi: 10.1109/LISAT.2015.7160197.

13. H. Zhang, J. Liu, D. Ma, and Z. Wang, Data-core-based fuzzy min-max neural network for pattern classification, IEEE Transactions on Neural Networks, vol. 22, no. 12 Part 2, pp. 2339–2352, Dec. 2011, doi: 10.1109/TNN.2011.2175748.

14. A. V. Nandedkar, and P. K. Biswas, A fuzzy min-max neural network classifier with compensatory neuron architecture, IEEE Transactions on Neural Networks, vol. 18, no. 1, pp. 42–54, Jan. 2007, doi: 10.1109/TNN.2006.882811.

15. P. K. Simpson, Fuzzy min-max neural networks—Part 1: Classification, IEEE Transactions on Neural Networks, vol. 3, no. 5, pp. 776–786, 1992, doi: 10.1109/72.159066.

16. A. Kulkarni, and N. Kulkarni, Fuzzy neural network for pattern classification, Procedia Computer Science, vol. 167, pp. 2606–2616, Jan. 2020, doi: 10.1016/J.PROCS.2020.03.321.

17. S. Mitra, and S. K. Pal, Fuzzy sets in pattern recognition and machine intelligence, Fuzzy Sets and Systems, vol. 156, no. 3, pp. 381–386, Dec. 2005, doi: 10.1016/J.FSS.2005.05.035.

18. http://www. kaggle.com/tourist55/alzheimers-dataset4-class-of images.

19. https://figshare.com/articles/dataset/brain_tumor_dataset/1512427.

20. B. S. Khehra, and A. P. S. Pharwaha, Comparison of genetic algorithm, particle swarm optimization and biogeography-based optimization for feature selection to classify clusters of microcalcifications, Journal of the Institution of Engineers: Series B, vol. 98, no. 2, pp. 189–202, 2017, doi: 10.1007/s40031-016-0226-8.

11 A Comprehensive Survey with Bibliometric Analysis on Recent Research Opportunities of Multimodal Medical Image Fusion in Various Applications

Manjiri A. Ranjanikar[1], Nilam Upasani[1], Asmita Manna[1], Jaishri M. Waghmare[2], Shimpy Goyal[3], Rachana Y. Patil[1], and Bharati P. Vasgi[4]
[1]Pimpri Chinchwad College of Engineering, Pune, Maharashtra, India
[2]Shri Guru Gobind Singhji Institute of Engineering and Technology, Maharashtra, India
[3]Bhagwan Parshuram Institute of Technology, GGSIPU, New Delhi, India
[4]Marathwada Mitra Mandals College of Engineering, Pune, Maharashtra, India

CONTENTS

DOI: 10.1201/9781003324430-13

11.1   INTRODUCTION

By combining numerous original images, image fusion technology can produce an output in scene description that is superior to any single input image; this is a technique to raise the output's quality. An essential tool for clinical medical decision making is multimodal medical image fusion (MMIF). Medical graphics typically fall into one of two categories: anatomical or functional. They are complementary and irreplaceable because they use diverse imaging techniques and can reflect the location of organs or lesions from various angles. Computed tomography (CT) and magnetic resonance imaging (MRI) images, which have great spatial resolution and can give information on the anatomical structure in the image, are the two types of images most commonly used to create anatomical images. Positron emission tomography (PET) and single-photon emission computed tomography (SPECT) images are the two types of functional images that are the most common. Despite having a poor spatial resolution, they can clearly show human tissue or metabolism as well as the state of an organ's blood flow. Doctors frequently use fusion images of anatomical and functional images to address clinical medical issues that are mirrored by the human body, organs, or cells. Fusion technology can be used for biomedical imaging in addition to the aforementioned typical medical images. Green fluorescent protein (GFP) and phase contrast (PC) are two popular biological imaging techniques. Image breakdown, establishing and executing fusion rules, and image reconstruction are the three basic stages of traditional image fusion. The fundamental goal of image decomposition is to extract the most important characteristics from the image; the quality of the fusion result can be influenced by how well the feature extraction tool works. In general, it is challenging to obtain all the necessary data from a single imaging modality to ensure clinical accuracy and the validity of the test for diagnoses. To create a new fused image with rich information that is trustworthy for clinical application, multimodal approaches merge medical images from several modalities.

Overcoming the limitations of prior studies, we provide a comprehensive assessment of multimodal medical imaging modalities, covering topics like the classification of medical image fusion techniques, freely available multimodal databases, and associated disorders. Spatial, frequency, decision-level fusion type, deep learning, hybrid, and sparse representation fusion are the six categories into which MMIF methods can be broken down. As a bonus, we also provide a brief overview of a few current studies covering multimodal image fusion for identifying various illnesses. Obtaining a fused image with as much supplementary information, the greatest quality, and the best visualization possible to aid in precise diagnosis and tailored therapy is the focus of this chapter. In a nutshell, this chapter aims to study the fundamentals of fusion imaging for medical purposes, and learn about the many types of medical imaging, how they compare, the key uses for medical image fusion, and the newest developments and future directions in this field. The following is the structure of this chapter. In the first section, we provide a brief overview of bibliometrics and its applications. In Section 11.2, we cover the groundwork for fusing medical images and the fusion procedure in detail. Some recent developments in the field of medical image fusion are discussed in Section 11.3. The final section provides a summary and recommendations for further research.

11.2 BIBLIOMETRIC INFORMATION AND PERFORMANCE ANALYSIS

Deep learning and machine learning approaches, in particular, are now frequently employed to automatically identify diseases from a variety of medical imagery. X-rays, CT, SPECT, ultrasound, MRI, infrared and ultraviolet, PET, and other imaging techniques are frequently employed to provide medical images utilized in diagnosis. Nevertheless, it is hard to extract all the crucial details and knowledge needed for an accurate diagnosis from a single medical imaging modality. Using many images for analysis will improve diagnostic precision and accuracy, but doing so will also increase processing time and storage requirements. Therefore, computer scientists are concentrating their efforts to combine several medical images to create one image with better information. Image fusion is a technique for integrating numerous images into a single image while preserving all the essential characteristics of the original images. Additionally, it is anticipated that the fusion of many images will result in the appearance of additional notable features. These extra features will make the diagnosing procedure much better. Over the past five years, an increasing number of researchers have been working on this medical image fusion due to the anticipated accuracy and precision. When the Scopus database is searched for papers on deep learning–based medical image fusion, approximately 1,050 publications published since 2013 are found. According to the Scopus database, Figure 11.1 illustrates the rising frequency of publications in this field.

Furthermore, a bibliometric analysis of nations, journals, authors, publications, and author keyword cooccurrences of recognized publications is undertaken in this study in addition to the year-by-year publishing. By starting with more general information, such as the major countries contributing research in this field, and moving on to more specific information, such as the most cited author or keywords coupling

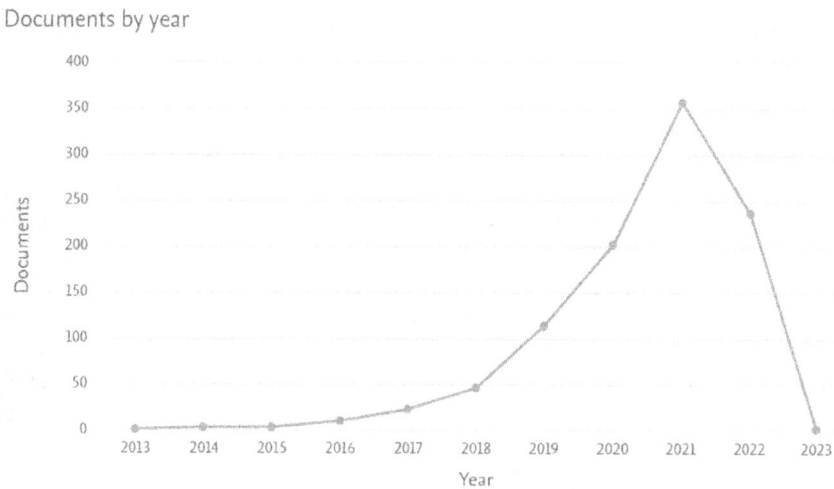

FIGURE 11.1   Year-wise publications in the "medical image fusion" domain since 2013.

TABLE 11.1
Total Link Strength of Top 10 Countries

Country	Document	Citation	Total Link Strength
China	472	3900	113
United States	151	2912	94
United Kingdom	55	924	53
Pakistan	34	536	51
Saudi Arabia	41	542	47
South Korea	24	266	31
Australia	30	457	28
India	136	898	28
Canada	21	491	16
Germany	26	353	16

of various publications, the results of the bibliometric analysis of the publications related to medical image fusion using deep learning would help readers to understand the relationships. The VOSViewer program is used to do the bibliometric analysis. If the nations from where these publications originated are examined, China holds the top spot with 472 publications, followed by the United States with 151 publications, and India with 136 articles. The United Kingdom, along with China and the United States, comes in the third position when the strength of all these journals' citation links is taken into account. Table 11.1 lists the top 10 nations based on total link strength.

In Figure 11.2, the bibliographic coupling of the top 10 countries is illustrated. Different colors in the diagram indicate different clusters where countries belonging to the same cluster are more likely to cite papers within the cluster or it can be said that publications belonging to a specific cluster is more related to each other. From this diagram, three different clusters can be identified: one comprising China and Australia; the second one comprising of United States of America, United Kingdom, Germany, and France and the third cluster comprising India, Saudi Arabia, Pakistan, South Korea, and Canada. Table 11.2 represents the bibliographic coupling of journals.

For identifying the journals with the highest number of publications, another analysis has been performed. Journals having at least 15 publications are considered for the analysis, and only 11 journals have passed this criterion. The journals with the most total link strength are chosen and arranged as per the total link strength as shown in Table 11.2. With 930 citations, 165 documents, and a total link strength of 2,246, *Lecture Notes in Computer Science* is the most popular one. Other popular journals are *Computer Methods and Programs in Biomedicine, IEEE Access, IEEE Journal of Biomedical and Health Informatics*, etc. Detailed year-wise distribution of documents as per sources is depicted in Figure 11.3.

In Figure 11.4, we see how this particular field of study is broken down into distinct subfields. Computer science, followed by engineering, mathematics, medicine, physics, astronomy, material science, and biochemistry, has the highest concentration of researchers.

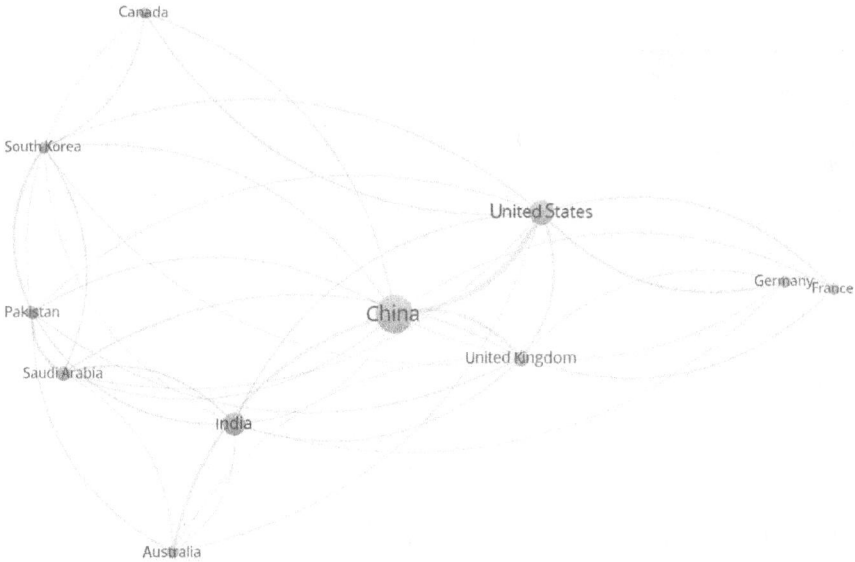

FIGURE 11.2   Bibliographic coupling of countries.

Figure 11.5 is a pie chart depicting the distribution of published documents across various document formats. Journal articles account for 51.5% of all publications on this subject, while conference papers make up 34.7%. It is anticipated that, in the coming years, a growing number of high-caliber journals will appear, all of which pertain to the present field of study.

Figure 11.6 shows the cooccurrences of the author's keywords in a network format. The minimal number of occurrences of a keyword is 20 as an inclusion criterion.

TABLE 11.2
Bibliographic Coupling of Journals

Journal Name	Citation	Documents	Total Link Strength
Lecture Notes in Computer Science	930	165	2,246
Computer Methods and Programs in Biomedicine	559	25	1,444
IEEE Access	388	25	1,181
IEEE Journal of Biomedical and Health Informatics	82	15	807
Proceedings of International Symposium on Biomedical Imaging	153	18	681
Progress in Biomedical Optics and Imaging	141	42	680
Computers in Biology and Medicine	190	15	648
Biomedical Signal Processing and Control	75	17	624
ACM Conference Proceedings Series	40	19	530
Communications in Computer and Information Science	15	19	464
Journal of Image and Graphics	20	19	3

Documents per year by source

Compare the document counts for up to 10 sources.   Compare sources and view CiteScore, SJR, and SNIP data

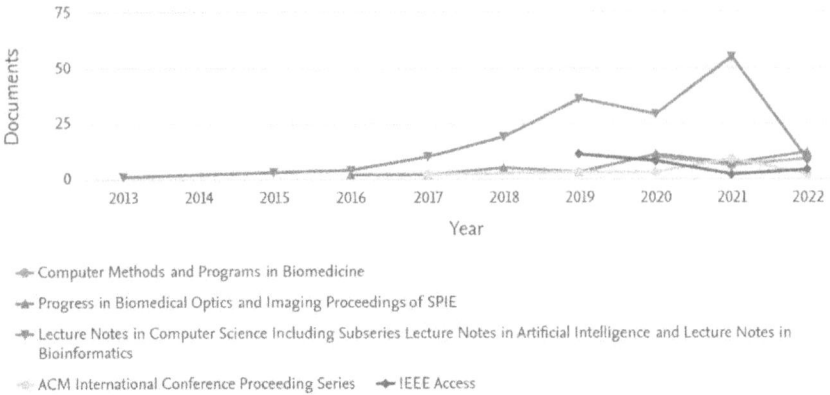

- Computer Methods and Programs in Biomedicine
- Progress in Biomedical Optics and Imaging Proceedings of SPIE
- Lecture Notes in Computer Science Including Subseries Lecture Notes in Artificial Intelligence and Lecture Notes in Bioinformatics
- ACM International Conference Proceeding Series   - IEEE Access

FIGURE 11.3   Year-wise distribution of documents by journals.

Out of 2,049 keywords, only 22 meet the threshold. In Figure 11.6, different colored clusters represent the more frequently connected keywords. The biggest cluster comprises keywords like deep learning, segmentation, classification, CNN, MRI, fusion, and image fusion. The second biggest cluster comprises keywords like computer-aided diagnosis, breast cancer, transfer learning, and COVID-19. Another cluster is formed with the keywords Convolution Neural Network, Feature Fusion, Medical Image Segmentation, Semantic Segmentation, Attention Mechanism, and U-Net.

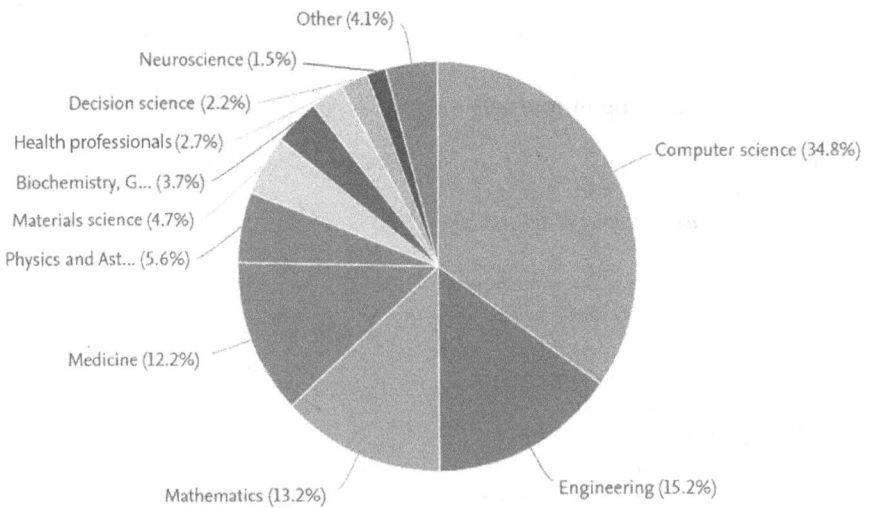

FIGURE 11.4   Publication details of the document by subject area.

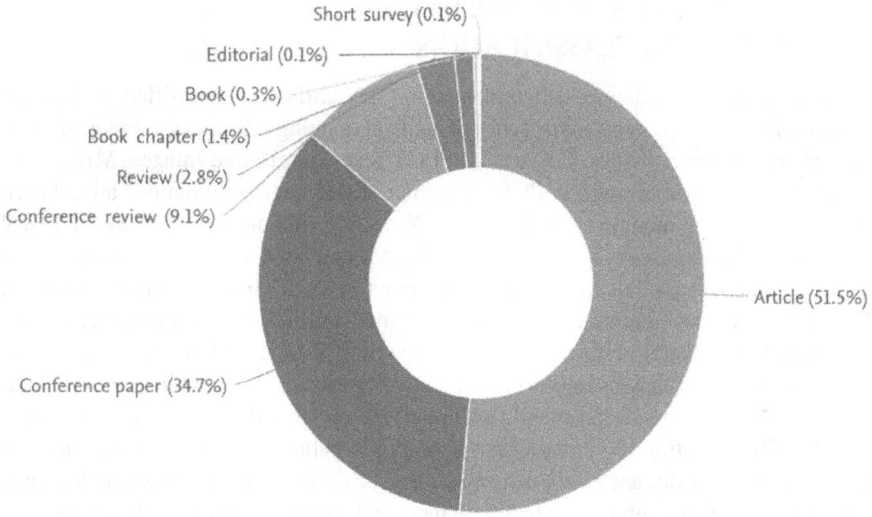

FIGURE 11.5   Publication details of the document by type.

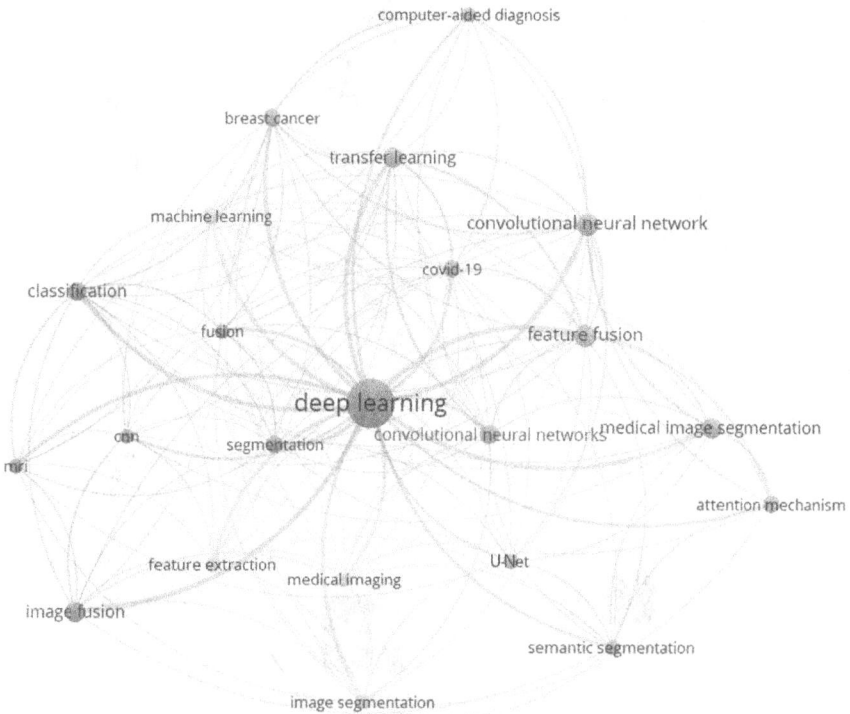

FIGURE 11.6   Bibliographic coupling of author keywords.

11.3   MEDICAL IMAGING MODALITIES
AND THEIR CLASSIFICATION

When it comes to medicine, different imaging modalities provide different data and features. Figure 11.7 depicts many types of medical imaging techniques employed in the field of biomedicine. X-rays, CT scans, SPECT scans, ultrasound images, MRI scans, infrared and ultraviolet images, PET scans, and other imaging modalities are all used in MMIF. Imaging modalities such as MRI, X-ray, CT, and ultrasound (US) can reveal not only the location, size, and appearance of the lesion but also the morphological and structural alterations it has caused in surrounding tissues. It's in the specifics, as it were. Figure 11.8 depicts a classification scheme for medical imaging modalities. Increased use of PET, functional magnetic resonance imaging (fMRI), and SPECT has allowed researchers to gain insight into tumor biology, soft tissue, and function. When medical image data (both structural and functional) are merged, they yield more insightful results. When treating the same organ in multiple patients, medical image fusion is essential for better disease monitoring and analysis. Remote sensing, machine learning, satellite surveillance, image contrast enhancement, image geometric adjustment, and medical imaging are just some of the many fields where image fusion techniques have

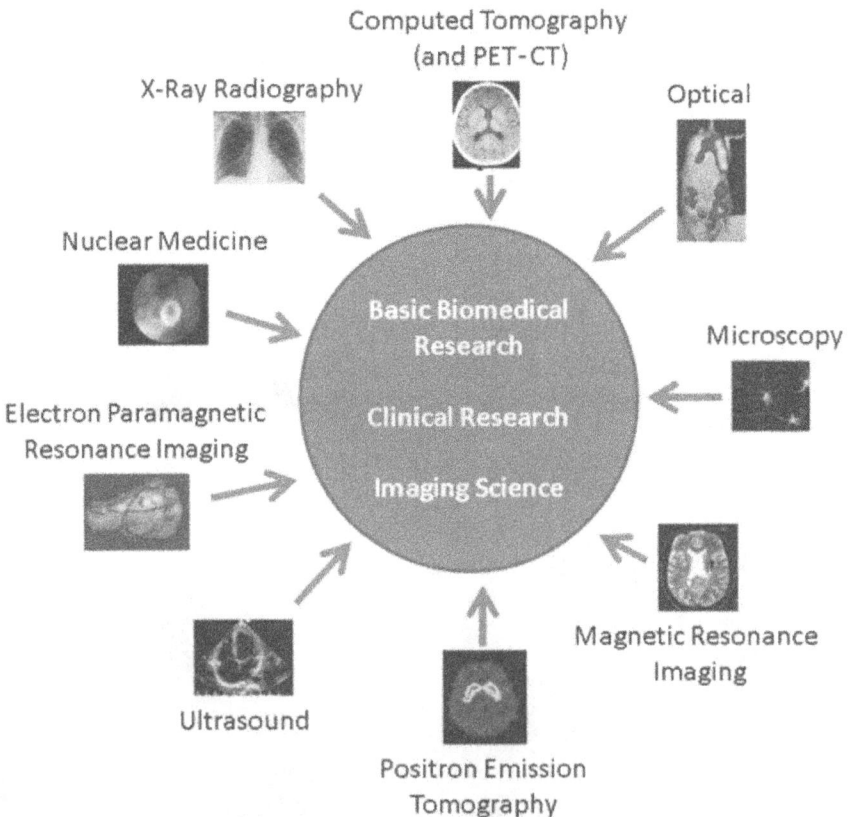

FIGURE 11.7   Medical imaging modalities used in biomedical research.

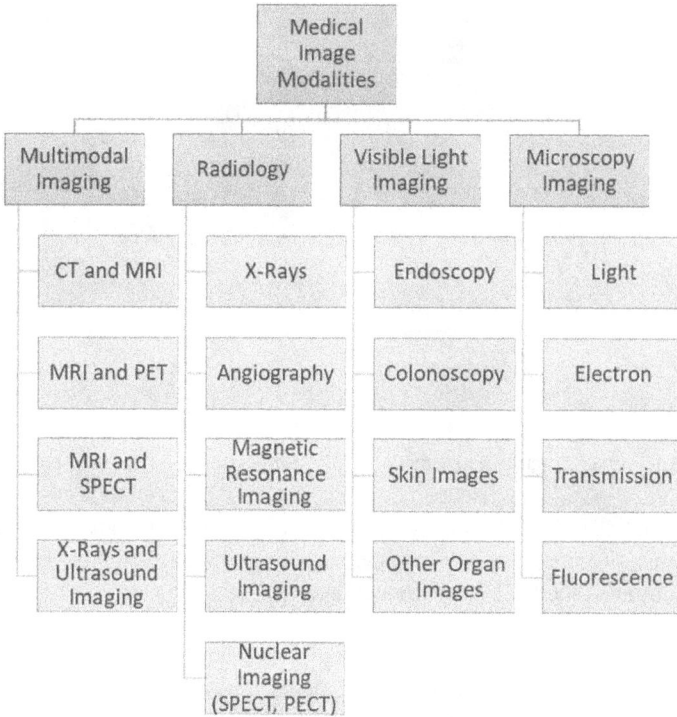

FIGURE 11.8 Classification of medical imaging modalities.

been successfully implemented to improve the detection of features that were previously invisible in a single image, such as malignancies, lesions, cancer cells, etc. Figure 11.8 explains the classification of medical imaging modalities. Additional clinical information can be extracted through the fusion of multimodal medical imaging pairings such as CT-MRI, CT-SPECT, PET-CT, MRI-PET, MRICT-PET, and ultrasound-X-rays. So, it's safe to say that a single image can't possibly convey everything that needs to be known. Therefore, MMIF is crucially required to capture all information in a single composite image, known as a fused image. When combined, these pieces of data are invaluable to doctors making a differential diagnosis. Reduced diagnostic hurdles are a major benefit of medical image fusion applications.

Recent technological developments have made digital image processing systems a practical tool for expanding a variety of industries, including machine vision, medical imaging, remote sensing, and the military. With these methods in place, it is possible to collect and analyze vastly more information. In image processing, the powerful method of image fusion is used to extract all the useful information from the source images and to reduce the growing volume of data. Image fusion's primary objective is to generate fresh images better suited for human and machine perception. When numerous images of a scene are combined into a single composite image, a process known as "image fusion," the essential aspects of each original image are preserved while also adding new information. The resulting fused image is more trustworthy and accurate in its depiction of a scene than any of the source images taken separately.

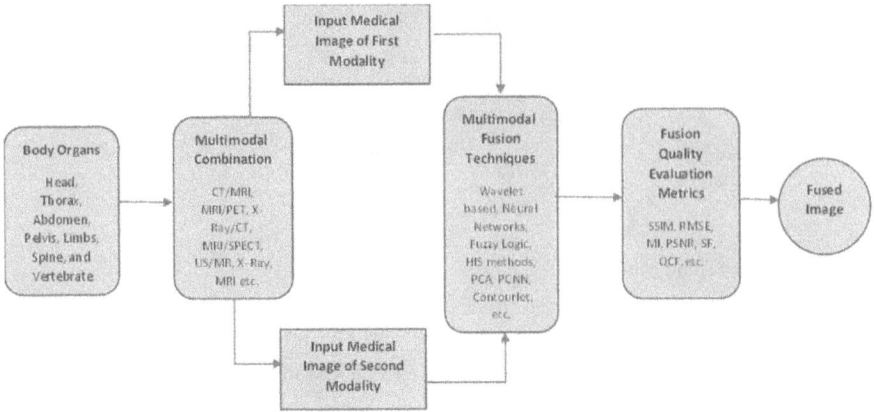

FIGURE 11.9   Overall multimodal medical fusion procedure.

Multimodal medical images benefit from the merging of redundant and complementary data since it improves accuracy and reduces ambiguity. Figure 11.9 depicts the overall multimodal medical fusion procedure.

Algorithms for fusing medical images have two steps. Both image registration and the fusion of key features from the registered images fall under this category. Figure 11.10 shows a simple image fusion model. The clinical track of events information obtained from two source images is typically complementary. It is frequently decided to appropriately incorporate the useful information obtained from the individual image. The first step in this fusion process is to align the spatially related modalities, which is accomplished via a method termed *registration*. The researcher first chooses the target body organ in the multimodal fusion method. The suitable fusion algorithm is then used to combine two or more imaging modalities. Performance metrics are necessary to verify the fusion algorithm. In the last stage, the fused image that is produced has more data on the body organ that was scanned than the input images did. As depicted in Figure 11.10, the image fusion technique is composed of several straightforward steps that work together to achieve the goal. Sample examples of medical imaging modalities under the fusion process are shown in Figure 11.11.

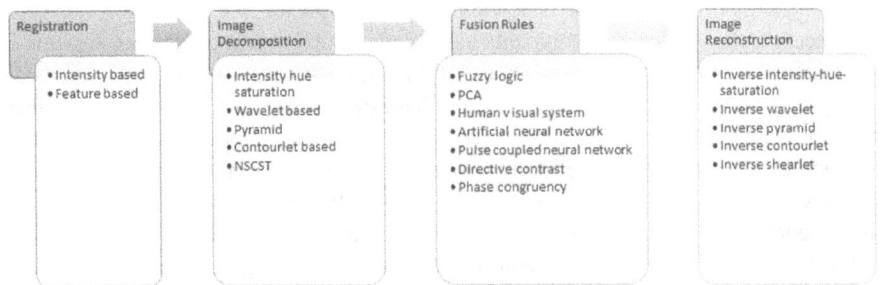

FIGURE 11.10   Medical image fusion step-by-step process.

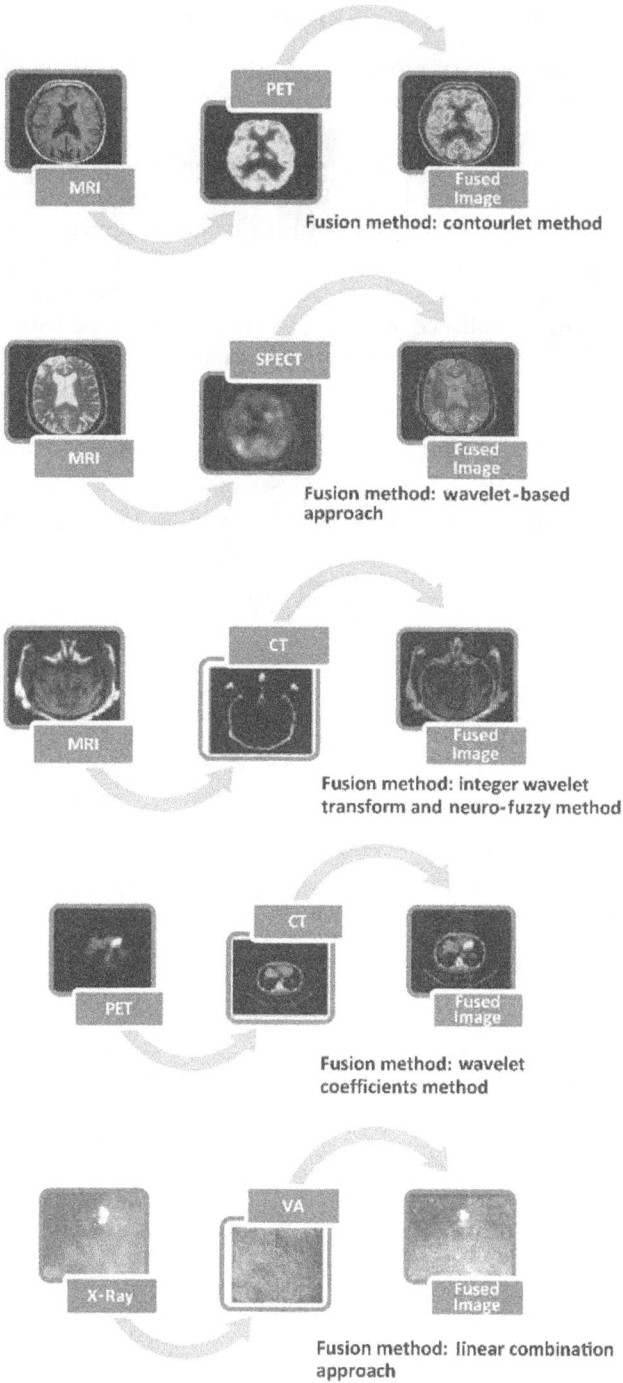

Fusion method: contourlet method

Fusion method: wavelet-based
approach

Fusion method: integer wavelet
transform and neuro-fuzzy method

Fusion method: wavelet
coefficients method

Fusion method: linear combination
approach

FIGURE 11.11   Sample examples of medical imaging modalities under the fusion process.

11.4 LITERATURE SURVEY OR RELATED WORK

Physicians and other medical professionals often use medical images for analyzing the abnormalities in different organs and for identifying diseases from such high-resolution images in a noninvasive manner. However, this manual analysis is a time-consuming process; therefore, computer scientists have come up with automated analysis from multimodal medical images. For getting a better understanding, they have come up with the idea of fusing multimodal medical images using several techniques like pixel-based fusion, frequency-based fusion, spatial fusion, sparse representation-based fusion, etc. As depicted in Figure 11.12, several types of research have been published in the last two decades in the domain of MMIF. In this section, a few well-cited and efficient techniques of multimodal image fusion have been studied and analyzed. Various image fusion techniques have already been compared, and the relative qualities and shortcomings of those techniques are discussed in multiple works by various authors so far [1–8]. However, those works are a bit old, and bibliometric analyses of the publications have not been included in those works. Thus, here we are presenting an analysis of the recent publications along with the bibliometric analysis.

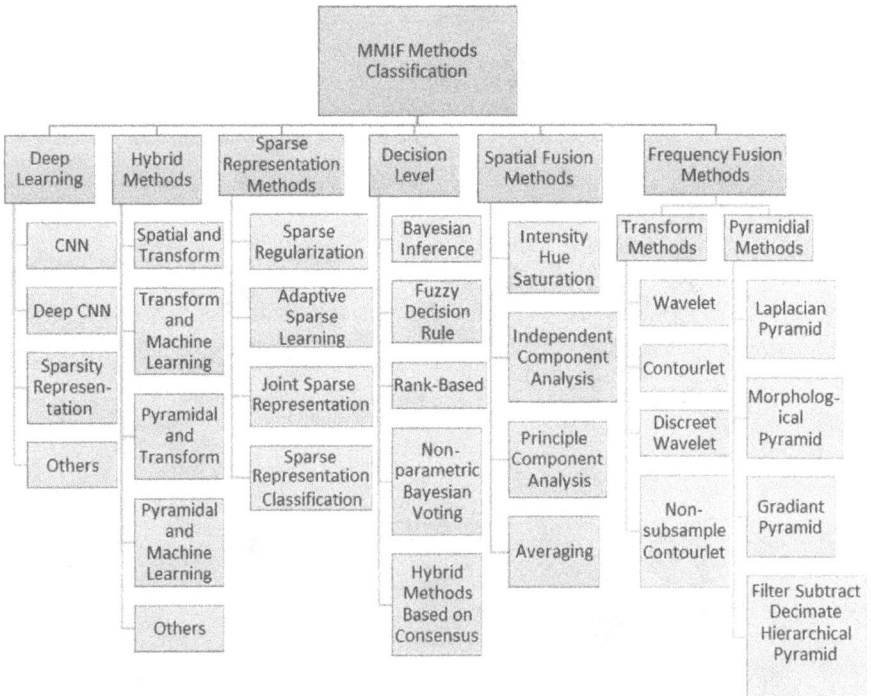

FIGURE 11.12 Classification of medical image fusion techniques.

11.4.1 Deep Learning–Based Method

The potential of deep learning technologies in the fields of pattern recognition and image processing has been intensively investigated. Since deep learning models can automatically extract the most effective characteristics from data, they can circumvent the troublesome nature of the manual design.

The adaptive pulse-coupled neural networks (PCNN) approach proposed by Xu et al. [9] and optimized with the quantum-behaved particle swarm optimization (QPSO) algorithm may merge medical images from different modalities. To create the fusion model, we first run the QPSO-PCNN model on two separate source images. For the PCNN model to discover the best parameters for the input images, the QPSO algorithm was used. Using a hybrid fitness function based on image entropy (EN), average gradient (AG), and spatial frequency (SF) was found to be the most effective way to enhance QPSO's productivity and quality. The fusion model's output, which might have been the pixel value or the trade-off value of the images, was then determined using the judgment factor based on the firing maps of the two source images. The final combined image is a result of the fusion model's calculations.

A two-scale hybrid layer decomposition approach was used by Singh et al. [10] to demonstrate a feature-level MMIF that maximized structural features while suppressing considerable noise and artifacts. The deconstructed base and detail layer fusing in the suggested method uses a convolutional neural network (CNN) with consistency verification and structural patch clustering (based on fuzzy c-means). The brightness and chrominance components that were taken from the source images and the final image are separated using a color space transform. The key features are then extracted from each deconstructed base layer component using a pretrained CNN model. To create the final fused image, the base layer, detail layers, and color components are all combined.

With the Laplacian pyramid and convolutional neural network reconstruction using a local gradient energy technique, Fu et al. [11] introduced an algorithm for fusing medical images that can significantly enhance edge quality. An initial step is using a convolutional neural network to reconstruct multimodal medical images. After that, the Laplacian pyramid is used during the segmentation and recombination steps. Experiments are necessary to find the best number of decomposition layers. The coefficients in each layer are fused using a local gradient energy fusion technique. Last but not least, the combined image is then output via Laplacian inverse transformation.

Zhang et al. [5] introduce the idea of image fusion as shown in Figure 11.13 and categorize the approaches according to the deep architectures they use and the types of fusions they can do. The current state of deep learning's application to image fusion tasks is then explored.

According to real-world requirements for medical diagnosis, Li et al. [12] suggested deep learning–based multimode medical image fusion. It is not limited to merely compensating for the shortcomings of single-page processing when it comes to MRI, CT, and SPECT image fusion, but may instead be applied to a wide variety of multimodal medical image fusion challenges in batch processing mode.

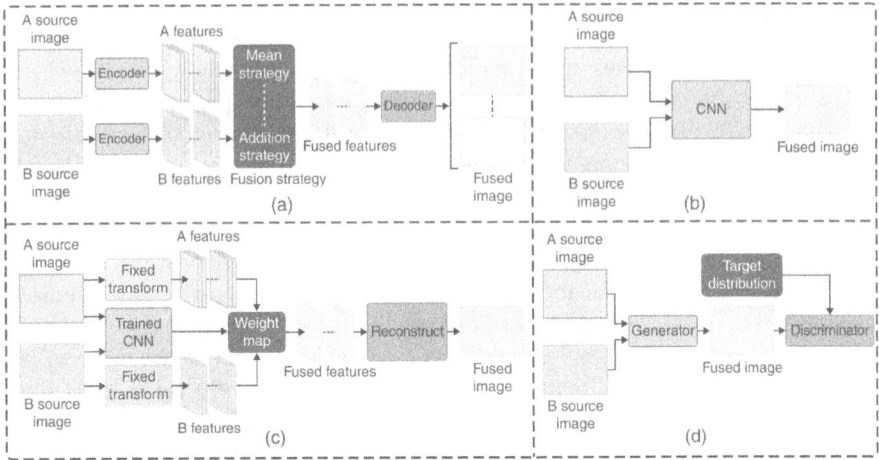

FIGURE 11.13   Different deep architectures for image fusion [5].

For merging anatomical-functional medical images, Li et al. [13] suggested a multiscale double-branch residual attention (MSDRA) network with separate modules for feature extraction, feature fusion, and image reconstruction. The image features were extracted using a module that chained together three identical MSDRA blocks.

11.4.2   SPARSE REPRESENTATION METHODS

Sparse representation has been shown to be an extraordinarily powerful statistical signal modeling method and has a good reputation in both theoretical research and practical applications. It's been quite successful in various image processing tasks, such as removing noise, increasing resolution, classifying images, etc. To create a more compact representation of the signal, a sparse representation model is utilized to express the signal in a specified overcomplete dictionary.

A segment graph filter (SGF) and sparse representation were proposed by Li et al. [14] as a method for medical image fusion sparse representation (SR). Edge information is incorporated into the fused image by decomposing the source images into a base image and a detailed image using the SGF. Following this, a fusion rule based on the normalized Shannon entropy is applied to the base images, while an SR-based fusion approach is applied to the detailed images. The final calculated image is the result of fusing the base and detail images together.

From traditional local and single-component SR-based methods to the most recent global and multicomponent SR-based methods, Liu et al. [15] provide an overview of the recent achievements and challenges in sparse representation (SR)–based medical image fusion.

Medical image fusion was proposed by Guo et al. [16] using convolutional sparse representation (CSR) and mutual information correlation. Nonsubsampled shearlet transform is used to separate the source image into a high-frequency subband and a low-frequency subband. High-frequency coefficient fusion employs CSR for the high-frequency subband. Mutual information correlation analysis is used to select the optimal fusion strategy for a certain region in the low-frequency subband. Here they analyze two types of medical image fusion issues: CT-MRI and MRI-SPECT.

A three-stage process for image fusion was developed by Yousif et al. [17], which relies on a mix of SR and Siamese Convolutional Neural Network (SCNN). First, the complete source image is fed into the traditional orthogonal matching pursuit (OMP), and the SR-fused image is then created by applying the max rule to better localize pixels. For each source image, we further reuse a novel technique of SCNN-based K-SVD dictionary learning. The method's nonlinear behavior has been demonstrated to be effective, leading to improved image detail extraction and transfer in the fused output and an overall increase in the sparsity characteristics of the output image. The final step, the fusion rule, takes the outputs of steps 1 and 2 and linearly combines them to form the effective quality.

Optimized sparse representation, as presented by An et al. [18], separates an image into a foreground and a background. In the next step, a sparse representation of the image's background is obtained by supercomplete dictionary learning. The suggested unsupervised deep learning image fusion method is made noise resistant by using this strategy. Finally, investigations utilizing this method reveal that the quality evaluation indicators of the fused image created by this method greatly surpassed those of both conventional machine learning and deep learning image fusion methods.

11.4.3 Decision-Level Methods

For predictive analytics, Ayesha et al. [19] provided a framework with varying degrees of generalizability for dealing with data of multiple natures. Effective characteristics have been extracted using dimensionality reduction methods for better analysis. The advantages of multimodal data have been highlighted in terms of their ability to boost the efficiency of predictive analytics across a range of fusion types.

The median filter is applied to get rid of noise in the final fused image, and Tirupal et al. [20] presented this method based on an interval-valued intuitionistic fuzzy set (IVIFS) for efficiently fusing multimodal medical images. Simulations are performed on a small number of data sets of multimodal medical images.

Multimodal medical image fusion was proposed by Nagaraja et al. [21] utilizing a novel hybrid metaheuristic technique. To begin, the weighted fast discrete curvelet transform (W-FDCuT) is applied to each of the images to be fused, separating them into high-frequency and low-frequency subbands. After the images have been broken down into subbands, the high-frequency subbands from each will be combined using an optimal Type-2 fuzzy entropy. For low-frequency subband fusion, however, an averaging approach is used. The final step in creating the fused image is to do the inverse W-FDCuT. Hybrid Jaya with sunflower optimization (HJ-SFO) is a metaheuristic methodology that improves the performance of W-FDCuT and Type-2 fuzzy entropy by increasing the value of the structural similarity index measure (SSIM), among other things.

11.4.4 SPATIAL FUSION–BASED METHODS

Challenges in pixel-level image fusion applications are analyzed in [22], where Li et al. provide a comprehensive overview of the state-of-the-art pixel-level image fusion systems with the following four applications: remote sensing, medical diagnosis, surveillance, and photography.

Bhatnagar et al. [23] proposed that a nonsubsampled contourlet transform (NSCT) serve as the basis for a new fusion framework for multimodal medical images. Low- and high-frequency components of the original medical images are combined after being transformed by NSCT. Low- and high-frequency coefficients are fused using two separate fusion rules based on phase congruency and directional contrast, respectively. When everything is ready, the inverse NSCT is performed using all composite coefficients to generate the fused image.

A new low-level feature-based approach to medical image fusion was proposed by Zhang et al. [24]. We use local binary pattern operators to break down the source images into a base layer and a detail layer to extract low-level information. Weight maps are built via saliency detection, which is then applied to the low-level features of the base and detail layers. Maintaining spatial coherence between the source images and their respective layers is accomplished through the fusion of a base layer and a detail layer using a weight map improved by fast-guided filtering. The final fused image is built by recombining the base and detail layers that were previously fused.

Combining the pixel-level nonlocal self-similarity (TS-PLNSS) prior with the pixel-intensity properties of the image, Zhu et al. [25] suggested a two-stage image decomposition framework. At first, an adaptive thresholding process separates the source image into a texture layer, a structure layer, and a base layer, each representing a different scale. The properties of each layer are then taken into account when deciding on a fusion strategy. Among these is an optimization function that incorporates structural information and is made to save as much of the original image's prominent information as possible. The final step is image reconstruction, which yields the combined medical image.

11.4.5 WAVELET-BASED METHODS

The field of medical image fusion has exploded in popularity over the past few decades, particularly with Multi-Scale Transform (MST)-based approaches. MST-based fusion methods generally involve three main sequential processes: first, decomposing the pending source images into several subbands, which represent some feature information of the images, using complex operators; second, applying different fusion rules, based on the pixel level, to fuse the corresponding sub-bands; and third, inverse transformation to obtain the final fusion image. Discrete wavelet transforms- and Laplacian pyramid transform-based algorithms were among the first mainstream approaches. Similar organs from different images or environments are fused. Wavelet transformation has been used in several studies over the past 20 years to fuse MRI and CT images. Jean Morlet introduced the concept of wavelet transforms in 1982. There are three distinct kinds of wavelet transforms: orthogonal, biorthogonal, and nonorthogonal (A-trous). Many different approaches to medical image fusion have been developed to address the complex medical challenges revealed by combining images of different body parts, cells, tissues, and organs. Despite the limitations, image fusion procedures find widespread use in modern medical diagnosis and research.

By minimizing distortion with an empirical wavelet transform (EWT) representation and a local energy maxima (LEM) fusion algorithm, Polinati et al. [26] established an approach that integrates the supplementary data from many imaging modalities. According to the characteristics of the input image, EWT chooses the most appropriate basis functions. As a result, important details like edges, which are key in image fusion, are preserved.

To separate the images into high-frequency subbands and low-frequency subbands, Kumar et al. [27] proposed a method in which the images from the two modalities are first applied using optimal dual-tree complex wavelet transform (DT-CWT). Using a combination of the Salp Swarm Method (SSA) and the Beetle Swarm Optimization (BSO), a hybrid meta-heuristic algorithm called Hybrid Beetle and Salp Swarm Optimization (HBSSO) optimizes the DT-filter CWT's coefficients for enhanced performance. Also, the improved type-2 fuzzy entropy was used to combine the high-frequency subbands of the original images. A similar hybrid HBSSO is used to optimize both the upper and lower membership restrictions. Optimized type-2 fuzzy entropy will pick high-frequency coefficients without any input from the user. Additionally, the averaging method is used to fuse the low-frequency subimages. In addition, the final fused medical image can be obtained with the aid of inverse optimized DT-CWT on the combined image sets. Both the optimized DT-CWT and the optimized type-2 fuzzy entropy seek to maximize the SSIM.

Based on the discrete stationary wavelet transform (DSWT) and a radial basis neural network (RBFNN), Chao et al. [28] devised a method for image fusion. Before DSWT can process images, they must first be broken down into their component high-frequency and low-frequency subbands using a technique called two-level decomposition. They were able to extract seven fused components from the seven neural networks. The final fused image was created by inverse wavelet transform. The neural network was trained using a procedure that combined the adaptive gradient descent algorithm (AGDA) with the gravitational search algorithm (GSA).

Using a combination of NSCT and DTCWT, Alseelawi et al. [29] suggested a powerful way for fusing many medical images into one. Input multimodality medical images included CT scans, MRI scans, and PET scans. A neural network is proposed to build a weight map that includes the pixel-by-pixel motion information included in dual or more multimodality medical images. Medical image fusion is accomplished on a multiscale basis using medical image pyramids to improve human visual comprehension. The fusion mode for the decomposed coefficients is adaptively modified using a local comparison-based method.

To acquire high-frequency information from low-frequency input, Dharejo et al. [30] suggested a generative adversarial network (GAN) with deep multiattention modules. Here, they use wavelet transform (WT) and GANs to extract high-frequency details from low-frequency inputs. With WT, the Low Resolution (LR) image is segmented into different frequency bands, and the transferred GAN makes use of multi-attention and unsampled blocks to forecast the high-frequency components.

Table 11.3 summarizes the benefits and drawbacks of current methods. In addition, the accessible Multimodal Medical Image Dataset is described in full in Table 11.4.

TABLE 11.3
Advantages and Disadvantages of Existing Techniques

Technique	Advantages	Disadvantages
Spatial based	• Easiest implementation • Highly concentrated image results produced • Processing and sharpening capacity is quick, computationally efficient, and faster	• The fused image may not be sharp • Image contrast is diminished by the blurring effect • The final algorithm requires a more complicated procedure than the pixel-level technique
Frequency based	• For reducing spectral distortion, it performs better than standard fusion methods • Produces higher SNR than standard pixel-level techniques • Both high spatial resolution and decent quality spectral components are included in the fused image • For multifocus images, excellent detailed image quality is obtained	• The final fused image may contain less spatial resolution • Fusion requires a more complicated procedure than that of pixel-level techniques • Generated fused images are more or less identical
Deep learning	• Optimization of image fusion is easier due to the self-learning environment of deep learning • Input data focus on fusing high-dimensional data to produce a feasible solution • The methodology can be customized according to the requirements • Compared to other fusion techniques, this technique is capable of producing a high-quality image from multiple input images	• Based on the dynamic process with complex parameters • Many challenges like local extremum, misidentification, and pace of training convergence need to be addressed • More time and hardware are required to train the fusion model • Does not give accurate results for small data sets of images
Hybrid based	• Complementary detailed information is extracted from input images • Clarity, texture, contrast, brightness information are improved in the fused image • Hybrid techniques prevent difficulties at the pixel level such as too sensitive noise and blurring • Artifacts are minimized in the resulting image	• Requires detailed knowledge of each technique; otherwise, nonuniform images may be produced • Typically complex and inherently time-consuming techniques • Difficult to implement in large data sets
Sparse representation	• Factors like SR coefficient improve the final image significantly • Retains the visual information better and improves the contrast of the image compared to other techniques • Information related to the structure of images and other extensive details are preserved	• Minimum details are preserved in the fused images • High susceptibility to misregistration • Sometimes produces visual artifact results in the fused image

(Continued)

TABLE 11.3 *(Continued)*
Advantages and Disadvantages of Existing Techniques

Technique	Advantages	Disadvantages
Decision level	• The quantity of superfluous and unclear information is reduced • Accuracy is increased by including the information content that is linked to each pixel in the image, which improves more than with feature-level fusion	• The methods get increasingly difficult to master • The methods are more time consuming and complicated

The following summarizes additional multimodal medical data sets:

- Center for Invivo Microscopy (CIVM), Embrionic and Neonatal Mouse (H&E, MR)
- Laboratory of Neuro Imaging (LONI) image data archive
- Radiology (ultrasound, mammographs, X-Ray, CT, MRI, fMRI, etc.)
- Collaborative Informatics and Neuroimaging Suite (COINS)
- The Cancer Imaging Archive (TCIA)
- Alzheimer's Disease Neuroimaging Initiative (ADNI), http://adni.loni.ucla.edu/
- Open Access Series of Imaging Studies (OASIS), http://www.oasis-brains.org/
- Breast Cancer Digital Repository
- Mammography, http://marathon.csee.usf.edu/Mammography/Database.html
- Mammographic Image Analysis Society (MIAS) minidatabase
- Mammography Image Databases: 100 or more images of mammograms with ground truth

TABLE 11.4
Available Multimodal Medical Image Dataset

Dataset	Modalities	Body Organ(s)	Format	Link
OASIS [OASIS-1, OASIS-2, OASIS-3]	MRI and PET	Brain	Nifti	https://www.oasis-brains.org/
TCIA	Mammography, X-rays, US, CT, MRI, PET, SPECT	Brain, chest, lungs, breast, abdomen, kidney, heart, neck	Dicom	http://www.med.harvard.edu/AANLIB/
BrainWeb Atlas	CT, MRI, PET, SPECT	Brain	GIF	http://adni.loni.usc.edu/
ADNI	MRI, FMRI, PET	Brain		https://www.cancerimagingarchive.net/
MIDAS	CT, MRI, SPECT, PET, US	Heart, brain, bones, head, liver	Dicom Raw, Mhd, hdr	

- NLM HyperDoc Visible Human Project color, CAT, and MRI image samples – over 30 images
- CT Scans for Colon Cancer
- [BreastScreening] UTA4: Breast Cancer Medical Imaging DICOM Files Dataset & Resources (MG, US, and MRI)
- [MIMBCD-UI] UTA7: Breast Cancer Medical Imaging DICOM Files Dataset & Resources (MG, US, and MRI)
- [Facebook AI + NYU FastMRI] includes two types of MRI scans: knee MRIs and brain (neuro) MRIs, containing training, validation, and masked test sets
- BCNB: Early Breast Cancer Core-Needle Biopsy WSI Dataset

11.5   CONCLUSION AND FUTURE DIRECTION

In this chapter, a comparative study of different image fusion techniques is presented. Along with the comparative study, a bibliometric survey has also been presented. The bibliometric survey would help researchers to channelize their research as per the identified popular keywords, identify the journals to publish their research work, and find out the most popular publications in this domain while the comparative study of different available techniques would guide them to understand the present state-of-the-art of MMIF research for the medical images. Researchers may work to overcome the shortcomings identified from various approaches to MMIF. From the identified strengths and weaknesses of those studies, it is understood that the research in the medical image fusion domain is still in the budding phase. Almost all available techniques available for medical image fusion have some flaws, and improvements can be done in many areas. Considering the shortcomings of existing techniques, it can be commented that advanced MMIF techniques and hybridization of the existing techniques to improve the results of the fused images are the need of the hour. As there currently exists a lack of suitable image representation methodologies and generally recognized fusion assessment criteria, future studies can focus on (a) the effectiveness of image fusion techniques, particularly with advanced deep learning techniques; (b) the implementation of evolving methods to enhance image areas of interest before the fusion process; and (c) creation of new multiscale decomposition techniques for fusing images from different sources. Since precise ground truth is lacking in most image fusion challenges, evaluating the quality of the fused output is tough. Furthermore, we need to construct no-reference metrics with better descriptive capabilities. Enhancing the resulting fusion image quality could compensate for restricted imaging modalities and heavy noise. Approaches should be determined for addressing issues such as image noise, high computing costs, and measurement discrepancies between images acquired using different medical imaging modalities. Another area of concern is to collect data and build a trustworthy data set of medical images of organs like the larynx, eyes, and ears – the areas where very limited work has been done so far. Optimization of huge data sets before applying fusion techniques is another area of concern that future researchers can dig into. Appropriate noise removal using advanced techniques before starting with the fusion process to improve the performance is also an area where research is needed.

REFERENCES

1. Swathi, P. S., M. S. Sheethal, and Vince Paul. "Survey on multimodal medical image fusion techniques." *International Journal of Science, Engineering and Computer Technology* 6, no. 1 (2016): 33.
2. Yadav, Satya Prakash, and Sachin Yadav. "Fusion of medical images using a wavelet methodology: A survey." *IEIE Transactions on Smart Processing & Computing* 8, no. 4 (2019): 265–271.
3. Faragallah, Osama S., Heba El-Hoseny, Walid El-Shafai, Wael Abd El-Rahman, Hala S. El-Sayed, El-Sayed M. El-Rabaie, Fathi E. Abd El-Samie, and Gamal G.N. Geweid. "A comprehensive survey analysis for present solutions of medical image fusion and future directions." *IEEE Access* 9 (2020): 11358–11371.
4. Huang, Bing, Feng Yang, Mengxiao Yin, Xiaoying Mo, and Cheng Zhong. "A review of multimodal medical image fusion techniques." *Computational and Mathematical Methods in Medicine* 2020 (2020).
5. Zhang, Hao, Han Xu, Xin Tian, Junjun Jiang, and Jiayi Ma. "Image fusion meets deep learning: A survey and perspective." *Information Fusion* 76 (2021): 323–336.
6. Hermessi, Haithem, Olfa Mourali, and Ezzeddine Zagrouba. "Multimodal medical image fusion review: Theoretical background and recent advances." *Signal Processing* 183 (2021): 108036.
7. Tirupal, T., B. Chandra Mohan, and S. Srinivas Kumar. "Multimodal medical image fusion techniques–a review." *Current Signal Transduction Therapy* 16, no. 2 (2021): 142–163.
8. Tawfik, Nahed, Heba A. Elnemr, Mahmoud Fakhr, Moawad I. Dessouky, Abd El-Samie, and E. Fathi. "Survey study of multimodality medical image fusion methods." *Multimedia Tools and Applications* 80, no. 4 (2021): 6369–6396.
9. Xu, Xinzheng, Dong Shan, Guanying Wang, and Xiangying Jiang. "Multimodal medical image fusion using PCNN optimized by the QPSO algorithm." *Applied Soft Computing* 46 (2016): 588–595.
10. Singh, Sneha, and Radhey Shyam Anand. "Multimodal medical image fusion using hybrid layer decomposition with CNN-based feature mapping and structural clustering." *IEEE Transactions on Instrumentation and Measurement* 69, no. 6 (2019): 3855–3865.
11. Fu, Jun, Weisheng Li, Jiao Du, and Bin Xiao. "Multimodal medical image fusion via laplacian pyramid and convolutional neural network reconstruction with local gradient energy strategy." *Computers in Biology and Medicine* 126 (2020): 104048.
12. Li, Yi, Junli Zhao, Zhihan Lv, and Jinhua Li. "Medical image fusion method by deep learning." *International Journal of Cognitive Computing in Engineering* 2 (2021): 21–29.
13. Li, Weisheng, Xiuxiu Peng, Jun Fu, Guofen Wang, Yuping Huang, and Feifei Chao. "A multiscale double-branch residual attention network for anatomical–functional medical image fusion." *Computers in Biology and Medicine* 141 (2022): 105005.
14. Li, Qiaoqiao, Weilan Wang, Guoyue Chen, and Dongdong Zhao. "Medical image fusion using segment graph filter and sparse representation." *Computers in Biology and Medicine* 131 (2021): 104239.
15. Liu, Yu, Xun Chen, Aiping Liu, Rabab K. Ward, and Z. Jane Wang. "Recent advances in sparse representation based medical image fusion." *IEEE Instrumentation & Measurement Magazine* 24, no. 2 (2021): 45–53.
16. Guo, Peng, Guoqi Xie, Renfa Li, and Hui Hu. "Multimodal medical image fusion with convolution sparse representation and mutual information correlation in NSST domain." *Complex & Intelligent Systems* 9 (2022): 1–12.
17. Yousif, Ahmed Sabeeh, Zaid Omar, and Usman Ullah Sheikh. "An improved approach for medical image fusion using sparse representation and Siamese convolutional neural network." *Biomedical Signal Processing and Control* 72 (2022): 103357.

18. An, Feng-Ping, Xing-min Ma, and Lei Bai. "Image fusion algorithm based on unsupervised deep learning-optimized sparse representation." *Biomedical Signal Processing and Control* 71 (2022): 103140.
19. Ayesha, Shaeela, Muhammad Kashif Hanif, and Ramzan Talib. "Performance enhancement of predictive analytics for health informatics using dimensionality reduction techniques and fusion frameworks." *IEEE Access* 10 (2021): 753–769.
20. Tirupal, T., B. Chandra Mohan, and S. Srinivas Kumar. "Multimodal medical image fusion based on interval-valued intuitionistic fuzzy sets." In *Machines, Mechanism and Robotics*, pp. 965–971. Springer, Singapore, 2022.
21. Nagaraja Kumar, N., T. Jayachandra Prasad, and K. Satya Prasad. "An intelligent multimodal medical image fusion model based on improved fast discrete curvelet transform and type-2 fuzzy entropy." *International Journal of Fuzzy Systems* 25 (2022): 1–22.
22. Li, Shutao, Xudong Kang, Leyuan Fang, Jianwen Hu, and Haitao Yin. "Pixel-level image fusion: A survey of the state of the art." *Information Fusion* 33 (2017): 100–112.
23. Bhatnagar, G., Q. Wu, and Z. Liu. "Directive contrast based multimodal medical image fusion in NSCT domain." *IEEE Transactions on Multimedia* 15, no. 5 (2013): 1014–1024.
24. Zhang, Yongxin, Chenrui Guo, and Peng Zhao. "Medical image fusion based on low-level features." *Computational and Mathematical Methods in Medicine* 2021 (2021).
25. Zhu, Rui, Xiongfei Li, Yu Wang, and Xiaoli Zhang. "Medical image fusion based on pixel-level nonlocal self-similarity prior and optimization." In *International Conference on Database Systems for Advanced Applications*, pp. 247–254. Springer, Cham, 2022.
26. Polinati, Srinivasu, and Ravindra Dhuli. "Multimodal medical image fusion using empirical wavelet decomposition and local energy maxima." *Optik* 205 (2020): 163947.
27. Kumar, N. Nagaraja, T. Jayachandra Prasad, and K. Satya Prasad. "Optimized dual-tree complex wavelet transform and fuzzy entropy for multi-modal medical image fusion: A hybrid meta-heuristic concept." *Journal of Mechanics in Medicine and Biology* 21, no. 3 (2021): 2150024.
28. Chao, Zhen, Xingguang Duan, Shuangfu Jia, Xuejun Guo, Hao Liu, and Fucang Jia. "Medical image fusion via discrete stationary wavelet transform and an enhanced radial basis function neural network." *Applied Soft Computing* 118 (2022): 108542.
29. Alseelawi, Nawar, Hussein Tuama Hazim, and Haider TH Salim ALRikabi. "A novel method of multimodal medical image fusion based on hybrid approach of NSCT and DTCWT." *International Journal of Online & Biomedical Engineering* 18, no. 3 (2022).
30. Dharejo, Fayaz Ali, Muhammad Zawish, Farah Deeba, Yuanchun Zhou, Kapal Dev, Sunder Ali Khowaja, and Nawab Muhammad Faseeh Qureshi. "Multimodal-boost: Multimodal medical image super-resolution using multi-attention network with wavelet transform." *IEEE/ACM Transactions on Computational Biology and Bioinformatics* (2022).

Part III

Medical IOT and Recent Trends

12 Big Data in IoT for Healthcare Application

Nilam Upasani[1], Deepali Joshi[2], Sanika Upasani[3], and Swayam Pendgaonkar[3]
[1]Pimpri Chinchwad College of Engineering, Pune, India
[2]Vishwakarma Institute of Technology, Pune, India
[3]Symbiosis Institute of Technology, Pune, India

CONTENTS

12.1 INTRODUCTION

As a result of the affordable rates of Internet service providers and electronic devices, there is a drastic increase in the data generation rate, which accounts for multimodal data in the form of text, images, videos, etc. This Big Data can be utilized to create data-driven predictive models in various fields. Revolution in the sensor technology, which is the backbone of Internet of Things (IoT), has caused the blending between the IoT and Big Data. Multiple ubiquitous devices interconnected together for data exchange resulted in the emerging field of IoT. One of the crucial aspects in the world of Big Data and IoT is data management. Various IoT-based applications such as remote patient healthcare monitoring, smart transport, grid systems, energy smart meters, smart cities, etc., generate massive amounts of data, which need to

DOI: 10.1201/9781003324430-15

be handled wisely. One of the prominent areas where these technological advances can be utilized for the benefit of society is healthcare. This is the need of the hour because of the unpredictability of life due to stress and unhealthy lifestyles. Every person should get the medical support and services 24×7 seamlessly, irrespective of their geographical location, which is the objective of IoT in healthcare. For efficient treatment of patients, the history as well as the real-time data of the patient should be available at the fingertips of the healthcare specialist. At the same time, the patient should be able to make an intelligent choice of the specialist by considering the history of treatment of patients. In practice, it would be a win–win situation for both. The healthcare specialists can effectively evaluate the physical conditions of patients remotely with the help of various health monitoring devices such as temperature monitors, electrocardiograms, blood glucose level monitors, etc. The data generated from these devices can be analyzed using Big Data analytics to diagnose serious diseases in their early stages to help save lives. Patients can be equipped with small sensors on the ill portion of the body part and remotely monitored continuously in critical situations. This would ensure the safety of patients and improve the quality of healthcare services. We make sincere practice to explore the state-of-the-art improvements in the healthcare domain due to advances in IoT in generating important data points and Big Data in storing and analyzing these data to find interesting results in terms of patterns and predictions.

Innovation in healthcare can be experienced with the development of deep learning, artificial intelligence, machine learning, edge analytics and smart sensorial things, with the integration of cloud computing [1, 2]. The data-centered application that empirically changes the communication and operation of the current healthcare networks is electronic health records (EHR). The EHR is a digital file consisting of the private information of patients (name, age, address, photo, etc.) and their health parameters (previous surgeries, blood type, existing diseases, vaccinations, etc.). One of the most important features for integrating cloud services in healthcare is maximizing cost efficiency [3]. Our proposed architecture suggests advancements in intensive patient care using smart sensors, an emergency notification system, and a clinical predictive model.

12.2   INTERNET OF THINGS AND BIG DATA: AN OVERVIEW

The IoT is a network of tens of millions of interconnected physical devices creating opportunities for the interaction between the physical and digital worlds [4]. The devices such as radio-frequency identification (RFID) sensor networks, actuators, global positioning system (GPS) devices, radar, and satellites provide rich information about themselves and their surroundings to the dedicated computing facilities. The IoT environment enables data exchange between all the sources of data that results in reducing human intervention, improving the process efficiency and economic benefits. The history of IoT is discussed in the next section.

12.2.1   IoT History

The idea of connected devices has existed since the early 1800s. The Internet, which is one of the most significant elements of IoT, was introduced as a part of the

Defense Advanced Research Projects Agency (DARPA) in 1962 and advanced into the Advanced Research Projects Agency Network (ARPANET) in 1969. The commercial service providers allowed public use of ARPANET in the 1980s that has evolved into our Internet. The Department of Defense started using GPS in early 1993, with a system of 24 satellites that was followed by the privately owned, commercial satellites.

The term "Internet of Things" was officially named by Kevin Ashton, cofounder of MIT's Auto-ID Center, in 1999 during his work at Procter & Gamble. He suggested using RFID technology to tag the IOT devices. The term actually started getting extensive attention in 2010. Other technologies, such as barcodes, QR codes, and digital watermarking, are also used to tag the devices [5, 6].

One more important element of IoT is IPV6, the most recent version of the Internet Protocol (IP), which has become the draft standard in 1998 and an Internet standard in 2017. It provides remarkably huge address space to accommodate an abundant quantity of devices. Software-defined networking (SDN), a new concept in network operation along with IPv6 addressing, allows us to reach the requirements standardized by fifth-generation (5G) wireless communications [7].

12.2.2   GENERAL ARCHITECTURE OF IoT

IoT: It is a collection of devices having unique identities and an on/off switch that are interconnected with intelligent interfaces on the Internet in specific contexts. IoT is likely to go beyond machine-to-machine (M2M) communications and offer advanced connectivity of devices, services, and systems. It covers a variety of protocols, applications, and domains. This revolution is expected to bring automation in nearly all fields, including advanced applications such as healthcare.

Things: Things are a wide range of interconnected devices like automobiles with built-in sensors, biochip transponders on farm animals, field operation devices that help firefighters in search and rescue, heart monitoring implants, etc.

There is no single reference architecture of IoT, as it includes an extremely wide range of devices, technologies, and applications. The basic architecture of IoT describing the four essential stages is shown in Figure 12.1.

I. Sensors/actuators

Sensors or actuators are used to interact with the digital world and physical world. Any device that provides inputs about object or environment under measurement is termed a sensor. The specific input could be heat, light, moisture, pressure, motion, or any other environmental phenomena. An actuator is a device that is used to move or control a system or environment. For the detailed analysis of data, it should be moved into a cloud- or data center–based system with extensive processing power that can bring various sources of data together. In the case of the immediate requirement of information for quick decisions, processing power can be made available on the sensors/actuators; however, that would limit the depth of insight.

The use of assistive technology, and in particular the adoption of cutting-edge healthcare sensors and equipment, has become more important as the

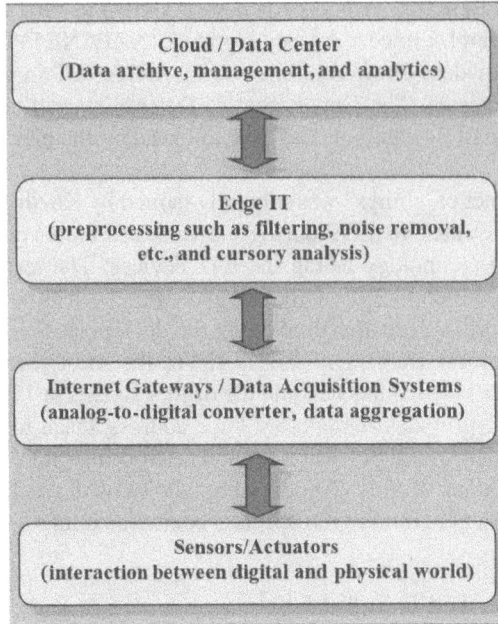

FIGURE 12.1 IoT architecture.

world's population ages [8]. The focus on IoT-based remote health monitoring systems is one technique that has received significant research attention. IoT-based systems in the medical area must convert sensor data into real-time clinical feedback. This strategy takes a wide range of factors into account, including data mining and learning as well as detecting, sending, processing, and storing [9].

II. Internet gateways

Internet gateways/data acquisition systems normally sit in close proximity to the sensors/actuators. Sensors generate the data in analog form. The analog-to-digital converter converts it into digital streams for further processing. The data acquisition systems (DASs) aggregate the abundant amount of data generated by the huge number of sensors. The Internet gateway routes the digitized and aggregated data over the Internet to the next stage for further processing.

III. Edge IT

The data, such as filtering, noise removal, etc., are preprocessed here before they move on to the cloud or data center. The cursory analysis of data can also be done here for faster response. Normally the edge IT is located closer to the sensors so as to reduce the burden on the core IT infrastructure, as the large data can consume network bandwidth and swamp the data center resources.

IV. Data center/cloud

The traditional backend data center or cloud-based system facilitates the in-depth analysis of data. The data are managed and stored securely here. The data from varied resources including the sensor data get combined to get deeper understanding. This process takes longer to get results, and hence it is used where feedback isn't urgent. Mobile apps and web-based applications available on cloud provide tools for further exploration and analysis through dashboards and visualizations.

Smart phones, tablets, PCs, and other smart devices are used as the controlling devices.

12.2.3 Blending of Big Data with IoT

Every picture we take, tweet we make, status we update, and video we upload contribute to the ocean of Big Data. An enormous amount of data is produced in the IoT environment from varied sources. Blending Big Data and IoT together would make it possible to harness that data to get insights and make decisions. The research challenge is to transform the data generated by these connections to knowledge to solve unsolved problems and make a positive impact on our lifestyle. Moreover, it must be done in a scalable and cost-effective manner so as to benefit the society. Blending of Big Data and IoT is shown in Figure 12.2.

IoT and Big Data can make wonders together in synchronization with each other. IoT devices play a major role in data gathering in various applications and transmit the data over the cloud through the Internet and other communication mechanisms like ZigBee, Bluetooth, Wi-Fi, etc. This huge amount of data is then transferred to Big Data architecture so as to make it accessible and ready for analysis. The Big Data analytics algorithms can now generate predictions and visualizations, study the recent trends from the precious data, and make quick and efficient decisions.

12.2.4 Opportunities, Challenges, and Applications of Big Data and IoT

IoT and Big Data are complementary technologies. In addition to that, they greatly impact each other. The growth of IoT would place more demands on Big Data

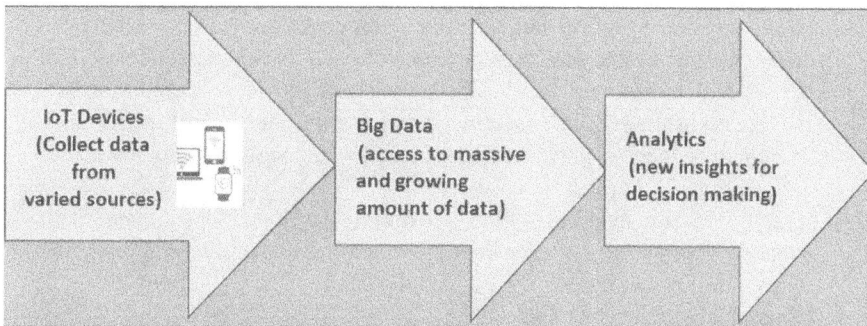

FIGURE 12.2 Blending of IoT and Big Data.

capabilities. Brought together, these two technologies would create opportunities in various fields, described as follows:

   I. The data generated can be used to find the trends and patterns of user behavior that would help to make the decisions. The decision making can be supported by the insights derived from predictive modeling techniques. Data visualization is available at the user's fingertips due to multiple open-source tools like Elastic search, R, etc.

  II. The advent of open-source, cloud-based technologies like Hadoop have significantly reduced the operating cost of Big Data generated through IoT applications. It has also provided cross-domain availability of the data to design smart applications, which was not possible in traditional isolated systems.

 III. Adequate algorithmic support of various analytical techniques is a backbone for blending Big Data and IoT together. Besides, the analytical techniques can work more effectively with the abundant data available using IoT.

 IV. Mission critical systems in IoT such as remote robotic surgery, industrial machineries in smart factories, enterprises with market agility, remote radar systems, etc., need real-time processing of the data. The Big Data architecture like Hadoop processes the data in a distributed manner to make the retrieval and analysis more efficient.

IoT data have special characteristics like heterogeneity, variety, noise, real-time processing, and rapid growth, which distinguishes it from normal Big Data. The IoT devices emit data in real time and hence have to be acted upon early so as to reap benefits out of it. The usage of these two technologies together opens new challenges for the research community. Following are the challenges that will seek the attention of the researchers in the near future [10, 11]:

   I. Decision-making algorithms will shift from the central server to the local devices so as to implement quick decisions in a real-time environment. The challenge is to provide more processing power to the lightweight local devices.

  II. In the context of big IoT data, privacy and security are the main challenges in storing and processing huge amounts of data. The theft or unauthorized access of personal user data has become a core problem. There has to be a protection of the sensitive information of users from external interference. It demands more stringent communication protocols and authentication procedures.

 III. Traditional data security solutions are mainly developed for stationary data, whereas recent data requirements are changing dynamically in real time. Thus, there is a dire need to develop advanced security solutions to handle dynamically increasing data.

 IV. Heterogeneity of the various autonomous devices connected poses challenges in the type and form of data generated and even their communication mechanism. These devices should be able to connect universally and must have a standard identification number similar to an IP address for our computing machines.

V. The machine learning algorithms have to be tuned so as to handle data from big IoT data architectures. The algorithms must be competent to handle heterogeneous communication, real-time exploration, extraction, and integration processes.

VI. Integrating varied data types is an intricate task in merging different systems or applications together. In this case, it becomes more complex because of heavy noise, the fast- and ever-growing nature of the data.

Big Data provides data storage and processing for the various IoT applications. The major opportunities of Big Data and IoT are centered in healthcare, transportation, enterprises, smart cities, consumer applications, etc. The detailed applications of these two technologies are discussed as follows.

I. Smart healthcare

The growing consumer demand for proactive health monitoring has created big scope for smart healthcare. The physical conditions of patients can be monitored continuously in critical situations with the help of various health monitoring devices such as temperature monitors, electrocardiograms, blood glucose level monitors, etc. The history of the patient and the current data of treatment can be made available at the healthcare specialist's fingertips to detect diseases. The data can be analyzed to diagnose serious diseases in their early stages to help save lives. The activities of elderly can be monitored continuously with the help of motion sensors, microphone, real-time streaming data, etc., and an alert can be sent to caretakers if something goes wrong.

II. Smart transportation

The aim is to make smarter and safer use of transport networks. Various technologies such as security CCTV systems, car navigation, container management systems, number plate recognition, traffic signal control systems, etc., are used as the monitoring and controlling systems for traffic congestion. Such systems find the optimal route based on the real-time conditions and then reroute the traffic, adjusting speed limits, signal timing, and prompt guide to an empty parking space. It can also lessen the number of road accidents by discovering the potentially hazardous situations based on the history of road mishaps.

III. Smart grid

Smart grids rapidly produce data that are used to track the current power consumption changes so as to efficiently manage the electricity and guarantee a reliable power supply that resists power leakages. The data are collected from several sources, such as the power utilization habits of users, energy consumption data measured by widespread smart meters, phasor measurement data for situational awareness, etc. [12]. The analytics is also advantageous for enterprises, universities, multinational corporations, retail stores, and hospitals to predict future supply needs.

IV. Smart enterprise

Smart enterprise can help the enterprise to make on-the-fly decisions on pricing, support deployments, logistics, and sales. It can continuously monitor customer needs to create new business verticals or to provide additional services on top of the traditional ones. IoT and Big Data together can improve the overall workers' security and safety by continuously monitoring the key performance indicators (KPIs) of health and safety.

V. Surveillance monitoring

For enhancing the security of restricted areas, many sensitive and unremarkable sensors could be deployed in that area. Any unauthorized access or potential attacks could be detected using Big Data analytics and alarm accordingly.

VI. Intelligent home

The IoT and Big Data can be used to make the homes smart to enable efficient resource management and provide complete comfort and security to the user. The home environment can be fitted with motion sensors for monitoring access control, lighting control, temperature monitoring, HVAC (heating, ventilation, and air conditioning) control, etc. Analytics can be used to spot unauthorized entry, fire, or leak detection, etc.

VII. Smart farming

Smart farming applications can enable continuous monitoring of soil and crop health, animal behavior, storage conditions, machinery in use, etc., to maximize the productivity and sustainability of agricultural systems.

VIII. Habitat monitoring

The behavior of endangered species could be monitored continuously with the small, nonintrusive sensors attached with them. Big Data analytics can be used to find the abnormal behavior of the species if any and provide a detailed observation of individuals and groups.

IX. Environmental monitoring

For these types of applications, temperature and humidity sensors can be installed in harsh regions to monitor the natural environment. The location and time of occurrence of events can be foreseen using predictive modeling techniques.

X. Consumer applications

There are many consumer applications of IoT and Big Data together. Personal assistants such as Alexa, Google Assistant, Siri, etc., can make ones' life very contented.

12.3 BIG DATA IN IoT FOR HEALTHCARE

The healthcare industry is mainly responsible to provide medical services and insurance, develop pharmaceuticals, and manufacture medical equipment. The major trends and challenges describing the state of healthcare in the twenty-first century are discussed in the next section.

12.3.1 Recent Trends in Healthcare

The recent trends and key challenges in this field are as follows:

I. The healthcare industry is in great distress as chronic diseases are on a rise at the same time the cost of healthcare services is continuously increasing. The basic challenge is that everyone should get healthcare treatment at the cheapest cost as their fundamental right.

II. The medical support and services should be seamlessly available 24×7 irrespective of the geographical location of the patient.

III. Patients expect seamless processes and transparency of data. The challenge is to keep them abreast by taking care of their concerns and continuously updating them. Moreover, patients and media can demand detailed investigations of wrong site surgeries or any medication errors.

IV. Patients demand quality of care based on which they normally decide with whom they should engage for the healthcare services.

V. Events like a pandemic such as the recent COVID-19 poses a rigorous challenge to the healthcare industry. The impact of the COVID-19 pandemic on mental health, workload, and well-being of healthcare workers has been an alarming issue [13].

We can improve physician efficiency and patient care by satisfying these needs with the help of recent technologies. The next section describes the significance of IoT and Big Data in healthcare and also throws light on the research advancements in this domain.

12.3.2 IoT in Healthcare

IoT, with its mission-critical nature, has brought a complete revolution in the treatment and diagnosis of disease, equipment maintenance, and the way hospitals operate. It would largely improve the quality and effectiveness of medical services, especially important for those requiring constant supervision such as patients with chronic conditions or the elderly. IoT would enable easily accessible, highly personalized, and on-time healthcare services for everyone.

The next decade may well see improved processes and patient care with IoT. The IoT would bring revolution in the following healthcare solutions:

I. Advanced patient care

By means of wearable sensors and service solutions, the patients' data can be monitored remotely in real time. Various health monitoring devices can be used to collect the data and Big Data to visualize it using charts and diagrams.

Sensors can be added to medicines that enable patients to receive reminders and physicians to keep accurate track of their treatment and whether patients are adhering to their treatment plans. An example is ingestible sensors, in which the pill gets dissolved in the stomach and gives a signal that is gathered up by the sensor worn on the body, which passes the received data to the mobile app. Another example would be the inhaler equipped with sensors that can continuously send alerts of the amount of insulin to the patient and physician. A sensor can be implanted below the patient's skin suffering from diabetes. It would communicate with a smart transmitter, which in turn sends blood glucose levels to smart devices, such as a mobile app on the patient's phone or tablet. The contact lenses embedded with noninvasive sensors can also be used to get the glucose levels of diabetes patients using their tears. Sensors can also be used to continuously monitor various parameters related to the heart diseases, such as blood fat, blood pressure, blood glucose, heart rate, pulse rate, etc. In case of any abnormalities, alerts can be sent to the physician, caretaker, or cardiac vans for medical service.

Patients can wear a health tracker for up to seven days prior to any major treatments for diseases like cancer. If required, the tracker can be carried constantly for numerous months over the time period of various treatments to study the side effects of treatments, if any. Using a variety of data collected through these trackers, diagnosis and treatment can be enhanced for several conditions. Sensors can also be used for receiving and tracking usual symptoms of rheumatoid arthritis and other quality-of-life measures. It is also useful in monitoring the symptoms of psychosis, hypertension, and depression.

Telemedicine exists in the healthcare services market for a long period of time, and yet only recently, with the advent of 4G technologies like wireless devices, smart phones, online video conferences, and wearables, was it able to show its full potential. That is, using technology to deliver remote clinical services.

Physicians can offer proactive care and significantly reduce the need for hospitalization.

II. Smart hospital

Smart hospitals can offer functions such as electronic medical record management, smart alerts and notifications, smart phone–based assistant applications for caregivers, track equipment usage and services, etc.

a. Track treatment

The data collected from patient monitoring devices throughout a hospital are analyzed to provide physicians with better visibility into patient's vitals. The physicians and caregivers can remotely monitor and configure an automated drug delivery system. Emergency alerts can be given when required. Various sections of the hospitals such as labs, intensive care units (ICUs), and operation theaters, can be interconnected. That will help to effectively track the current status and location of the patient in the hospital and also the treatment schedule. Furthermore, the patients can also track their treatment process, communicate with physicians, and give timely feedback using smart consoles.

b. Track services

The real-time monitoring of the services such as housekeeping, inventory, security, etc., would help to improve the overall standards of the medical facilities. The workforce of the hospital can be managed effectively using real-time staff location, leave status, and competence data.

IoT assures the predictive maintenance of critical medical devices by fixing potential problems before they occur. The devices can be monitored continuously for faults and prevent malfunctions. Maintenance of the essential equipment will make them available when patients need them urgently. IoT also enables a remote installation or update of the required software/firmware on the devices.

Moreover, inventory of all the medical devices can be maintained, assets can be tracked, and the devices can be configured and controlled remotely. Tracking of usage of different equipment in the hospital can be done to ensure availability and transparency in the purchase process. For example, RFID and other tagging technologies can be used for pharmacy inventory management.

IoT can assist tracking and managing medicine and other supplies in an efficient way to help the hospital staff to spend more time with patients rather than searching and managing the things.

Building's environmental characteristics, such as temperature, noise, pressure, humidity, etc., can be regulated as per the requirement of the hospital environment.

12.3.3 HEALTHCARE ANALYTICS USING BIG DATA

Big Data architecture like Hadoop is very well accepted in the industry as it reduces operational and storage costs radically and handles enormous data without any change required in commodity hardware. In the healthcare industry, data are generated at two sources: sensors and humans. These data are becoming bigger as there is lots of new IoT-enabled equipment installed in hospitals generating data in various formats. Sensitive patient-driven data are also available that is in natural language and usually in unordered format consisting of reports, prescriptions, and data from imaging systems. Thus, healthcare is one of the most promising areas where Big Data can be used. The advantage of healthcare analytics using Big Data would be in terms of forecast outbreaks of epidemics, keeping away from preventable diseases, lowering costs of treatment, and improving the quality of life. In this section, we discuss the need of Big Data in healthcare: what are the challenges for its implementation? Why and how is it needed? In the subsequent section, we elaborate on various opportunities for Big Data healthcare systems that impact our lives.

Big Data analytics, intelligently used, can create business value and provide competitive advantage to any organization. Compared with many other industries, healthcare has been a late adopter. Nevertheless, there is a rapid increase in adoption of this technology in the healthcare domain, and it has potential to have a rapid growth and significant impact.

Following section explains the necessity of Big Data in healthcare.

I. Advanced patient care
   a. Disease prediction: Spread of contagious diseases can be observed and thus controlled by analysis of social logs of the patient from a particular area or province. This helps in preventive care measures taken by

the government in due time. The diseases like swine flu, dengue, and Chikungunya can be prevented in due time.

b. Predictive analytics in healthcare: In particular cases of patients with complicated medicinal histories, suffering from numerous conditions, Big Data predictive analytics is used to aid medical professionals take Big Data–informed decisions within instants and improve patients' treatment. Recently developed tools would also be able to determine, giving an example, a patient who is prone to diabetes and will thereby be suggested to use weight management or go through additional screenings that are based on millions of records of the patients.

c. Real-time alerting: In hospitals, clinical decision support (CDS) software analyzes a patient's history and current status immediately, enabling medical experts to make prescriptive decisions based on the suggestions provided. An example of such software is Asthma-polis, which has begun the use of inhalers with built-in GPS trackers in order to predict asthma variations both for a larger population as well as at an individual level. These data along with data from the Centers for Disease Control and Prevention (CDC) are being used in order to provide better treatment plans for asthmatics [14].

d. Big Data in cancer treatment: For diseases like cancer that can be linked to human genes, where a single gene record has about 20K features, Big Data analytics is particularly helpful. Medical researchers can analyze enormous volumes of data on cancer patient treatment plans and survival rates to identify therapies and trends with the best real-world success rates. For instance, scientists can look at tumor samples in biobanks that are connected to the patient's medical files. The utilization of these data has allowed researchers to discover trends that will improve patient outcomes, such as how certain mutations and cancer proteins respond to various treatments.

e. EHR: This is a well-known use of Big Data in the healthcare industry. Every patient has a digital record that includes information about their demographics, allergies, lab test results, medical history, and more. Healthcare providers from the public and private sectors can access the data, which is shared through secure information systems. Each record is made up of a single editable file, allowing the doctors to make changes over time without worrying about data duplication or paperwork. By sending out reminders and alerts when a patient has to obtain a new lab test or monitor medicines, EHRs can be used to determine whether a patient has been following a doctor's directions. Even though EHRs are a fantastic idea, several nations have not yet adopted them.

II. Smart hospital

a. Enhancing patient service experience: Physician decisions are now increasingly becoming evidence based, as they rely on clinical and research data in contrast to exclusively their schooling and professional opinion. Detection of diseases can be done at an early stage based on the clinical historical data available. Dosage of drugs can be optimized so as to avoid side effects and complete recovery and therefore reduce the cost for the prescription. Various algorithms like similarity analysis, clustering, trend analysis, and classification can be used to perform the described tasks.

b. Hospital's feedback monitoring: Many patients/relatives write reviews and share their experiences about the hospitals' doctors and services provided on social media. The selection of hospitals can be made based on such reviews. Government can also keep a watch on whether its norms and regulations are followed or not by analyzing such posts.

c. Using health data for analyzing trends and strategic planning: The University of Florida used free public health data and Google Maps to visualize information through heat maps that are focused on multiple issues, such as chronic diseases and population growth. Researchers tallied these data with the availability of medical services in the most heated areas. The results derived from this permitted them to increase more care units to most challenging areas and review their healthcare delivery strategy. Hence strategic planning allows the use of Big Data in healthcare.

d. Scheduling staff and resources: This is an operational problem in hospitals which is efficiently handled in Paris using time series analysis. This analysis helped the researchers to monitor pertinent trends in admission rates. Then machine learning could be used to determine the most precise algorithms that foretold future admissions patterns and manage the staff accordingly.

This new treatment approach indicates a greater need for Big Data analytics in healthcare facilities.

12.3.4   OPEN RESEARCH CHALLENGES OF USING BIG DATA AND IoT IN HEALTHCARE

The recent technological advancements in the healthcare industry have enabled proactive care and also helped to manage the healthcare administrations, treatments, and equipment usage more efficiently. Though, there are challenges in this field [15–17].

1. Security: Although the quality of services and cost are of key concern to patients, security and privacy of data doesn't fall far behind. As a result, the medical data available on cloud platforms should be secured with top privacy policies.

     The Health Insurance Portability and Accountability Act of 1996 (HIPAA) is United States legislation for safeguarding medical information by providing data privacy and security. The privacy of data on the cloud can be ensured by complying with HIPAA. It must also comply with all the state and federal laws.

The challenge with the health monitoring devices is the lengthy development process, which includes security concerns and testing periods. Therefore, the manufacturers take more time to bring them into the market.

2. Data integration: One of the major problems in using Big Data in healthcare is that the medical data are obtained from varied sources governed by different administrative departments, hospitals, and states. Compilation of these data sources requires creating a new schema of infrastructure where all data providers work together with each other.

3. Advancements in techniques: Healthcare needs to be at par with other businesses that already have shifted from standard regression-based methods to more future-oriented methods like machine learning, predictive analytics, and graph analytics by applying new data analysis strategies and tools. Besides, availability of tools and techniques adopted in other industries can be an inspiration for the health industry to cope with this demand of utilizing Big Data in the healthcare industry early.

12.4 PROPOSED SCHEME: IoT ARCHITECTURAL MODEL FOR INTENSIVE PATIENT CARE USING A PREDICTIVE MODEL

Emergency situations in healthcare require punctilious attention under a second of timespan. Humans might take some time to respond, which is why we use IoT devices. These devices can communicate with each other and help save lives.

The proposed architecture shown in Figure 12.3 portrays how IoT devices can use the hospital database to help with reducing the manual labor to devise new

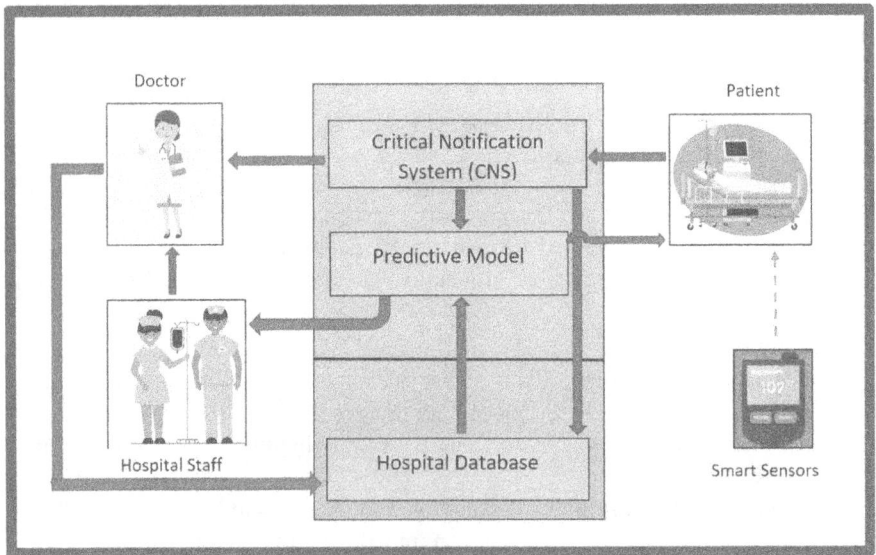

FIGURE 12.3 Proposed scheme: IoT architectural model for intensive patient care using a predictive model.

prescriptions for similar dosage. It starts with the sensors on the patient. These sensors measure various life-essential parameters including heartbeat, blood pressure (BP), EKG, temperature, etc. The following sensors can be used. For temperature-sensing applications, a fully printed carbon nanotube (CNT) based on negative temperature coefficient (NTC) thermistor has been developed. For heartbeat detection, an optical sensor can be used in which infrared light is transmitted by the infrared sensor (IR LED TX) to the fingertip and then reflected light on a photodiode RX sensor and converted into a suitable signal. The pulse waves and reference BP values can be used to do the partial least squares regression (PLSR) [18–20].

These real-time data are sent to the hospital database, which then stores the data and forwards a copy to the machine learning–based predictive model. This predictive model [21] will help the doctors with multiple things like dosage determination, illness confirmation based on various symptoms, likely future scopes for betterment or worsening of current conditions, etc.

A critical notification system (CNS) is the emergency situation notification system that immediately informs the connected doctors and hospital personnel on the CNS platform. This system works on two concepts: remote patient monitoring [22] and critical alert systems. The patient under care is connected to the CNS using smart sensors. These smart sensors, as defined earlier, will measure changes in the life-essential parameters, and as soon as they identify a change outside the defined range, the sensors use the RFID-tags technology to relay those signals to the CNS, which then relays them to pager-like devices given to the doctors and hospital staff. Thereby, immediate action can be taken. These sensors, the CNS, and the hospital database along with the predictive model form the hospital IoT network. The CNS then secondarily sends the sensor change signals to the predictive model, thus helping it further with the cause. The network API is used to check the data in the sensor unit. The hospital database is constantly updating with latest CNS data and predictive model predictions. This IOT architecture can also help doctors when there is a pandemic like the recent COVID-19, where most common symptoms could have been treated with simple prescriptions from the doctor.

12.5 HEALTHCARE SYSTEM IN INDIA

One of India's biggest service sectors is healthcare [23, 24]. The challenges faced by the sector are considerable, from handling rural and urban zones, to the need to reduce mortality rates, ensuring accessibility of trained medical personnel, need to provide medical health insurance, building better physical infrastructure, etc. There has been an increase in both noncommunicable diseases, including chronic diseases and communicable/infectious diseases.

The Health Management Information System (HMIS) is the government's primary healthcare system for administrative purposes. The HMIS data are used at both subdistrict and national level on a monthly basis to monitor the primary healthcare program at various administrative levels.

The National Family Health Survey (NFHS) records the effectiveness of public healthcare and child, maternal, and geriatric health conditions at an interval of six years via sampled population surveys. The NFHS is a large-scale, multiround survey conducted in a representative sample of households throughout the country.

Various government bodies like the National Centre for Disease Informatics and Research (NCDIR), a wing under the Indian Council of Medical Research (ICMR), are accountable for numerous disease records in India. The motive of the National Transplant Registry is to gather data related to the transplants from several centers in India and to collect the data often to find out the quantity of essential demographic statistics of Indian patients going through transplants, transplants being done in the country, patient survival after transplants, the immunosuppressive regimens used by several centers, complications during management, short/long-term results, donor profiles, etc. Big Data and IoT together can bridge the gap of supply and demand of organs faster.

The health intelligence wing of the Directorate General of Health Services (DGHSs) is called The Central Bureau of Health Intelligence (CBHI). It is a vital establishment that deals with analysis gathering, compilation and distribution of data on health conditions in India, covering several health aspects including health resources, health status, utilization of health services, etc.

The Centre for the Development of Advanced Computing (C-DAC) portrays a vital role in the design and development of the health management system in India [25]. It has designed and developed a versatile HMIS in a variety of models like SaaS (Software as a Service) over the cloud infrastructure and the conventional standalone hospital version. A hospital's workforce is empowered to perform their duties effectively and efficiently along with streamlining the treatment flow of patients using real-time HMIS. It is designed using a unique amalgamation of a "patient-centric and medical staff–centric" paradigm, providing benefits to both healthcare providers and patients. Additionally, C-DAC has developed a novel idea for the statewide application of HMIS across a number of public hospitals, including district hospitals, superspecialty hospitals, and area hospitals. Over 40 hospitals in India now use the HMIS developed by C-DAC. C-DAC has developed numerous products, including e-Sushrut, eSwasthya, Medical Document Semantic Analyzer, ERP solution for health delivery in the SaaS model, HMIS solutions with special features for cancer care in this area, and telemedical systems that allow patients in remote locations to engage in live consultation with doctors located elsewhere. Health informatics via mobile technologies (HIMT) applications are divided into three main areas: emergency services, health awareness, and preventive care and treatment.

Distributed EHR is an important application. A distributed EHR store is a secure, reliable, scalable, distributed healthcare information store that replaces or complements current healthcare data storehouses. It collects medical records from varied healthcare systems available in healthcare facilities spread over a hospital, group of locations and hospitals, region, or nation. It is established on a fail-safe, highly redundant, and secure system framework. It provides a base for developing applications on top.

To store and exchange health records including medicines, wellness parameters, lab test results, medical images, etc., a personal health record locker is offered. It is a cloud-based system for managing personal health records (PHR) for Indian citizens. The features include a comprehensive dashboard for tracking one's health along with the saving and storage of personal health records like lab test results, prescriptions, and medical images. Additionally, it offers the ability to sync wellness information from smart phone applications, activity trackers, and other devices as well as the sharing of health records with doctors, family, and friends. Personal Health Record Management System (PHRMS) has been connected with Aadhaar and Digilocker.

In addition to this, C-DAC is working on various applications using Big Data analytics and IoT. Among the applications are a decision support system for an automatic EEG analyzer for neurological disorder detection named Ayusoft, medical image analyzer for cervical cancer, diabetic retinopathy identification software for timely intervention, a computer-aided detection (CAD) system for mammograms, and eSmear image acquisition software for cervical smears. ICare@Home introduces health games that are a perfect mixture of health entertainment and education for everyone.

12.6 CONCLUSION

In this chapter, we have seen the possible avenues that Big Data and IoT can craft together and thus touch everyone's life and make the world a better place to live in. The handshake of these two technologies signifies the revolution of the new era in automation and prominently has a lot of potential to impact various domains. We have mainly highlighted their application in the healthcare domain, including the issues and challenges. Blending of these two technologies in healthcare would enable easily accessible, cost-effective, highly personalized, and on-time healthcare services for everyone. Things will change rapidly if the challenges highlighted in this chapter are met. We have also focused on the existing applications and future possible research paths to explore. Finally, we proposed an IoT architectural model for intensive patient care using a predictive model and discussed a case study of the healthcare systems in India.

REFERENCES

1. Rahman, A., M. S. Hossain, N. A. Alrajeh, and F. Alsolami. "Adversarial examples-security threats to COVID-19 deep learning systems in medical IoT devices." IEEE Internet of Things Journal 8, no. 12 (2021): 9603–9610.
2. Hossain, M. S., S. U. Amin, M. Alsulaiman, and G. Muhammad. "Applying deep learning for epilepsy seizure detection and brain mapping visualization." ACM Transactions on Multimedia Computing, Communications, and Applications 15, no. 1 (2019): 1–17.
3. Singh, Suruchi, Bhatt Pankaj, K. Nagarajan, Neha P. Singh, and Veer Bala. "Blockchain with cloud for handling healthcare data: A privacy-friendly platform." Materials Today: Proceedings 62 (2022): 5021–5026.
4. Vermesan, O., Friess, P., Guillemin, P., Gusmeroli, S., Sundmaeker, H., Bassi, A., Jubert, I.S., Mazura, M., Harrison, M., Eisenhauer, M., and Doody, P. 2022. "Internet of things strategic research roadmap." In *Internet of things-global technological and societal trends from smart environments and spaces to green ICT* (pp. 9–52). River Publishers.
5. "From M2M to the Internet of Things: Viewpoints from Europe." Techvibes. 7 July 2011. Archived from the original on 24 October 2013.
6. Sristava, Lara. "The Internet of Things – Back to the Future (Presentation)." European Commission Internet of Things Conference in Budapest – via YouTube, 16 May 2011.
7. Dawadi, Babu R., Danda B. Rawat, Shashidhar Ram Joshi, and Pietro Manzoni. "Towards Smart Networking with SDN Enabled IPv6 Network." ArXiv abs/2203.01528 (2022): n.p.

8. Leal-Junior, Arnaldo G., Camilo A.R. Diaz, Letícia M. Avellar, Maria José Pontes, Carlos Marques, and Anselmo Frizera. "Polymer optical fiber sensors in healthcare applications: A comprehensive review." Sensors 19, no. 14 (2019): 3156.

9. Nguyen, H. H., F. Mirza, M. A. Naeem, and M. Nguyen. "A review on IoT healthcare monitoring applications and a vision for transforming sensor data into real-time clinical feedback." 2017 IEEE 21st International Conference on Computer Supported Cooperative Work in Design (CSCWD), 2017, pp. 257–262. doi: 10.1109/CSCWD.2017.8066704.

10. Marjani, Mohsen, et al. "Big IoT data analytics: Architecture, opportunities, and open research challenges." IEEE Access 5 (2017): 5247–5261.

11. Ahmed, Ejaz, et al. "The role of big data analytics in internet of things." Computer Networks 129 (2017): 459–471.

12. Hashem, I.A.T., V. Chang, N.B. Anuar, K. Adewole, I. Yaqoob, A. Gani, E. Ahmed, and H. Chiroma. "The role of big data in smart city." International Journal of Information Management 36, no. 5 (2016): 748–758.

13. Jonsdottir, I.H., A. Degl'Innocenti, L. Ahlstrom, C. Finizia, H. Wijk, and M. Åkerström. "A pre/post analysis of the impact of the COVID-19 pandemic on the psychosocial work environment and recovery among healthcare workers in a large university hospital in Sweden." Journal of Public Health Research 10, no. 4 (2021 Jul 14): 2329. doi: 10.4081/jphr.2021.2329.

14. http://www.ingrammicroadvisor.com/data-center/7-big-data-use-cases-for-healthcare

15. Raghupathi, Wullianallur, and Viju Raghupathi. "Big data analytics in healthcare: Promise and potential." Health Information Science and Systems 2, no. 1 (2014): 3.

16. Basco, J. Antony, and N. C. Senthilkumar. "Real-time analysis of healthcare using big data analytics." IOP Conference Series: Materials Science and Engineering 263, no. 4. IOP Publishing, Bristol, England, 2017.

17. Sun, Jimeng, and Chandan K. Reddy. "Big data analytics for healthcare." Proceedings of the 19th ACM SIGKDD International Conference on Knowledge Discovery and Data Mining, ACM, 2013.

18. Turkani, Vikram S., Dinesh Maddipatla, Binu B. Narakathu, Bradley J. Bazuin, and Massood Z. Atashbar. "A carbon nanotube based NTC thermistor using additive print manufacturing processes." Sensors and Actuators A: Physical 279 (2018): 1–9.

19. Shirzadfar, H., M.S. Ghaziasgar, Z. Piri, and M. Khanahmadi. "Heart beat rate monitoring using optical sensors." International Journal of Biosensors and Bioelectronics 4, no. 2 (2018): 48–54.

20. Katsuragawa, Y., and H. Ishizawa. "Non-invasive blood pressure measurement by pulse wave analysis using FBG sensor." 2015 IEEE International Instrumentation and Measurement Technology Conference (I2MTC) Proceedings, 2015, pp. 511–515. doi: 10.1109/I2MTC.2015.7151320.

21. Uddin, S., A. Khan, M. Hossain, and M.A. Moni. "Comparing different supervised machine learning algorithms for disease prediction." BMC Medical Informatics and Decision Making 19 (2019): 281.

22. Hilty, D.M., C.M. Armstrong, A. Edwards-Stewart, M.T. Gentry, D.D. Luxton, and E.A. Krupinski. "Sensor, wearable, and remote patient monitoring competencies for clinical care and training: Scoping review." Journal of Technology in Behavioral Science 6, no. 2 (2021): 252–277. doi: 10.1007/s41347-020-00190-3.

23. Cloud-Based Citizen-Controlled Integrated Personal Health Record. https://myhealthrecord.nhp.gov.in

24. Archenaa, J., and E.A. Mary Anita. "A survey of big data analytics in healthcare and government." Procedia Computer Science 50 (2015): 408–413.

25. https://www.cdac.in/index.aspx?id=health_info

13 Automatic Detection of Diabetic Retinopathy to Avoid Blindness

Smita Das[1], Sushanta Das[2], Saptarshi Debray[3],
Madhusudhan Mishra[3], and Swanirbhar Majumder[2]
[1]MBB College, Agartala, Tripura, India
[2]Tripura University (A Central University),
Tripura West, Tripura, India
[3]NERIST (Deemed to be University), Doimukh,
Arunachal Pradesh, India

CONTENTS

13.1 INTRODUCTION

An active microvascular condition of diabetes mellitus called diabetic retinopathy (DR) causes blurred vision, floaters, and difficulties seeing colors and sometimes results in permanent vision loss. Clement cases may be treated with cautious management of diabetes. Advanced cases may need surgery or laser treatment. So, early detection of DR is very important.

According to the World Health Organization, diabetes will be the seventh-worst global cause of death by 2030 [1]. So, DR detection requires discussion and analysis of the associated techniques and findings.

The retinal fundus images are mainly used for the analysis and detection of DR, and this analysis is done by the Asia Pacific Tele-Ophthalmology Society 2019 Blindness Detection (APTOS 2019 BD) data set [2]. This image data set includes 3,662 samples that were gathered from various rural Indian populations. The data were compiled by India's Aravind Eye Hospital. To gather the retinal image samples for fundus photography, the hospital technicians visited rural areas of India. These fundus images were gathered over a long period of time in various environments and conditions. After that, a team of medical professionals evaluated and classified the samples collected using the International Clinical Diabetic Retinopathy Disease Severity Scale (ICDRSS). This data set was collected to study the capability of AI and Big Data analytics to enhance diagnostics for improved patient care delivery to stop blindness.

The retinal abnormalities in DR also include cotton wool spots, hemorrhages, retinal neovascularization, exudates, microaneurysms, etc., which are clearly shown in Figure 13.1. The manual identification of retinal abnormalities is a time-consuming task, but the automatic identification technique offers timely and accurate detection of the abnormalities. The identification of ophthalmologic diseases depends primarily on the characteristics of retinal blood vessels, including their length, width, and branching structures. Some of the contributing elements that mess up the extraction procedure are uneven brightness of vessels and the irregular contrast of the retinal image throughout the accession process. The qualities of blood vessels, such as their size, shape, and gray level, may also be confused by some surrounding factors with the same characteristics. The extraction of vessels is also hampered by other issues such as lack of image contrast, signal noise, image intensity, etc. [3]. As a result, this chapter will help ophthalmologists assess fundus images to find DR.

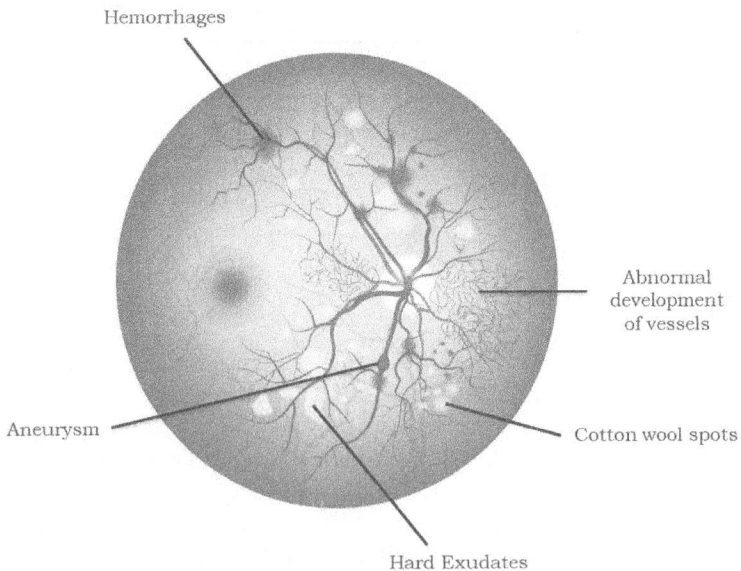

FIGURE 13.1 DR-affected retina.

When doing automatic processes, the system directly generates the result after processing the fundus image. A lot of research is required because these techniques are improving so quickly. In [4], Khojasteh et al. used a technique to identify microaneurysms, exudates, and hemorrhages using the expected output of a convolutional neural network (CNN). Li et al. developed an approach in [5] that makes use of a deep CNN. To detect exudates, Mateen et al. in [1] developed a pretrained CNN architecture. In [6], Shinde et al. proposed Le-Net architecture for validation of input fundus image and detection of Region of Interest by applying the brightest spot algorithm. In [7], Lin et al. introduced Comprehensive Artificial intelligence Retinal Expert (CARE) by using CNN. In [8], Bulut et al. used CNN networks such as Visual Geometry Group (VGG), AlexNet, ResNet, and Xception. In [9], Abitbol et al. used the CNN classifier to distinguish fundus images between different vascular diseases and healthy controls. In [10], Dong et al. developed a DL algorithm, named the Retinal Artificial Intelligence Diagnosis System (RAIDS), to detect retinal diseases simultaneously. To study this relevant topic exposes the relevance and originality of the question associated with this research topic. It identifies areas to prevent duplication; recognize contradictions like disputes in previous studies, openings in research, and open queries left from earlier research; and increase statistical knowledge related to the research topic. So, this chapter will give a comprehensive study on deep learning (DL) approaches using Inception-v3 models for the detection of DR by giving an illustration of various performance assessments for detection of DR like precision, specificity, sensitivity, accuracy, etc. In this chapter, our contributions are as follows:

- Introduction to DR
- Discussion on DL techniques in DR
- Special focus on CNN
- Elaboration on Inception-v3 technique of CNN applied on DR images
- Results obtained with this technique
- Conclusion

13.2   DEEP LEARNING APPROACH

DL is a combination of artificial intelligence (AI) and machine learning (ML) that replicates the way a normal human being learns about a certain thing and acquires certain forms of knowledge. See Figure 13.2. DL is a prime aspect of data science that requires predictive and statistical modeling of data. It also requires an excessive amount of data. In ML, we need to do the feature extraction, training of the model, and hyperparameter tuning by ourselves; in DL, all of that is done by itself. In simple words, DL is a self-operating true response model. We can see that traditional ML algorithms are linear, while DL algorithms are assembled in a hierarchy of increasing complexity and abstraction. Each layer in the hierarchy proposes a nonlinear transformation to the input and applies what it discovers to produce an analytical model as output. The process continues until the output has passed an admissible measure of accuracy and loss [11].

There are a lot of DL algorithms available for utilization by anyone. The top ten most popular of them are CNN, recurrent neural networks, long short-term memory

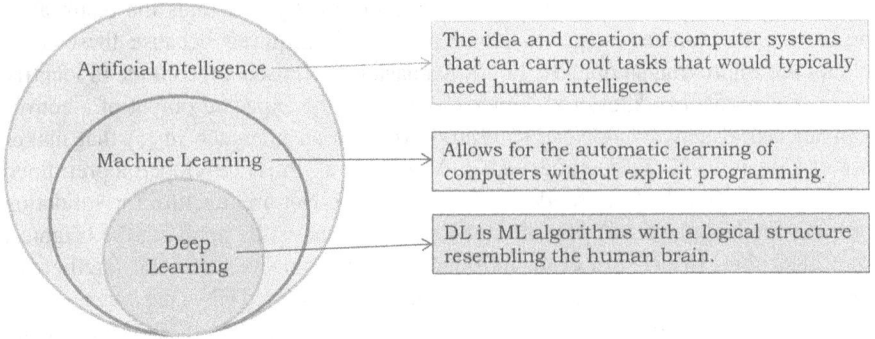

FIGURE 13.2   Hierarchy of DL, ML, and AI.

network, generative adversarial networks, radial basis function networks, self-organizing maps, multilayer perceptrons, deep belief networks, restricted Boltzmann machines, and Autoencoders.

In this chapter, CNN is implemented to detect DR in fundus images. CNN is a subtype of neural network that is primarily used for image and speech recognition applications. The built-in convolutional layer of CNN decreases the high proportions of images without losing their information. The main advantage of CNN is that it detects the essential features automatically without the help of any human supervision. Another important characteristic of CNN is its capability to utilize spatial correlation in data. The CNN topology is parted into various learning stages formed of a combination of the subsampling layers, nonlinear processing units, and convolutional layers. The preprocessing requirement in CNN is much less than that of other methods. While in other methods feature-based filters are generated manually, with extensive training, CNN can learn all these filters by themselves. That is why CNN is suitable for this use case.

13.3   CNN ARCHITECTURE

CNN mainly contains three types of layers, fully connected (FC) layers, pooling layers (PL), and convolutional layers (CL). Once all these layers are assembled, the convolutional neural network architecture will be established. Additionally, the activation function and the dropout layer parameters are needed to create CNN [12]. The basic CNN architecture is shown in Figure 13.3.

13.3.1   CONVOLUTIONAL LAYER

The primary purpose of this layer is to pull out the different features from the raw images. The computation process of this layer is carried out between the input image and a particular sized filter. The dot product is taken between the filter and the input image's components. The result is known as the feature map (FM), and it gives details about the image, including its edges and corners. This FM is later pushed to the next layers to teach them additional matters from the input image. Once the

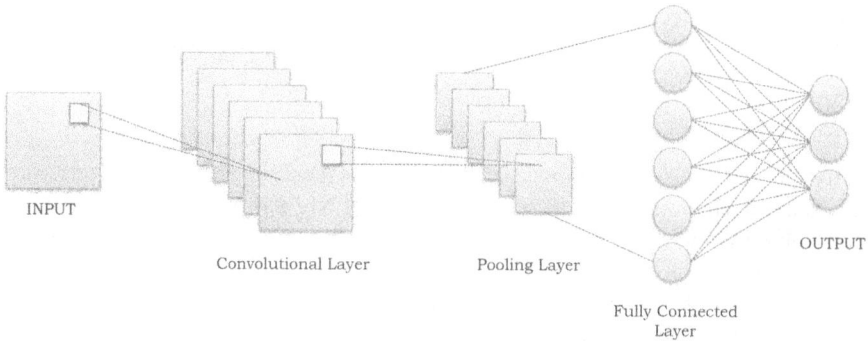

FIGURE 13.3 Convolutional neural network architecture.

convolution operation has been applied to the input, CNN's convolution layer passes the output to the next pooling layer. CNN's convolutional layers are very useful since they guarantee the spatial relationship between the pixels is intact.

13.3.2 POOLING LAYER

A pooling layer often comes next to the CL. The main goal of this layer is to save on computational costs by decreasing the size of the convolved FM. This is done independently on each feature map and by reducing the links between layers. Basically, it is a summary of the features produced by a convolution layer. The largest component in max pooling is collected from the FM. The average pooling calculates the components of a predefined sized image portion. Sum pooling computes the total sum of the predefined section's components. Typically, the fully connected layer and convolutional layer are connected by the pooling layer. This CNN approach allows the networks recognize the features on their own by generalizing the characteristics extracted by the convolution layer. This assists in decreasing computations within a network.

13.3.3 FULLY CONNECTED LAYER

The FC layer contains neurons with their weights and biases. It is utilized to correlate different neurons in between two various layers. These layers make up the final few layers of any CNN and are often located before the final output layer. In this, the input from the previous layers is flattened and supplied to the FC layer. The leveled vector is then put through a few additional FC layers, and the standard operations on computational functions happen. The classification procedure starts to take place at this point. This layer in CNN decreases human supervision.

13.3.4 DROPOUT LAYER

When a particular model works so well on training data but has a negative effect when applied to new data, this is called *overfitting*. Normally, overfitting in the training data set can result from all features being connected to the FC layer. To solve the issue, a dropout layer is introduced, where a small number of neurons are separated from the network during training and the output is a reduced-size model.

13.3.5 ACTIVATION FUNCTIONS

Activation functions are the most crucial elements of the CNN architecture. Activation functions are employed to discover and approximate any class of continuous and complex link between network variables. In simple words, it decides which information should shoot in which direction. This network adds nonlinearity to the networks. The Softmax, ReLU, tanH, and sigmoid functions are a few examples of regularly used activation functions. Each of these operations has a particular use. Softmax functions and sigmoid are preferred for binary classification of the CNN model, whereas Softmax is typically employed for multiclass classification. In a CNN model, activation functions determine whether a neuron is active or not. It determines via mathematical processes whether the input to the work is significant or not for prediction.

13.4 THE PROPOSED CNN TECHNIQUE

In this section, the proposed technique Inception-v3 based on CNN to detect diabetic retinopathy is presented. It features a network that is deeper others. It is less expensive to compute. As a regularizer, it employs auxiliary classifiers. An Inception network provides high-performance output with the efficient use of computer resources along with a small increase in computational load. It can use various sizes of convolutional filters to extract features from input data at different scales. The particulars of fundus image data set APTOS-2019 BD used for this study is shown in Table 13.1 [13].

13.4.1 ARCHITECTURE OF INCEPTION-V3

The Inception-v3 CNN architecture basically uses factorized 7×7 convolutions, label smoothing, and an auxiliary classifier [14]. Its error rate is lower than its predecessors. The use of auxiliary classifiers, effective grid size reduction, factorization into smaller convolutions, and spatial factorization into asymmetric convolutions are all performed by this algorithm. The basic architecture of Inception-v3 is shown in Figure 13.4.

The Inception-v3 architecture is built one layer over another [15], as follows:

- **Factorized convolution:** As it decreases the quantity of parameters used in the network, it aids in decreasing computing efficiency of Inception-v3. It also evaluates network effectiveness.

TABLE 13.1
Particulars of Images in the Data Set

Data Set	Total Number of Images	Training	Testing	Classes
APTOS-2019 BD	3,662	80%	20%	2

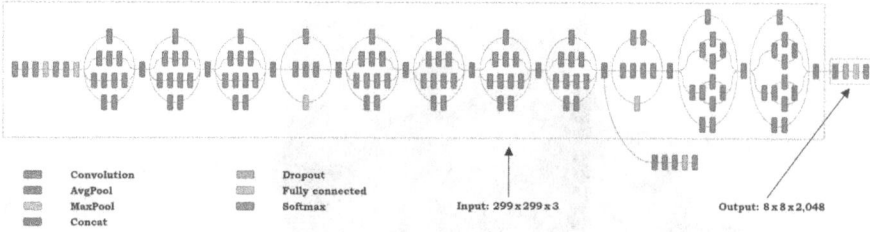

Convolution
AvgPool
MaxPool
Concat

Dropout
Fully connected
Softmax

Input: 299 x 299 x 3

Output: 8 x 8 x 2,048

FIGURE 13.4 Basic architecture of Inception-v3

- **Smaller convolutions:** Training is unquestionably sped up by swapping out larger convolutions for smaller ones. Consider a 5 × 5 filter that has 25 parameters; the two 3 × 3 filters that replace it have only 18 (3*3 + 3*3) parameters [16].
- **Asymmetric convolution:** A 1 × 3 convolution followed by a 3 × 1 convolution might be used in place of the 3 × 3 convolution. The number of parameters would be a little bit greater than the suggested asymmetric convolution if the 3 × 3 convolution is changed to a 2 × 2 convolution [16].
- **Auxiliary classifier:** During training, a little CNN is introduced between the layers, and the resulting loss contributes to the main network's loss. The auxiliary classifier in Inception-v3 serves as a regularizer.
- **Grid size reduction:** Pooling techniques are typically used to reduce grid size.

13.4.2 IMPLEMENTATION OF THE INCEPTION-V3 USING PYTHON

This experiment makes use of the integrated development environment (IDE) PyCharm Community Edition 2020.3.5 x64. See Figure 13.5.

The Inception-v3 model by default takes the input of image 299 × 299 pixels and three color channels. So, the image data that were read from the data set were converted into a resolution of 299*299 pixels and appended to a corresponding array.

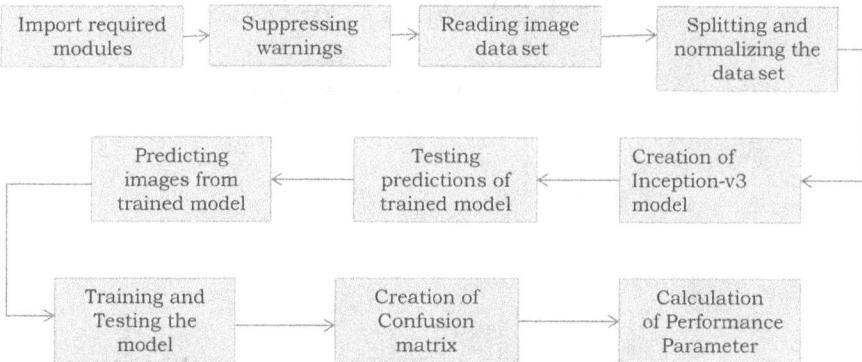

FIGURE 13.5 Steps of implementation of Inception-v3 model.

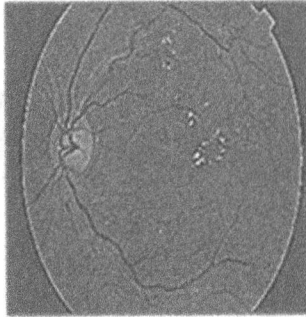

FIGURE 13.6   Non-DR image.

We can take any patient's fundus eye images and use the center slice as input to the program to predict whether the person has DR or not. The model's prediction is then printed as a graphical user interface (GUI) output. See Figure 13.6.

The confusion matrix (CM) of the model can be shown either in a simple command line (CLI) or through a GUI output with visual aids that help the user understand the confusion matrix effortlessly. Figure 13.7 depicts the CM of the model.

The precision, sensitivity, specificity, and accuracy of the confusion matrix can be calculated using the formulas (13.1)–(13.4), respectively:

$$\text{PRECISION} = \frac{TP}{TP + FP} \tag{13.1}$$

$$\text{SPECIFICITY} = \frac{TN}{TN + FP} \tag{13.2}$$

$$\text{SENSITIVITY} = \frac{TP}{TP + FN} \tag{13.3}$$

$$\text{ACCURACY} = \frac{TP + TN}{TP + FP + TN + FN} \tag{13.4}$$

PREDICTED DATA

		POSITIVE	NEGATIVE
ACTUAL DATA	POSITIVE	TRUE POSITIVE(TP)	FALSE NEGATIVE(FN)
	NEGATIVE	FALSE POSITIVE(FP)	TRUE NEGATIVE(TN)

FIGURE 13.7   Confusion matrix.

TABLE 13.2
The Training Achievement of the Presented Model on Five Different Epochs

Epoch	TL	TA	VL	VA
1/5	0.3813	0.8631	0.2470	0.8731
2/5	0.2395	0.9174	0.5086	0.8336
3/5	0.2310	0.9170	0.4972	0.7804
4/5	0.1825	0.9440	0.4098	0.9222
5/5	0.1657	0.9467	1.0188	0.6999

13.5 RESULTS AND EXPLANATION

The Inception-v3 model was trained first time for five epochs with batch size 8 and then ten epochs with batch size 16. We have done two experiments by using two different hardware configurations. The hardware configuration used for the first and second experiments are GPU: Nvidia RTX with 6 GB memory; Processor: Ryzen 9, 16 GB RAM GPU and GPU: 6 GB memory; and Processor: Intel Xeon (R) E-2224G and 16 GB RAM, respectively. Tables 13.2 and 13.3 depict the training and validation achievements like training loss (TL), training accuracy (TA), validation loss (VL), and validation accuracy (VA) of the first experiment on five and ten epochs, respectively.

Tables 13.4 and 13.5 depict the training and validation achievements of the second experiment on five and ten epochs, respectively.

The confusion matrix of the proposed model Inception-v3 for five and ten epochs with different hardware configurations is depicted in Figure 13.8a and 13.8b.

From the results produced by the Inception-v3 model with five and ten epochs with different hardware configurations, we can analyze the model's training and validation loss and accuracy. Figure 13.9a–d show the graphical analysis of the results.

Additionally, Table 13.6 depicts the performance of the model on five epochs and ten epochs with different hardware configuration.

TABLE 13.3
The Training Achievement of the Presented Model on Ten Different Epochs

Epoch	TL	TA	VL	VA
1/10	0.3632	0.9024	0.2560	0.9550
2/10	0.2377	0.9194	0.1334	0.9400
3/10	0.1717	0.9283	0.1535	0.9482
4/10	0.2309	0.9167	NaN	0.5157
5/10	0.2171	0.9307	0.4779	0.7517
6/10	0.2134	0.9075	0.6939	0.4843
7/10	0.1874	0.9112	0.2164	0.9550
8/10	0.1498	0.9529	0.2569	0.9127
9/10	0.1458	0.9590	0.1668	0.9413
10/10	0.1041	0.9642	0.1804	0.9659

TABLE 13.4
The Training Achievement of the Presented Model on Five Different Epochs

Epoch	TL	TA	VL	VA
1/5	0.4217	0.8576	0.6845	0.8199
2/5	0.2676	0.8925	0.5784	0.5962
3/5	0.2304	0.9174	0.1866	0.9345
4/5	0.2028	0.9314	0.2940	0.8868
5/5	0.2093	0.9259	0.4221	0.8909

TABLE 13.5
The Training Achievement of the Presented Model on Ten Different Epochs

Epoch	TL	TA	VL	VA
1/10	0.3652	0.8867	0.2359	0.9236
2/10	0.2180	0.9232	0.3087	0.9031
3/10	0.1939	0.9382	0.1167	0.9714
4/10	0.1400	0.9546	0.3524	0.8909
5/10	0.1140	0.9635	0.1432	0.9550
6/10	0.1134	0.9648	0.3041	0.9209
7/10	0.1063	0.9642	0.1754	0.9673
8/10	0.0996	0.9706	0.1294	0.9673
9/10	0.0731	0.9764	0.1282	0.9714
10/10	0.0591	0.9799	1.3560	0.8540

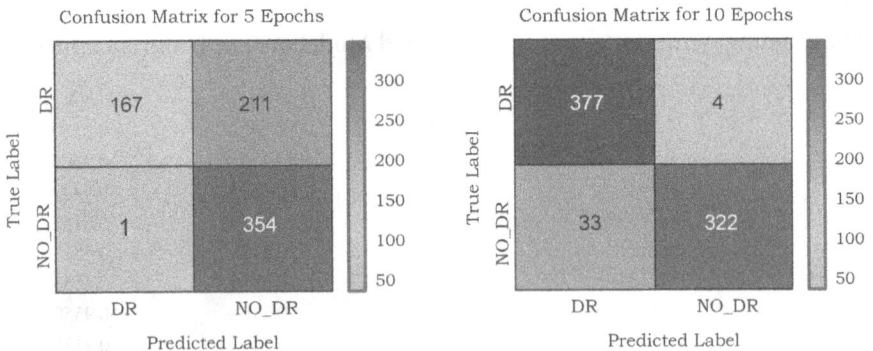

(a)

FIGURE 13.8(a)   Confusion matrix of first experiment.

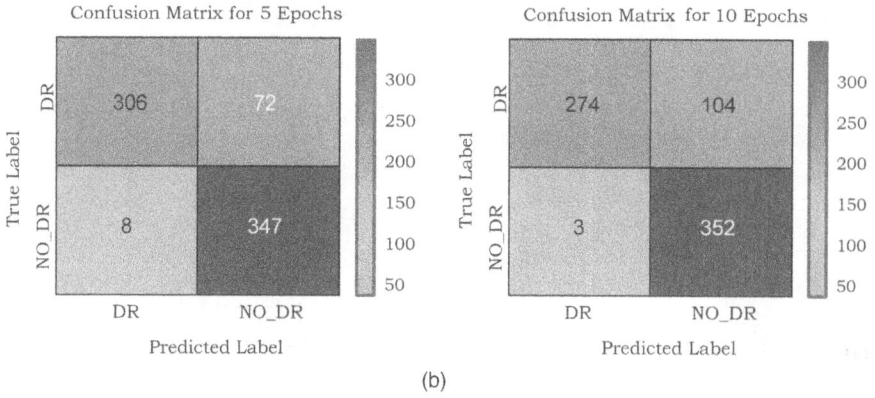

(b)

FIGURE 13.8(b) Confusion matrix of second experiment.

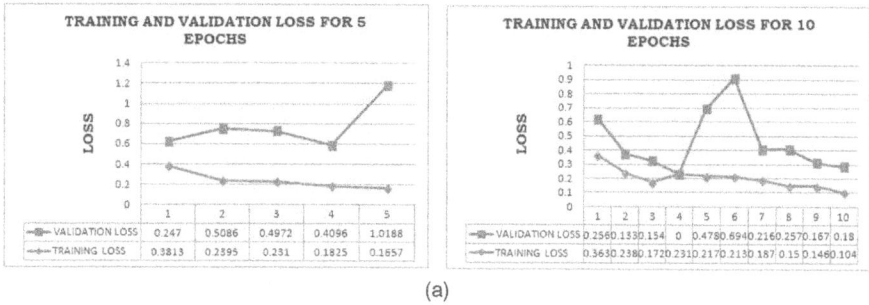

(a)

FIGURE 13.9(a) Training and validation loss for five and ten epochs of first experiment.

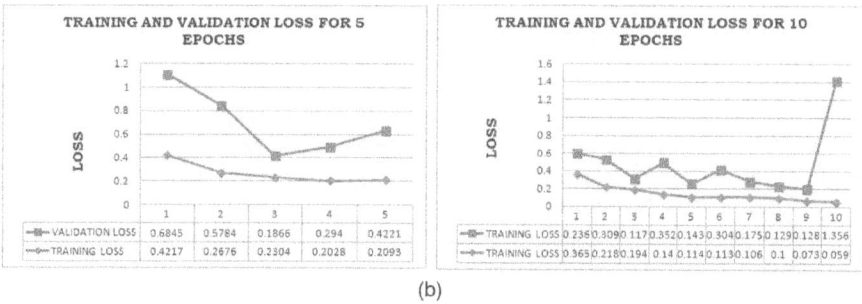

(b)

FIGURE 13.9(b) Training and validation loss for five and ten epochs of second experiment.

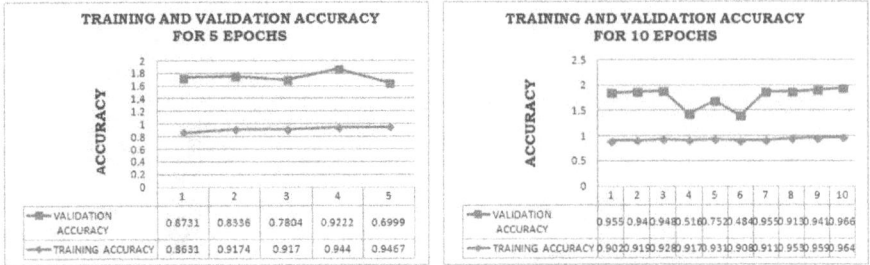

(c)

FIGURE 13.9(c)   Training and validation accuracy for five and ten epochs of first experiment.

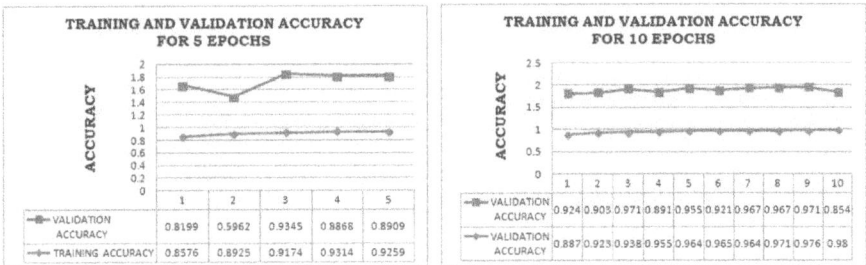

(d)

FIGURE 13.9(d)   Training and validation accuracy for five and ten epochs of second experiment.

TABLE 13.6
Performance of the Proposed Model

Epochs	Hardware Description	Sensitivity	Specificity	Precision	Accuracy
5	GPU: Nvidia RTX with 6 GB memory; processor: Ryzen 9 and 16 GB RAM	0.6794	0.0047	0.6265	0.7107
10	GPU: Nvidia RTX with 6 GB memory; processor: Ryzen 9 and 16 GB RAM	0.4626	0.8918	0.9877	0.9495
5	GPU: 6 GB memory; processor: Intel Xeon (R) E-2224G and 16 GB RAM	0.5313	0.1000	0.8281	0.8908
10	GPU: 6 GB memory; processor: Intel Xeon (R) E-2224G and 16 GB RAM	0.5623	0.08540	0.7719	0.8540

The comparative analysis shows that the performance of the proposed model varies with epoch sizes as well as hardware configuration. With the changes in epoch size from five to 10, we have changed batch size also from eight to 16. In the first experiment, accuracy was increased from 0.7107 to 0.9495 when epoch and batch size were changed. But, in the second experiment accuracy decreased from 0.8908 to 0.8540 when the epoch size was increased.

13.6 CONCLUSION

DR detection needs a discussion and a thorough analysis of the related approaches and results [17]. This chapter introduces the Inception-v3 model, which is an important component in DR detection. The experiment reveals that no single technique is appropriate for many eye disorders and that each patient's vascular degradation is unique. Future research will concentrate on hybrid-based strategies that will remove the drawbacks of the current retinal vascular extraction method [18]. So, our future work will involve feature extraction utilizing transform domain with convolutional neural networks, followed by image resizing and thresholding. These methods will be examined on online databases. Different performance metrics, such as sensitivity, specificity, and accuracy, will be utilized to assess the suggested approach.

REFERENCES

1. Mateen M, Wen J, Nasrullah N, Sun S, Hayat S. (2020). "Exudate Detection for Diabetic Retinopathy Using Pretrained Convolutional Neural Networks." Hindawi Complexity, 2020:11. doi: 10.1155/2020/5801870.
2. https://2019.asiateleophth.org
3. Kumar K, Samal D, Suraj S. (2019). "Automated Retinal Vessel Segmentation Based on Morphological Preprocessing and 2D-Gabor Wavelets." Advanced Computing and Intelligent Engineering, pp. 1–12. doi: 10.13140/RG.2.2.35652.07044.
4. Khojasteh P, Aliahmad B, Kumar DK. (2018). "Fundus Images Analysis Using Deep Features for Detection of Exudates, Hemorrhages and Microaneurysms." BMC Ophthalmology, 18:288. doi: 10.1186/s12886-018-0954-4.
5. Li YH, Yeh NN, Chen SJ, Chung YC. (2019). "Computer-Assisted Diagnosis for Diabetic Retinopathy Based on Fundus Images Using Deep Convolutional Neural Network." Hindawi Mobile Information Systems, 2019:1–14. doi: 10.1155/2019/6142839.
6. Shinde R. (2021). "Glaucoma Detection in Retinal Fundus Images Using U-Net and Supervised Machine Learning Algorithms." Intelligence-Based Medicine, 5:100038. doi: 10.1016/j.ibmed.2021.100038.
7. Lin D, Xiong J, Liu C, Zhao L, Li Z, Yu S, Wu X, Ge Z, Hu X, Wang B, Fu M, Zhao X, Wang X, Zhu Y, Chen C, Li T, Li Y, Wei W, Zhao M, Li J, Xu F, Ding L, Tan G, Xiang Y, Hu Y, Zhang P, Han Y, Li JPO, Wei L, Zhu P, Liu Y, Chen W, Ting DSW, Wong TY, Chen Y, Lin H. (2021). "Application of Comprehensive Artificial Intelligence Retinal Expert (CARE) System: A National Real-World Evidence Study." Lancet Digital Health, 3:486–495. http://www.thelancet.com/digital-health.
8. Bulut B, Kalın V, Gunes BB, Khazhin R. (2020). "Deep Learning Approach for Detection of Retinal Abnormalities Based on Color Fundus Images." 2020 Innovations in Intelligent Systems and Applications Conference (ASYU), pp. 1–6, doi: 10.1109/ASYU50717.2020.9259870.

9. Abitbol E, Miere A, Excoffier JB, Mehanna CJ, Amoroso F, Kerr S, Ortala M, Souied EH. (2022). "Deep Learning-Based Classification of Retinal Vascular Diseases Using Ultra-Widefield Colour Fundus Photographs." BMJ Open Ophthalmology, 7:e000924. doi: 10.1136/bmjophth-2021-000924.

10. Dong L, He W, Zhang R, Ge Z, Wang YX, Zhou J, Xu J, Shao L, Wang Q, Yan Y, Xie Y, Fang L, Wang H, Wang Y, Zhu X, Wang J, Zhang C, Wang H, Wang Y, Chen R, Wan Q, Yang J, Zhou W, Li H, Yao X, Yang Z, Xiong J, Wang X, Huang Y, Chen Y, Wang Z, Rong C, Gao J, Zhang H, Wu S, Jonas JB, Wei WB. (2022). "Artificial Intelligence for Screening of Multiple Retinal and Optic Nerve Diseases." JAMA Network Open, 5(5):e229960. doi: 10.1001/jamanetworkopen.2022.9960.

11. https://machinelearningmastery.com/what-is-deep-learning

12. https://www.upgrad.com/blog/basic-cnn-architecture

13. https://www.kaggle.com/datasets/mariaherrerot/aptos2019

14. Khokale SR, Bhalsing A, Bagul D, Ugale A, Borse N. (2022). "Leaf Disease Detection Using Transfer Learning." International Journal of Scientific Development and Research (IJSDR), 7(5):59–63. www.ijsdr.org.

15. https://iq.opengenus.org/inception-v3-model-architecture

16. https://blog.paperspace.com/popular-deep-learning-architectures-resnet-inceptionv3-squeezenet

17. Das S, Majumder S. (2022). Overview and Analysis of Present-Day Diabetic Retinopathy (DR) Detection Techniques. Approaches and Applications of Deep Learning in Virtual Medical Care. A Volume in the Advances in Healthcare Information Systems and Administration Book Series. IGI Global chapter 3, pp. 52–80. doi: 10.4018/978-1-7998-8929-8.ch003.

18. Das S, Majumder S. (2021). "A Review on Pattern Recognition Based Retinal Blood Vessels Extraction Technique to Detect Diabetic Retinopathy (DR)." Proceedings of International Conference on Data Science and Applications ICDSA 2021, 2:69–80. doi: 10.1007/978-981-16-5348-3.

14 A Review on Wireless BAN to Measure the Respiration Rate Using SoC Architecture

H. R. Archana[1], H. H. Surendra[1], A. P. Jyothi[2], S. Lalitha[1], and K. N. Madhusudhan[1]
[1]Department of Electronics and Communication Engineering, B.M.S. College of Engineering, Bengaluru, Karnataka, India
[2]Department of Computer Science Engineering, Ramaiah University of Applied Sciences, Bengaluru, Karnataka, India

CONTENTS

DOI: 10.1201/9781003324430-17

14.1 INTRODUCTION – BACKGROUND STUDY

This era of constant miniaturization and high-speed communication between various systems has contributed to the development of intelligent systems. Wireless BAN forms one of the promising candidates to establish efficient and accurate medical treatments at times of emergencies. This makes it immensely useful for healthcare applications. The heterogeneous WSNs have some biological sensors that can be placed at any part of the body or through a wearable device.

BANs are short-range wireless networks intended to connect some low-power devices along with biosensors situated on the humanoid body to accumulate data by processing biological information over a range of time for continuous monitoring of health conditions [1]. In general, the BAN implementations can be done in three ways. It is necessary to retrieve the data from the sensors within the body to understand the physical and the physiological parameters that are transmitted to inter-body communication nodes [2, 3]. The incorporation of BAN along with WSN will help in remote monitoring of various body parameters [4].

A survey of different energy efficient protocols [5] is done for usage of suitable protocol to a particular application. The structure of sensors and its attributes examination can be acted in a finite element analysis based on the virtual recreation platform [6]. In the way of research toward WBANs, there arise various challenges like a suitable system architecture, power-efficient protocols, and appropriate routing methods [7].

Healthcare applications need to address various challenges like low power, limited computations, material constraints, robust nature, fault tolerance, scalability, interference, and security [8]. Data security forms another major challenge to allow monitoring of the respiratory rates of the patient remotely over the Ethernet using reconfigurable SoC for a sensor network under ZYNQ [9].

For applications related to imaging, image enhancement using MPSoC can be utilized [10]. The AXI4 protocol is used to enhance the speed of the signal received from the nodes to be transmitted to the highest tier [11]. There are different ways incorporated to measure the variations of the input signal, and they can be broadly classified as two methods: contact based and contactless [12]. Multiple issues at various junctions have to be considered in the complete design of the smart system [13]. Multistage clustering optimization for large-scale WSN can be considered for remote communication [14].

Multiple sensors can be integrated on to the same device by considering the same AXI interface, which can support multiple masters and multiple slaves [15]. Integration of WSN and SoC has diversified applications like agriculture, security, surveillance, and healthcare [16]. The concept proposed can be applied to pandemics such as COVID to monitor various parameters like temperature and pulse rate [17]. Topology routing is considered for time-critical real-time applications with enhancement in the network lifetime [18]. WSNs are integrated to the Internet through gateways to support the access of various networks. This can be achieved either through an independent network or hybrid network approach [19].

Data communication is established between the wearable device to the access point, which can be several meters away. The networks consume low power and can easily maintain the data security as the distance is shorter.

14.2 BAN IMPLEMENTATIONS

BAN implementations can be done in three ways: electric field communication, electric current communication, and electromagnetic communication.

14.2.1 ELECTRIC FIELD COMMUNICATION

This is a contactless approach that gives the output depending on the charges on the surface of the body.

14.2.2 ELECTRIC CURRENT COMMUNICATION

In this method, the person needs to make a contact with a source like electrodes, which generate charges through electronic equipment. The output depends on the trace currents detected in the wearers' body.

14.2.3 ELECTROMAGNETIC COMMUNICATION

In this case, the data transmission takes place at high frequencies generally in the ultrahigh frequency (UHF) band. For various applications, electric field communication forms the most promising technology in the recent advancements of healthcare.

14.3 LEVELS OF DISCRETION OF A BAN

Depending on the type of application and the level of implementation, an appropriate method can be employed. There are basically three levels of discretion for the analysis of a BAN, as shown in Figure 14.1.

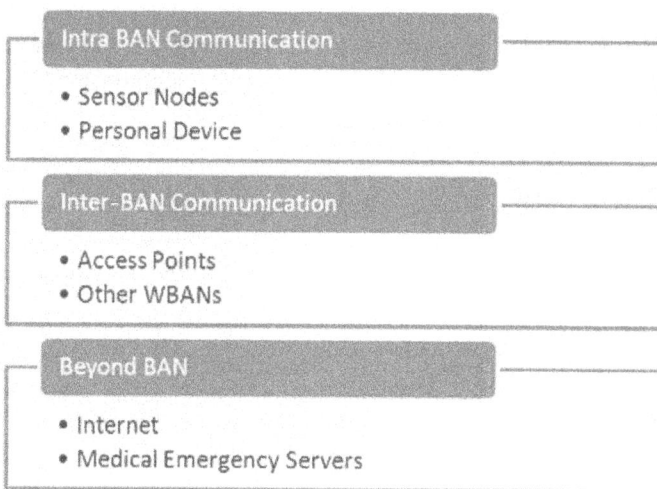

Intra BAN Communication
- Sensor Nodes
- Personal Device

Inter-BAN Communication
- Access Points
- Other WBANs

Beyond BAN
- Internet
- Medical Emergency Servers

FIGURE 14.1 Levels of discretion of a BAN.

First is the intra-BAN communication happening among the body sensors and master nodes which thinks about vitality, inactivity, and throughput boundaries. Second is the inter-BAN communication that utilizes the correspondence between the master nodes to at least one access point. This involves various wireless communications being employed, such as Zigbee, 3G, and Bluetooth. Third is beyond the implementation of the preceding methods, which is very much essential to gain the immediate attention of the authorized personnel to access and remotely monitor the patient's medical data with the help of a cellular network or Internet.

14.4 INTRABODY COMMUNICATION

This comprises the first level, which basically retrieves the data measured by the sensors continuously for various physical and physiological parameters. In intrabody communication, the body acts as a medium through which the signals are received at the device placed on the human body. Several mathematical models for the body were proposed on this ideology. The main purpose of a BAN is to monitor the various parameters of humans, like heart rate, mobility, and insulin levels, and communicate the variations to personnel at the nearest site. This can minimize the rates of heart attacks or stroke and also avoid frequent visits of the patients to the hospitals, which can in turn reduce unnecessary expenses to the patient.

14.5 CASE STUDY: RESPIRATION RATE USING THE MICROELECTROMECHANICAL SYSTEM

Advancement in the microelectromechanical system (MEMS) and wireless communication networks has paved a way for enormous scope, low force, multiutilitarian, and ease systems. Its usage in healthcare is most appreciated in the form of wearable systems, personal healthcare monitoring during mobility, monitoring the soldiers' well-being in the battlefield, and emergency medical care of old aged.

Relevance of an intrabody communication in measurement of respiration rate utilizing MEMS with capacitive pressure sensor plays a vital role. A small-scale framework for estimating rate of respiration using an electromechanical system-based capacitive nasal sensor person is created. Two comparative diaphragm-based designs are structured and essentially manufactured. To quantify the breath rate, mounting of sensors beneath both nostrils is done, so that the nasal wind current during motivation and termination affect the sensor diaphragm.

The planned square diaphragm design is avoided and, in this way, prompts a related change in the first capacitance esteem because of the nasal wind current. This adjustment in capacitance esteem is illustrated by a related dual test. To digitize the pressure data, the farad-to-volts conversion is intended for an accurate interface with the microelectromechanical system capacitive weight sensor, trailed by an enhancer and a differential cyclic analog-to-digital converter. The structured MEMS-based capacitive nasal sensor is equipped for recognizing ordinary breath of individual rate (18.5 ± 1.5 bpm).

It is imperative to screen the respiratory rate in an individual as it gives significant data viewing their respiratory framework execution just as a condition. It is the
quantity of breaths at regular time intervals. A typical respiratory rate at quiescent is
12 and its relating recurrence is 0.2 Hz. For the duration of recuperation from careful
sedation, narcotic agonists utilized for torment manage can back off the respiration
rate, prompting bradypnea (respiratory rate < 12) or apnea (suspension of breath for
an uncertain period), while aviation route obstacles will increment the respiratory
rate, causing tachypnea (respiratory rate > 30). The strategies normally utilized for
estimating respiratory rate are as per the following:

Visual perception
Impedance pneumography
Acoustic detecting
Fiber-optic detecting
Respiratory inductance plethysmograph
Nasal prongs

In the current examination, a MEMS-built capacitive breath rate sensor is structured in a finite element analysis (FEA)/boundary element analysis (BEA)-based
virtual plan reproduction stage. The investigation of the planned sensor is processed
in a similar reenactment programming. As the diaphragm diverts under a tension
burden, the portable plate of the capacitor encounters a similar measure of avoidance from the focal point of the diaphragm. In this manner, diaphragm avoidance is
promptly changed over to a capacitance change.

14.6   SENSOR WORKING AND DESIGN

A capacitive pressure sensor consists of two plates: static and portable. Both
plates are in square symmetry and parallel to each other. The static plate keeps
the portable plate inside of a conserved space. The deflection at diaphragm will
help in determining the capacitance. The change in capacitance depends on various factors like pressure and sensitivity of the plates. Virtual fabrication steps
can be done on an FEA/BEA-based platform with suitable mask and sacrificial
layers. The yield is considered with genuine breathed-out weight. The comparison of dynamic variation of respiration with the regular rate of respiration can
be carried out.

14.7   BLOCK DIAGRAM REPRESENTATION

A distinctive model is selected to reduce common-mode trouble. The correlated double-
sampling capacitance-to-voltage converter is designed for an exactitude interface.
It is with a microelectromechanical system capacitive pressure sensor, followed by
an amplifier and a differential cyclic analog-to-digital converter (ADC) to digitize
the pressure information. The output voltage is considered as the input for the next
calculation. Figure 14.2 represents the overall block diagram.

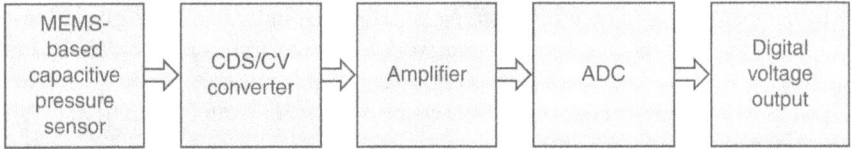

FIGURE 14.2   Block diagram representation.

14.8   PROPOSED HIERARCHICAL REPRESENTATION OF LAYERS OF BAN

The interrelativity of the different technologies can be understood better with the help of the hierarchical representation as shown in Figure 14.3.

14.9   WIRELESS BODY AREA NETWORKS

Advancement in the miniaturization of electronic devices, sensors, and growth in Wireless Communication (WC) led to the deployment of a wireless body area network (WBAN). WBAN works such that the device can be worn or implanted on any part of the body. The device senses and monitors the physiological changes and transmits these signals to the dedicated medical servers. Depending on the type of technology used, there are two classifications of mobile healthcare devices: wearable or implantable devices. Some of the wearable sensor devices include pulse oximeters, electrocardiogram (ECG) and electromyography (EMG) devices, and blood pressure (BP) monitoring devices. Implantable devices include glucose monitoring devices and neural stimulators, which send the signals in the form of electrical impulses to the brain or spine to treat diseases like Parkinson's and epilepsy.

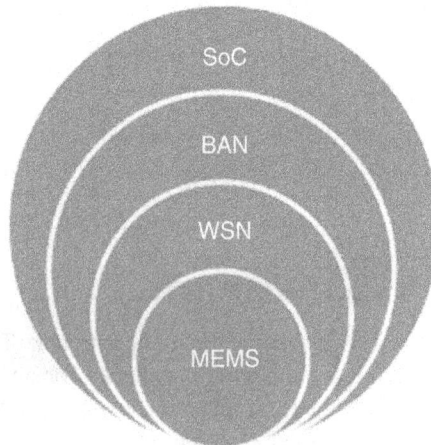

FIGURE 14.3   Proposed Hierarchical representation of layers of BAN.

14.10   WEARABLE DEVICES

The wearable devices can be in the form of a ring, like a pulse oximeter to measure the saturation levels of oxygen in the body. An ECG waveform generator produces the waveform depending on the propagation of electric signals through heart muscles as a variant of time. The variations in the generated pattern compared to a normal pattern indicate the problem of the patient.

Yet another application can be activity/motion detection with a biosensor device that integrates the functionality of an accelerometer and a gyroscope. A gyroscope helps to determine the variations in the angular velocity due to movements of an individual. The device helps to indicate if there are any uncontrolled motions of the person which in turn forms a symptom for Parkinson's disease.

A wireless electroencephalograph (EEG) is an application that helps in the detection of epilepsy and provides details about the rate of recovery in infected person. This sensor is equipped with the functions of data acquisition, signal conditioning, signal processing, and wireless communication. The wireless neural interface helps to gain data from two channels of wireless sensor networks.

14.11   RELEVANCE OF WBAN IN HEALTHCARE IMPLANTABLE DEVICES

Individuals suffering from type 1 diabetes can be monitored regularly with the variations in the insulin level, thus reducing the risk of hyperglycemic excursions. Monitoring the blood glucose levels can help in mitigating the risks of hypoglycemia with administered levels of insulin. The sensors can be implanted beneath the abdomen covered with a multilayered membrane. This can be embedded with a drug delivery system also, which ensures injection of insulin at appropriate levels at regular intervals depending on the generated readings.

14.12   PROTOCOLS USED IN BAN

Protocols play a major role in sensing the input, processing the data, and communicating to the access points. Hence power efficiency forms a key factor in BAN protocols. Most energy-efficient systems can be designed using medium access control (MAC) protocols.

Some works have been implemented on robust protocol stacks for multihop BAN, which is basically employed to avoid problems due to low-quality links. Link degradation might result in poor establishment of connectivity between the wireless gateways. Hence to reduce this problem, a time-division medium access (TDMA)-based MAC protocol is used. Other protocols that are used can be to control low-use peripherals with device drivers.

Streamlining the implementation of BAN, a standard IEEE 802.1.4 was created that laid out specifications for the allowable levels of radio power in the environs of human body. Well equipped with communication protocols like Bluetooth or Zigbee, the standard WBAN with master/slave architecture was designed that supports

WBAN. Later, IEEE 802.15.4 was developed, which worked on two access modes depending on active and inactive periods.

The TDMA-based MAC protocol thus became the most used one for WBAN networks. Network architectures play a very important role in communicating the signals received through body sensors and the access points. Multitier architectures support many data being gathered at the nodes and transmitted to a gateway that forms the interface and which is further transmitted to the highest tier, as shown in Figure 14.4. The MAC protocol provides an energy-efficient system and good synchronization.

Integrating AXI protocols provides higher speed of processing from the data origin nodes to the secondary tier or interface node. To enhance the speed of the signal received from the nodes to be transmitted to the highest tier, the AXI4 protocol can be incorporated.

The various data accumulated at the nodes indicate the sensor data that are used for determining multiple parameters. One of the nodes include the capacitive pressure sensor, which measures the change in capacitance due to variations in pressure of inhaled and exhaled air flow and converts this change in capacitance to an equivalent digital voltage.

WSNs provide confidentiality and authenticity without Internet access. Integrating IoT to WSN demands more security and utilization of available devices and workload

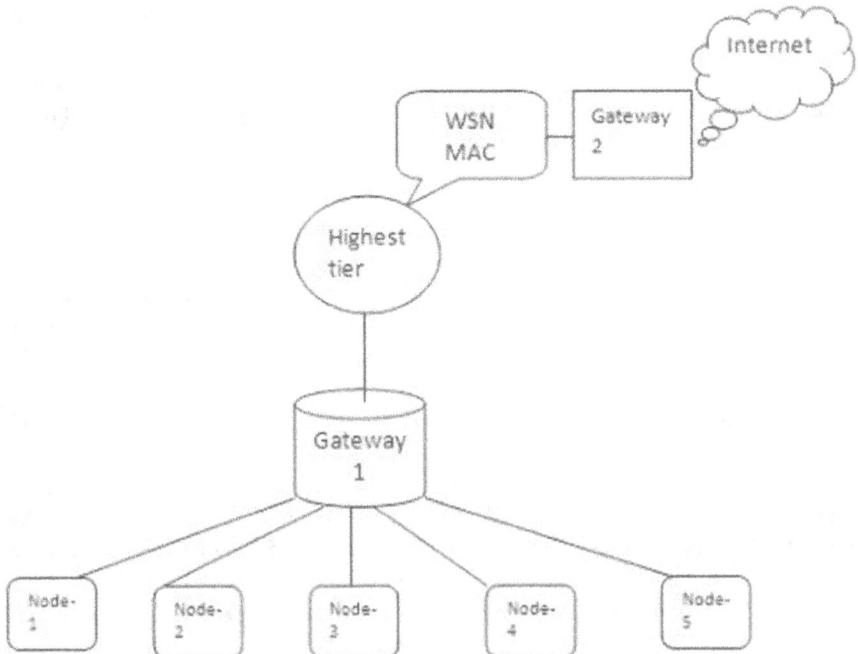

FIGURE 14.4 Multi-tier architecture.

distribution of the available resources. The IoT devices provide updates on the status of the data collected from the patient to the monitoring location through the cloud. The data monitoring is done remotely, and emergency conditions can be immediately addressed by the doctors.

14.13   WBAN TO MEASURE RESPIRATION RATE

Many application-specific WBANs are designed that poses problems in handling high-volume data obtained from sensors and communication systems of various physiological parameters in various applications like biotelemetry, hip guard, oximetry, and ECG monitoring. Respiration can be generally defined as the number of inhalations and exhalations per minute. Respiration rate generally differs in different age groups. Measuring the respiration rate is required to determine if the person has normal respiration or suffers from tachypnea, bradypnea, or apnea. These variations are sensed and transmitted using WBANs.

There is a need for measurement of variations in the respiratory rate during various physical activities or for patients who suffer from the aforementioned variations that form a very critical issue to be addressed. Working of a capacitive pressure sensor can be understood with the help of the representation shown in Figure 14.5. Use of capacitive pressure sensors indicates the variation in relative humidity. This is a contact-based approach. The dielectric material placed in between the plates has a property that relatively indicates the rise in the humidity content in the environment. The dielectric value varies depending on the amount of water content being absorbed.

The analog electronic circuit used helps in the transduction principle to obtain an equivalent electrical signal, proportional to the changes in the sensor values due to the inhale and exhale process. The acquired data are analyzed, and the output respiratory frequency (f_R) is determined. This in turn is given as input to WBAN. In this context, it is very much essential to note the coexistence along with the communication among the MEMS, sensor data (intra-), WBAN, and remote access points (inter-).

The respiratory rates accumulated by the sensors are transmitted through wireless links and processors. Wireless transceivers are employed at either ends' sensors or the access nodes of WBAN. Low-power MAC and implant communication with routing protocols plays a major role in designing the interactive system.

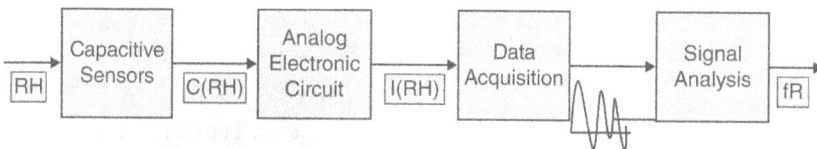

FIGURE 14.5   Representation of capacitive pressure sensors.

14.14   RECONFIGURABLE SoC

Reconfigurability is a term associated generally to system that gives rise to multiple changes dynamically. A flexible and reconfigurable data acquisition and transmission system can be employed in a WBAN SoC. System on a chip comprises of the integration of the sensors, processors, wireless modules for intracommunication, and a supportive unit to establish communication for inter-BAN.A Xilinx Zync-7000 APSoC. It is required to have a reconfigurable system in order to detect the faulty sensors at times, and the board helps in detection of hardware connectivity with the sensor data, which usually can be transmitted through Zigbee and software compatibility on the Linux platform to detect the instantaneous changes with the sensor data. Xilinx APSoC integrates a dual-core ARM Cortex processor and Xilinx 7–FPGA. The intra- and the intercommunication happen with the help of AXI protocol, which supports high-speed transmission of the acquired and processed information.

14.15   IMPORTANCE OF AXI PROTOCOL

Most of the SoC devices designed in the current scenario use the AXI-Advanced extensible Interface protocol. AXI is used with the Xilinx series devices as an interface with two sections, namely processing and programmable sections. AXI specifies how the various modules within the chip communicate among each other. The communication between individual modules takes place with the help of a handshake signal before the transmission of a signal. There are two segments, namely master and the slave, which can handle five channels to perform read and write operations. To transmit any control/ read or write signal it is necessary for both master and slave to issue a valid/ready signal. There are separate phases and channels that support the write/read processes. The identical channels between the master and the slave include read address, write address, read data, write data, and write response, as shown in Figure 14.6. AXI allows burst type communication, which facilitates continuous transfer of signals. Every data transfer will be complete by the generation of a write response signal.

AXI provides point-to-point interconnects with high bandwidth and allows low latency. It is used in applications comprised of interfacing IP blocks and SoC designs. The multiple masters and slaves can interface through interconnect and process the data by sending and receiving signals. AXI helps in improving the performance of the design when interfaced with multiple masters and slaves. For our application, the different signals from various sensors are considered masters, and the connectivity to be established through the WSN.AXI4 in particular supports a configuration consisting of 16 masters to 16 slaves. The main advantage of the protocol is it allows interoperability and good compliance.

14.16   INTERFACING AXI TO WSN MAC

The performance of a chip is assessed with the help of communication protocols, which normally is achieved with AMBA AXI4 protocols. The different interconnect protocols, namely Stream, Burst, and Lite, are used in AXI4, which helps achieve high performance. WSNs linked with various hardware accelerators and the processors with the help of AXI4 protocols as interfaces. Some diversified applications

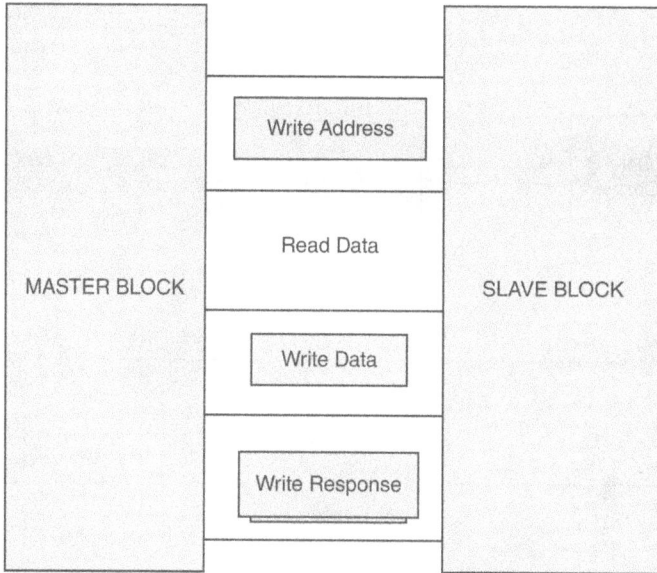

FIGURE 14.6 Channels interconnecting master and slave blocks.

of SoC WSN combination include precision agriculture, security, surveillance, and healthcare.

The AXI4 Stream interface is the most preferred for large data transfer between system components. AXI4 Stream interfaces the direct memory access (DMA), and the hardware accelerators are implemented on a Zync, where in the communication between them is bidirectional. The memory controller and the other components in the CPU support transfer of data from various sensors through electronic interface. Most of the SoC designs aim at increasing the frequency and memory bandwidth with the help of parallel processing of hardware accelerators. WSNs' SoC depend on exchange of data on a chip along with system components.

The interfacing of the AXI4 and WSN MAC protocol is depicted in Figure 14.7. The general blocks of AXI4 Stream comprise Dual Core ARM Cortex, DDR Memory Controller, Interface, DMA, and the Hardware Accelerator. The DMA is used to access information and transfer between DDR and WSN blocks. The transmissions between the individual blocks happen with the help of buses. The rate of processing is high, as AXI4 Stream supports huge data transfer. The data obtained at the higher tier form the source of input to the WSN MAC, which is addressed for processing through AXI4 Interface.

14.17 SINGLE-CHIP MEASURING AND TRANSMITTING THE RESPIRATION RATE AT HIGH SPEED

Chip is the outermost hierarchical layer that includes the other sublayers within, namely BAN, WSN, and the microelectromechanical system device. The signals obtained from microelectromechanical system sensors are processed by the BAN

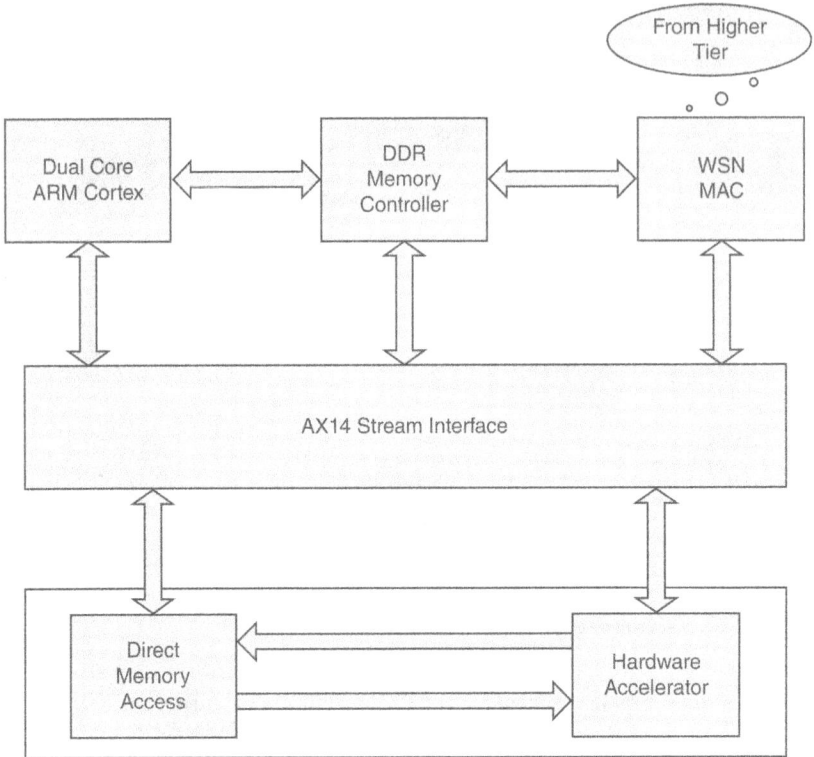

FIGURE 14.7   Representation of interfacing of AXI and WSN MAC.

layer, which employs high energy-efficient MAC protocols at the highest tier, which are compatible with the WSN. Different nodes can be mapped on to various sensors not limited to capacitive pressure sensors that measure the respiration rate. There can be other sensors to monitor the pulse rate, ECG, and heartbeat rate that can be confined for individual nodes. The WSN MAC protocol then communicates the fetched data from the highest tier to the memory controller and the AXI4 Stream interface. This is conveyed to the DMA to access the corresponding memory slot for functioning. Hardware accelerators not only support the process of increasing the speed of access with the components of SoC, like the processors, timers, and microcontrollers, but also reduce power consumption and increase efficiency.

Figure 14.8 represents a single chip that is comprised of various blocks and segments to perform the measurement of respiration rate with the help of capacitive pressure sensors in the microelectromechanical system device. The obtained signal as a respiratory frequency signal is then communicated through BAN, incorporating standard WSN protocols. The DMA and the hardware accelerators are a part of the AXI4 Stream that helps in storage and accelerating the processing of data acquired through WSN. The general-purpose SoC blocks contain the subblocks that perform general functions like the timer using clock generation, and the interrupt controller that helps

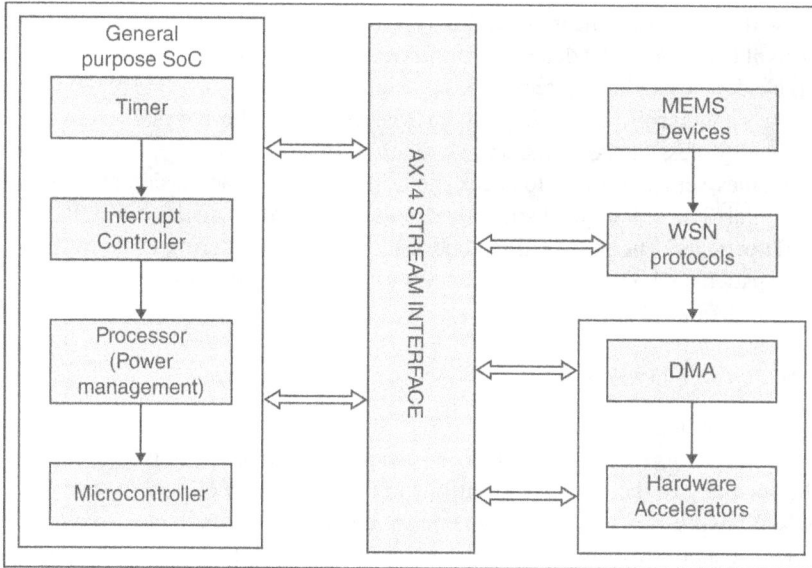

FIGURE 14.8   Single chip measuring and transmitting the respiration rate at high speed.

in generating interrupts based on the highest-priority signal from corresponding sensor inputs. The processor supports power and energy management of the entire SoC. The AXI Stream interface block acts as a bridge between both the inputs transmitted and processed and generates a suitable digital output obtained from memory. Employing the AXI4 protocol leads to high-speed interaction among the various IPs.

The different blocks represent different IPs for the functionality to achieve data monitoring of the respiration rate. The working of the device becomes more appreciable if multiple other sensors can be integrated in the microelectromechanical system block to perform other functionalities like heartbeat monitoring and pulse rate detection. With the help of a multiple masters/slave configuration, a maximum of 16 inputs and 16 outputs can be connected using AXI4.

14.18   APPLICATION OF THE WORK IN THE COVID-19 SCENARIO

There are multiple parameters that are to be assessed to determine the positivity of the coronavirus, like the symptoms of fever, cold, cough, and difficulty in breathing. To prescribe quarantine, it is necessary to assess the following parameters:

* Thermal scanning for fever
* Pulse oximeter for blood oxygen levels and pulse rate
* Blood sugar-level monitoring
* Blood pressure-level monitoring

The proposed method can be used to maintain the statistics of the comorbidity conditions of the patients, like kidney stones, diabetes levels, obesity, and thyroid, along with the measurement of variations in the respiration rate, which is one of the important features for the detection of the virus. The incorporation of the chip onto a wearable device can help in remote monitoring of the respiration rate of the patients. This plays a vital role in situations where even robust healthcare systems fail to assist healthcare professionals, PPEs, and ventilators. In such scenarios, remote monitoring becomes very important to check the criticality of the admission of a patient to the hospital. The technique also facilitates the healthcare assistance of self-isolated COVID patients. The proposed method also helps in monitoring of the respiratory rate for patients who have restricted access to healthcare professionals.

14.19   CONCLUSION

Integration of multiple domains like the microelectromechanical system, WSN, BAN, and SoC forms a major thrust of interconnecting technology. Advancements in the accuracy of the microelectromechanical system devices, and the use of compatible WSN protocols along with an energy-efficient BAN implemented on a single chip with a supportive AXI4 interface, mark the innovation of this technology compared to that of the other methodologies. Employing more sensors helps in monitoring various other parameters, as discussed previously. The proposal forms a more realistic solution to the COVID situation for remote monitoring of a patient's respiratory rate.

REFERENCES

1. Zhang, Guang He, Carmen Chun Yan Poon, Yuan Ting Zhang. "A Review on Body Area Networks Security for Healthcare." *ISRN Communications and Networking*, Vol. 2011, 2011. DOI: 10.5402/2011/692592
2. Negraa, Rim, Imen Jemilia, Abdelfettah Belghith. "Wireless Body Area Networks: Applications and Technologies." *Science Direct-Procedia Computer Science*, Vol. 83, 2016: 1274–1281. DOI: 10.1016/j.procs.2016.04.266
3. Stamenkovic, Zoran, Goran Panic. "A System-on-Chip for Wireless Body Area Sensor Network Node." 2008 11th IEEE Workshop on Design and Diagnostics of Electronic Circuits and Systems. DOI: 10.1109/DDECS.2008.4538770
4. Seyedi, Mirhojjat et al. "A Survey on Intrabody Communications for Body Area Network Applications." *IEEE Transactions on Bio-Medical Engineering*, Vol. 60, No. 8, 2013. DOI: 10.1109/TBME.2013.2254714
5. A.P., Jyothi, Usha Sakthivel. "Trends and Technologies Used for Mitigating Energy Efficiency Issues in Wireless Sensor Network." *International Journal of Computer Applications*, Vol. 111, 2015: 32–40. DOI: 10.5120/19521-1150
6. Chattopadhyay, Madhurima, Deborshi Chakraborty. "A New Scheme for Determination of Respiration Rate in Human Being Using MEMS Based Capacitive Pressure Sensor: Simulation Study." *International Conference on Sensing Technology* 2014. DOI: 10.13140/RG.2.1.4931.4727
7. Crosby, Garth V., Tirthankar Ghosh, Renita Murimi, Craig A. Chin. "Wireless Body Area Networks for Healthcare: A Survey." *International Journal of Ad hoc, Sensor & Ubiquitous Computing (IJASUC)*, Vol. 3, No. 3, 2012: 1–10.

8. Neves, Paulo, Michal Stachyra, Joel Rodrigues. "Application of Wireless Sensor Networks to Healthcare Promotion." *Journal of Communications Software and Systems*, Vol. 4, No. 3, 2008: 181–190.

9. Keerthana, K., R. Prashanthi. "Flexible and Reconfigurable SOC for Sensor Network under ZYNQ." *IJSTE – International Journal of Science Technology & Engineering*, Vol. 3, No. 1, 2016: 145–151.

10. H.R., Archana, Vasundara Patel K.S. "An Investigation Towards Effectiveness in Image Enhancement Process in MPSoC." *International Journal of Electrical and Computer Engineering (IJECE)*, Vol. 8, No. 2, 2018: 963–970.

11. Makni, Mariem et al., "Performance Exploration of AMBA AXI4 Bus Protocols for Wireless Sensor Networks." *2017 IEEE/ACS 14th International Conference on Computer Systems and Applications (AICCSA)*. DOI: 10.1109/AICCSA.2017.26

12. Massaroni, Carlo et al. "Contact-Based Methods for Measuring Respiratory Rate." *Sensors*, Vol. 19, 2019: 908.

13. Meharouech, Amira et al. "Moving Towards Body-to-Body Sensor Networks for Ubiquitous Applications: A Survey." *Journal of Sensor and Actuator Networks*, Vol. 8, No. 2, 2019: 27. DOI: 10.3390/jsan8020027

14. Jyothi, A.P., S. Usha. "MSoC: Multi-Scale Optimized Clustering for Energy Preservation in Wireless Sensor Network." *Wireless Personal Communications*, Vol. 105, 2019: 1309–1328. DOI: 10.1007/s11277-019-06146-y

15. Rajani, Smt. A., K. Sai Rameswari. "Design and Synthesis of AXI Slave Interface Memory Controller." *International Journal of Science, Engineering and Technology Research (IJSETR)*, Vol. 4, No. 12, 2015: 3306–3310.

16. Hempstead, Mark. "An Accelerator-Based Wireless Sensor Network Processor in 130 nm CMOS." CASES'09, October 11–16, 2009, Grenoble, France.

17. Massaroni, Carlo et al. "Remote Respiratory Monitoring in the Time of COVID-19." *Frontiers in Physiology*, Vol. 11, 29 May 2020. DOI: 10.3389/fphys.2020.00635

18. Jyothi, A.P., S. Usha. "Interstellar Based Topology Control Scheme for Optimal Clustering Performance in WSN." *International Journal of Communication Systems*, Vol. 33, 2020: e4350. DOI: 10.1002/dac.4350

19. LasyaSri, B., L. Nirmala Devi. "Integration Approaches and Challenges of WSN for IoT." *International Research Journal of Engineering and Technology*, Vol. 5, No. 5, May 2018: 1246–1248.

Part IV

Biomedical Signal Processing

15 Deep Feature Extraction for EEG Signal Classification in Motor Imagery Tasks

Rashmi S and Vani Ashok
Department of Computer Science & Engineering,
Sri Jayachamarajendra College of Engineering (SJCE),
JSS Science & Technology, University of Mysore,
Karnataka, India

CONTENTS

15.1 INTRODUCTION

The brain is the most complex information processing system known to human beings and is dedicated to performing visuomotor tasks. In recent research related to robotics, BCI systems draws the major attention due to its extensive application in neurology-related medical diagnoses. BCI acts as an interface between computers and the user's brain, interprets the brain's activity, and directs the external device to work accordingly. The MI-based BCI interprets motor cortex signals (brain signals related to movement of a body part) that are called as MI-EEG. These systems are very helpful for alleviating the patient's suffering from neurophysiological disorders like paralysis as they can be used to assist such patients to interact with external world or robotic devices such as wheelchairs.

The recent research related to the MI-EEG signal classification task has shown that the area requires domain knowledge of brain signal collection, signal processing for denoising, and pattern recognition and machine learning for feature extraction and classification. MI signals are basically voltage fluctuations of ionic current generated in brain cells when a person thinks of or imagines performing a certain action. The signals are captured using EEG machines, which consist of electrodes that are placed on the user's scalp. Signals captured using these electrodes are inherent to noise due to rapid fluctuations in the EEG signals [1]. The generated brain signals within the brain are measured using a device attached to scalp. The skull and skin regions interfere and contribute to a decrease in the signal quality. Also, it is a challenging task to decide which particular region of the brain is to be connected using electrodes to avoid a mixture of different intent signals being collected. These are factors contributing to inherent noise associated with EEG signals and are measured as signal-to-noise ratio (SNR). According to work by T. Ball et al. [2], approximately only 5% of the original brain signals are collected using the EEG devices. The low signal-to-noise ratio and the insufficient spatial resolution are due to the complex structure of the brain. Feature engineering and parameter selection, which includes filter type, passband, channel, frequency, etc., are considered major hurdles for efficient and accurate classification of EEG signals [3]. Deep learning approaches are best suited for EEG signals processing irrespective of aforementioned challenges [4]. Several deep learning approaches are proposed to accurately classify the MI-EEG signals, which is needed for efficient operation of BCI systems.

Multiple existing methods have been studied and analyzed for EEG signal feature extraction and classification. The important methods that are used for MI-EEG classifications are dimensionality reduction algorithms like linear discriminant analysis (LDA) [5], machine learning algorithms like SVM [6], Naive Bayes (NB) [7], and in recent deep learning frameworks like CNN, RNN, and deep belief network (DBN). An optimized SVM as a pattern recognition method for EEG classification was proposed by Miao et al. [8]. This method reported performance of 85.9% by the use of squirrel search algorithm. The method proposed by Dose [9] using temporal and spatial convolutional layers for feature extraction and fully connected layers for feature classification has achieved mean accuracy of 80.10% for a global two-class classifier and 86.13% for a subject-specific classifier. The average accuracy on group-level classification of 97.28% is achieved by Lun et al. [10] using a convolutional neural network. In their experiments, they also demonstrated that the CNN classification method with minimal electrode can obtain high accuracy. Recent studies include use of RNN for accurate signal classification. Fusion methods like combination of CNN and long short-term memory (LSTM) by Yang et al. [11] have shown promising results in concurrent learning of spatial information and temporal correlation from EEG signals. One more similar study by Xiang Zhang et al. [3] also shows that a combination of spatial and temporal features extracted from EEG signals can be combined using autoencoding techniques to eliminate background artifacts. These features can be effectively used as input to ensemble tree-based classification structures.

The study of spatial (intrasample) and temporal (intersample) variations have revealed that a combination of both resulted in better classification. Hence, the proposed framework extends the idea of fusing the spatial and temporal feature maps for effective EEG classification. Even though deep learning frameworks are used for direct intent classification in most of the related work studied, their use as feature extraction methods is not explored and experimented with more widely. The present work is an attempt to showcase the difference between classification performance when deep learning methods are used alone and in a combination of deep learning with machine learning algorithms.

15.2 MATERIALS AND METHODS

This section explains the proposed MI-EEG signal classification model using deep learning and machine learning algorithms. Section 15.2.1 describes MI-EEG data used for the experiment. In Section 15.2.2, the baseline methods used in the experiment are explained. Sections 15.2.3 and 15.2.4 describe spatial feature extraction by the CNN deep neural network and temporal feature extraction by the RNN deep neural network respectively. Section 15.2.5 explains the different classification algorithms tested for the combined features map from CNN and RNN models.

15.2.1 DATA SET

MI-EEG is the data collected during the mental process of imagining performing a certain action [11, 12]. The brain signals generated during this course of actions or imaginations are captured using the EEG device. The publicly available benchmark MI-EEG signal data set from the PhysioNet eegmmidb (EEG motor movement/ imagery) database is used for the proposed work [13, 14]. The BCI200 EEG system is used to collect these data [15, 16], and 64 channels/electrodes are used to record the brain signal fluctuations at a 160 Hz sampling rate. For the current experiment, 28,000 labeled EEG data collected from 10 different persons are used. The signals were acquired during motor imagery movement and real movement. The raw data from PhysioNet were not well structured, and they were collected in trials having different time lengths. Hence the raw data that are resampled and filtered by Xiang Zhang et al. [3, 17, 18] are used in the proposed work. Each row in the data corresponds to signal values collected from 64 channels. The actions are labeled as 0, 1, 2, 3, and 4, as shown in Table 15.1. Images in the table are the actions imagined by the subjects during which EEG signals are collected.

TABLE 15.1

The Motor Imagery Tasks and Their Corresponding Labels in Signals Data

Task					
Intent	Eye closed	Left hand	Right hand	Both hands	Both feet
Labels	0	1	2	3	4

The EEG data sample representation having 64 columns of signal readouts from the EEG signal capturing device and the 65th column having intent or label information (ground truth) is shown as the following matrix representation:

$$V_{28000,65} = \begin{bmatrix} v_{1,1} & v_{1,2} & v_{1,3} & \cdots & v_{1,64} & l_1 \\ v_{2,1} & v_{2,2} & v_{2,3} & \cdots & v_{2,64} & l_2 \\ v_{3,1} & v_{3,2} & v_{3,3} & & v_{3,64} & l_3 \\ \vdots & \vdots & \vdots & & \vdots & \vdots \\ v_{28,000,1} & v_{28,000,2} & v_{28,000,3} & \cdots & v_{28,000,64} & l_{28,000} \end{bmatrix}$$

where $v_{i,j}$ is individual signal value with i ranging from 1 to 28,000 and j ranging from 1 to 64. The corresponding label value is converted to one hot encoding, which is again a vector of 5 binary values. The binary value 1 is placed in the vector position corresponding to the integer value of the intent and rest of the values to 0. The entire 28,000 such vectored data are divided in the ratio of 3:1 for training and testing. The low SNR and high dimensionality, which is due to the number of electrodes used and the duration for which data are recorded, make EEG data classification difficult. Deep neural networks are best suited for such data handling as it involves a bulk amount of data processing and there is no preprocessing required to automatically learn the complicated features from the bulk data [19].

15.2.2 BASELINE METHOD

The proposed method is based on the idea of combining spatial and temporal features extracted from two deep learning models, CNN and RNN [3]. In the selected baseline method chosen, the stacked feature maps constructed using temporal and spatial feature models are again trained using autoencoding to eliminate background noise and other artifacts. Autoencoding is proposed as feature adaptation method, and multiclass classification accuracy of 95.53% is obtained from this experiment. The proposed method is deviated from the baseline method by fine-tuning the CNN and RNN architecture for feature extraction. The use of autoencoding is eliminated, instead of which classification algorithms are experimented to justify that machine learning algorithms themselves sufficient for feature classification.

15.2.3 FEATURE EXTRACTION BY CNN

The CNNs are class of deep learning architecture majorly used in image recognition and classification. Even though they are best suited for two-dimensional data processing like images, recently they are used in other problem domains like EEG signal classification. The vectored data are treated as a two-dimensional matrix (time and channel). Due to their convolving nature in data processing, CNNs are said to be best suited to extract spatial correlation in the EEG signals. The one-dimensional vectored EEG data are convolved using CNN filters, and then pooling layers are employed to reduce the dimensionality. The series of such convolution and pooling stages repeats, and at the end fully connected layers are used to classify the signals

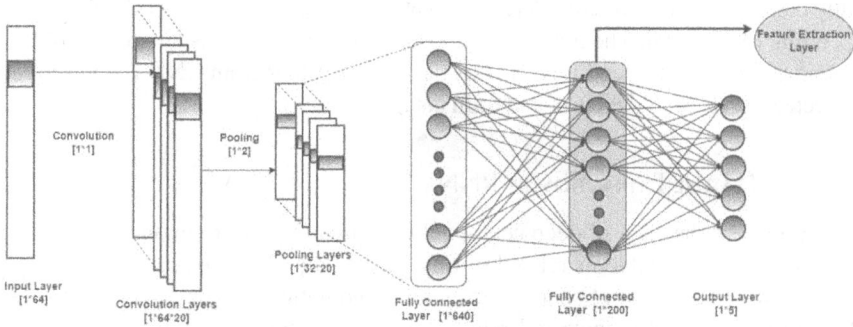

FIGURE 15.1   Proposed CNN architecture for spatial feature extraction.

to corresponding intents. The CNN architecture used in the proposed solution is as given in Figure 15.1.

As in the case of images, CNNs are used to exploit the spatial relationship between the pixel values. In the proposed context, they are used get the spatial connection between the EEG real values. The network consists of an input layer, a single convolution layer with a pooling layer, two fully connected layers, and finally the output layer. The EEG signal data of dimension [1*64] is considered an input layer. The raw input data are convolved using convolutional filters. As shown in Figure 15.1, a total of 20 convolutional filters are used to get [1*64*20] dimensional data at the first hidden layer. The depth of data from input to the first convolution layer changes to 20. The convolution filters of dimension [1*1] are used with stride value of [1*1]. The size of the resultant vector after an individual convolutional operation remains the same due to zero padding. The gray boxes in the input layer of Figure 15.1 show the convolution filtering operation on the input sample. The rectified linear unit (ReLu) activation function is used after the convolution operation. The next transformation operation is pooling. The pooling filter of size [1*2] is employed to reduce the dimension of convoluted signals. The max pooling operation is used to prevent overfitting [20]. Pooling operation reduces the dimension to [1*32*20]. The high-level feature extraction done in the previous layers are now flattened to a single vector. That is, the data in the form [1*32*20] are flattened to [1*640]. The two fully connected layers further processes the data. The first fully connected layer has neuron count equal to the dimension of the data from the flattening operation, which is 640, whereas size of the second fully connected layer has the neuron size equal to 200. Sigmoid activation is used after the first fully connected neural network layer operation. In these neuron counts, the number of layers and operations are carefully decided after several trials of network tuning. The last layer is the output layer, which consists of five neurons each for individual MI-EEG tasks, as mentioned in Table 15.1. The SoftMax activation function for multiclass scenarios is used. The cross-entropy is used to calculate the error and is optimized using the AdamOptimizer back-propagation algorithm with a learning rate value of 0.004. CNN here is trained to classify the EEG signals to corresponding tasks. But the last layer, which is directly operated with the output layer, will carry the maximum spatial feature information for accurate classification of the EEG data. Hence data at second fully connected layer are considered the spatial feature map of size [1*200] of corresponding EEG signal. The model is trained until it reaches a constant plateau of 89% classification accuracy, and then 200 spatial feature values from CNN framework are collected for all EEG data (test and train data).

15.2.4 FEATURE EXTRACTION BY RNN

The RNNs are the class of deep neural network architecture commonly used to predict the results of problems related to time series data or sequential data. They are well known in the field of speech recognition and natural language processing [21, 22] as they exploit the temporal relationship in sequential data. In the context of EEG raw data, RNNs are employed to extract intersample relevance of the EEG real values to classify them as belonging to a particular action or task. The idea behind using RNN is that they can efficiently extract the sequential co-relation in the signals as their structure helps in remembering the past inputs for time series data. The general structure RNN consists of an input layer, hidden layers, and an output layer. The network architecture of RNN in the proposed solution is as shown in Figure 15.2. It consists of five hidden layers, of which the last two layers are made up of LSTM [23–25] cells.

The calculation flow between first three hidden layers is simple. The data flow transformation operation from layer L_i to layer L_{i+1} with weight matrix W_{ij} and bias B_i is given in Equation (15.1). Consider the data flow calculation between input layer and hidden layer 1. The matrix multiplication operation is performed as shown in Equation (15.2), where HL stands for hidden layer, IL stands for input layer, and WM stands for weight matrix.

$$L_{i+1} = \left(L_i * W_{ij} \right) + B_i \tag{15.1}$$

$$HL\left[1*1*100\right] = \left(IL\left[1*1*64\right] \right) * WM\left[64*100\right] + Bias\left[1*100\right] \tag{15.2}$$

The last two layers in the proposed structure consist of LSTM cells. LSTMs are the variation introduced in the RNN to prevent a vanishing gradient and

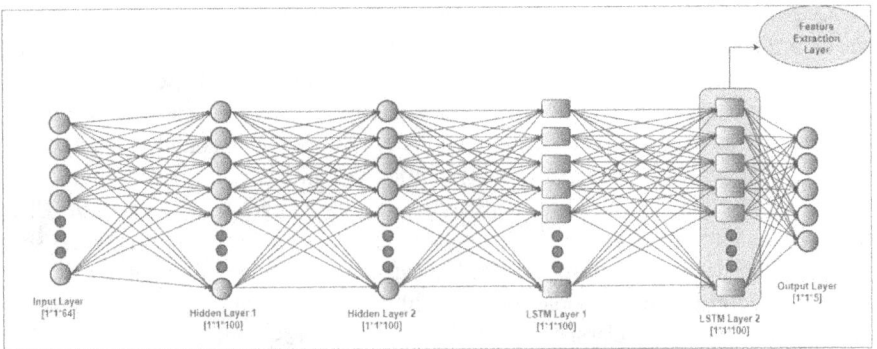

FIGURE 15.2 Proposed RNN architecture for temporal feature extraction.

TABLE 15.2
The Basic LSTM Cell Operations Performed at the Individual Gate Level

Gates	Equations
Forget gate (F_i)	$F_i = \sigma[T(X_{(i-1)(j)}, X_{(i)(j-1)})]$
Input gate (I_i)	$I_i = \sigma[T(X_{(i-1)(j)}, X_{(i)(j-1)})]$
Output gate (O_i)	$O_i = \sigma[T(X_{(i-1)(j)}, X_{(i)(j-1)})]$
Modulation gate (M_i)	$M_i = \tanh[T(X_{(i-1)(j)}, X_{(i)(j-1)})]$
State or memory of jth cell at i^{th} layer (S_{ij})	$S_{ij} = [F_i \odot S_{(i)(j-1)}] + [I_i \odot M_i]$
Value j^{th} cell at i^{th} layer after LSTM operation ($X_{(i)(j)}$)	$X_{(i)(j)} = O_i \odot \tanh(S_{(i)(j)})$

overfitting problem, and they are more accurate than RNNs. The basic LSTM cells are employed, which consist of an input gate, forget gate, modulation gate, and output gate. The data flow calculation is implemented according to the equations mentioned in Table 15.2.

The expression $T(X_{(i-1)(j)}, X_{(i)(j-1)})$ in all the gates denotes the operation in Equation (15.3). W, W' represents weights corresponding to the individual gates, and b represents the bias.

$$T\left(X_{(i-1)(j)}, X_{(i)(j-1)}\right) = X_{(i-1)(j)} * W + X_{(i)(j-1)} * W' + B \qquad (15.3)$$

At the end, we have the output layer, which gives the classification results using the feature maps extracted from the hidden layer's neurons. The SoftMax activation function is employed at the last layer. Cross-entropy is used for cost estimation, and the AdamOptimizer algorithm is used for weight correction with a learning rate value of 0.005. The last LSTM layer that is directly connected to the output layer will carry maximum temporal features extracted from EEG time series data. Hence, vectored data from the last LSTM are considered a temporal feature map. This layer consists of 100 neurons; hence 100 temporal feature values are learned for individual EEG signals. The model is trained until it reaches a consistent value of 94% accuracy in classification. Then the feature map is saved for all training and testing data, which can then be used as data for other classification algorithms.

15.2.5 FEATURE FUSION AND CLASSIFICATION USING THE MACHINE LEARNING ALGORITHM

The intent feature map collected using a CNN deep feature learning network and RNN deep feature learning network is fused together to make a single feature map. The two individual vectors of size [1*200] (in the case of CNN) and [1*100] (in the case of RNN) are stacked together to make a single vectored data of size [1*300]. This feature map is constructed for all EEG data samples and are further used to classify them into five motor imagery actions. Several machine learning classification algorithms are used classify the feature maps. Results of the same with a running time comparison are quoted in the results section. The schematic representation of the end-to-end architecture is shown in Figure 15.3.

SVM is a supervised machine learning algorithm used for both classification and regression applications. Earlier works have used SVM for EEG signal classification and achieved remarkable results [26, 27]. In the proposed work, SVM is extended for multiclass classification using a "one versus the rest" algorithm using the radial basis function (RBF) kernel to classify the EEG feature map.

In a decision tree model, a tree-like structure is learned from the training data and is used to predict the classification results of the test data. The process of learning follows the recursive partitioning of the data features using information gain. The test data follow the tree path to get classified into its category. The high-dimensionality data processing concept of the decision tree makes it suitable for EEG feature classification [28]. Instead of using the EEG signals directly to train the decision tree, features learned from the deep learning frameworks are used to train the tree.

Extreme gradient boosting (XGBoost) is an ensemble algorithm that allows users to train the model using set of hyperparameters that help to avoid misclassification even in presence of skewed data distribution in the training data. The most important

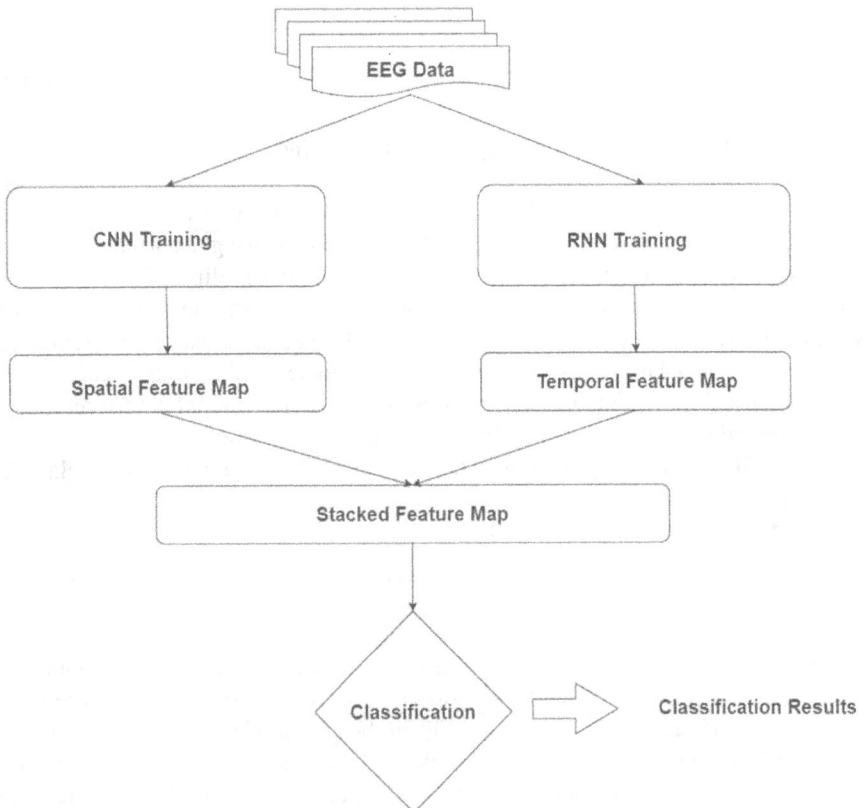

FIGURE 15.3   The decomposition of the proposed EEG signal classification structure.

factor behind the success of XGBoost is its scalability in all scenarios [29]. The existing EEG classification methodologies using XGBoosting have achieved very good classification accuracy using feature optimization [30].

Adaptive Boosting (AdaBoost) is another ensemble-based approach to build a strong classification model from week classification models. The individual week learners are added to one Adaboost model to correct the misclassification existing and the process repeats until a strong Adaboost model is built. This algorithm in combination with genetic algorithm has achieved remarkable result in Emotion recognition using EEG signals [31].

The k-nearest neighbors (KNN) algorithm is associated with less training time and high predictive power. The algorithm categorizes the new data based on maximum similarity with data stored during the training time. In the proposed work, three nearest neighbors (k = 3) are used to measure similarity. KNN has been used for binary classification of EEG signals [32], but in the proposed work, it is used to solve multiclass problems.

Naive Bayes is probabilistic classifier used to classify high-dimensional data into categories such as text classification. The algorithms work on the concept of likelihood and posterior probability with the assumption that the feature maps are independent of each other. The performance of this algorithm on EEG data is analyzed in work a by J. Machado et al. [33]. The Gaussian Naïve Bayes model is used in the proposed work to predict the intent classes.

15.3 RESULTS AND DISCUSSION

The TensorFlow framework is used to implement the model. TensorFlow is the open-source platform available to implement deep learning algorithms. The experiment was conducted on a machine with an NVIDIA TESLA K80 Titan 1X with 12 GB of RAM. Out of 28,000 EEG samples, 21,000 samples were used for training and 7,000 EEG samples were used for testing. Train and test data are shuffled before each run. In each epoch, 7,000 samples are fed to neural networks for training. Training the CNN model took approximately 95 seconds for 3,000 iterations, and training the RNN model took approximately 7 seconds for 200 iterations. The CNN model training gave 89% classification accuracy, whereas the RNN model gave 94% classification accuracy. When the feature maps of both CNN and RNN are stacked and trained using SVM algorithm, the classification accuracy increases to 98.16%, which shows that spatial and temporal feature maps carry the information that will further boost accuracy when given as an input to the machine learning modules. Along with SVM, several other machine learning algorithms are tested. The results of the same with running time are compared in Table 15.3.

It is inferred from Table 15.3 that SVM gives the highest classification accuracy compared to all other algorithms. The second best is the KNN classifier, but execution time for KNN classifier is considerably high for real-time operation of the EEG classification. The execution time of the SVM classifier can further be reduced to 14 seconds when the linear kernel is used instead of the RBF kernel, but classification accuracy reduces by 0.7% with the linear kernel. The confusion matrix and evaluation for the SVM classifier is listed in Tables 15.4 and 15.5.

TABLE 15.3

EEG Fusion Feature Map Classification Results with Different Machine Learning Algorithms

Machine Learning Algorithm	Classification Accuracy	Training Time (in Seconds)	Testing Time (in Seconds)
SVM	98.24%	22	20
Decision tree	95.65%	11	<1
XGBoost	96.82%	240	<1
AdaBoost	91.30%	118	41
KNN	97.70%	103	90
Naive Bayes	95.11%	8	7

TABLE 15.4

EEG Fusion Feature Map Classification Confusion Matrix and Evaluation Matrix for the SVM Classifier

Diagonal Average 98.24%		Prediction						Evaluation		
		1	2	3	4	5	Total	Precision	Recall	F1-Score
Ground	1	2,340	4	5	2	2	2,353	0.97	0.99	0.98
truth	2	27	1,237	1	5	5	1,275	0.98	0.97	0.97
	3	11	7	1,035	1	0	1,054	0.99	0.98	0.99
	4	6	7	3	1,047	3	1,066	0.99	0.98	0.99
	5	21	9	2	2	1,218	1,252	0.99	0.97	0.98
	Total	2,405	1,264	1,046	1,057	1,228	7,000			

TABLE 15.5

Comparison of Classification Results of Proposed Framework with Other Methods

Literature	Method	Data Set	Classification Results
G. Xu et al. [34]	VGG-16 CNN	BCI Competition IV	74.2%
Zhang et al. [3]	CNN+RNN+Autoencoder+XGBoost	Physionet eegmmidb	95.53%
Wang et al. [35]	1D-AX with LSTM network	Dataset 2A of BCI Competition IV	71%
J. Yang et al. [11]	DWT+CNN+LSTM	Physionet MI EEG	87.36%
X. Lun et al. [10]	CNN	Dataset 2A of BCI Competition IV	97.28%
H. Dose et al. [9]	CNN	Physionet MI EEG	87.98%
Proposed method	CNN+RNN+SVM	Physionet eegmmidb	98.2%

In addition, we have also compared the proposed methods results with other existing methodologies, and the same are listed in Table 15.5. Our proposed method gives greater performance results compared to other methods that are based on deep learning (including transfer learning).

15.4 CONCLUSION

The proposed work is based on a novel deep learning fusion method to extract a feature map for accurate and efficient classification of MI-EEG intent signals into corresponding tasks or actions. The main insights of the chapter involve exploiting the spatial and temporal relationship between EEG signal samples; comparing how temporal and spatial feature maps contribute to signal classification; and using machine learning algorithms to boost the classification results when trained using stacked feature maps. The results find that the classification accuracy was increased by 2.7% compared to baseline method chosen. Also, it is concluded from the results that the time efficiency obtained shows that the proposed methodology can be used to design a real-time BCI system for subject-specific EEG data. The aim of increasing the classification accuracy by using deep learning methods as feature extraction techniques is achieved with improved time efficiency. It is also concluded that the autoencoding as proposed in the baseline method can be eliminated without affecting the overall performance of the framework.

The same work can be extended to other MI-EEG signal data sets, particularly those that are not subject specific. Also, feature extraction methods can be further explored with other deep learning frameworks like DBN, restricted Boltzmann machine (RBM), generative adversarial networks (GAN) and gated recurrent units (GRU)-based RNN models.

REFERENCES

1. G. Repovs, Dealing with noise in EEG recording and data analysis, Informatica Medica Slovenica, vol. 15, no. 1, pp. 18–25, 2010.
2. T. Ball, M. Kern, I. Mutschler, A. Aertsen, and A. SchulzeBonhage, Signal quality of simultaneously recorded invasive and non-invasive EEG, Neuroimage, vol. 46, no. 3, pp. 708–716, 2009.
3. Xiang Zhang, Lina Yao, Quan Sheng, Salil Kanhere, Tao Gu, and Dalin Zhang, "Converting Your Thoughts to Texts: Enabling Brain Typing via Deep Feature Learning of EEG Signals," doi: 10.1109/PERCOM.2018.8444575, 2018.
4. Alexander Craik, Yongtian He, and José Contreras-Vidal, Deep learning for electroencephalogram (EEG) classification tasks: A review, Journal of Neural Engineering, vol. 16, doi: 10.1088/1741-2552/ab0ab5, 2019.
5. Raoof Masoomi, and Ali Khadem, "Enhancing LDA-based discrimination of left and right hand motor imagery: Outperforming the winner of BCI Competition II," Knowledge-Based Engineering and Innovation, doi: 10.1109/KBEI.2015.7436077, Nov 2015.
6. Sai Chong Yeh, Mokhtar Norrima, and Prasad Girijesh, Automated classification and removal of EEG artifacts with SVM and wavelet-ICA, IEEE Journal of Biomedical and Health Informatics, vol. 22, no. 3, pp. 664–670, 2018.

7. M. Miao, H. Zeng, A. Wang, C. Zhao, and F. Liu, Discriminative spatial-frequency-temporal feature extraction and classification of motor imagery EEG: An sparse regression and weighted naïve Bayesian classifier-based approach, Journal of Neuroscience Methods, vol. 278, pp. 13–24, 2017.

8. Miao Shi, Congcai Wang, Xian-Zhe Li, Mingqiang Li, L. Wang, and Neng-gang Xie, EEG signal classification based on SVM with improved squirrel search algorithm, Biomedical Engineering/Biomedizinische Technik, vol. 66, pp. 137–152, 2020.

9. H. Dose, J. S. Møller, S. Puthusserypady, and H. K. Iversen, "A Deep Learning MI - EEG Classification Model for BCIs," 26th European Signal Processing Conference (EUSIPCO), pp. 1676–1679, doi: 10.23919/EUSIPCO.2018.8553332, 2018.

10. X. Lun, Z. Yu, T. Chen, F. Wang, and Y. Hou, A simplified CNN classification method for MI-EEG via the electrode pairs signals, Frontiers in Human Neuroscience, vol. 15, no. 14, p. 338, doi: 10.3389/fnhum.2020.00338, 2020.

11. J. Yang, S. Yao, and J. Wang, Deep fusion feature learning network for MI-EEG classification, IEEE Access, vol. 6, pp. 79050–79059, doi: 10.1109/ACCESS.2018.2877452, 2018.

12. Gert Pfurtscheller, Christa Neuper, and C. Neuper, Motor imagery and direct brain-computer communication, Proceedings of the IEEE, vol. 82, no. 7, pp. 1123–1134, doi: 10.1109/5.939829, 2001.

13. https://archive.physionet.org/cgi-bin/atm/ATM.

14. A. L. Goldberger, L. A. N. Amaral, L. Glass, J. M. Hausdorff, P. Ch. Ivanov, R. G. Mark, J. E. Mietus, G. B. Moody, C.-K. Peng, and H. E. Stanley, PhysioBank, PhysioToolkit, and PhysioNet: Components of a new research resource for complex physiologic signals, Circulation, vol. 101, no. 23, pp. e215–e220. https://archive.physionet.org/pn4/eegmmidb/, 2000.

15. http://www.schalklab.org/research/bci2000.

16. G. Schalk, D. J. McFarland, T. Hinterberger, N. Birbaumer, and J. R. Wolpaw, BCI2000: A general-purpose brain-computer interface (BCI) system, IEEE Transactions on Biomedical Engineering, vol. 51, no. 6, pp. 1034–1043, 2004.

17. https://github.com/xiangzhang1015/Deep-Learning-for-BCI.

18. X. Zhang, L. Yao, X. Wang, J. J. M. Monaghan, D. Mcalpine, and Y. Zhang, A survey on deep learning-based non-invasive brain signals: Recent advances and new frontiers, Journal of Neural Engineering, vol. 18, no. 3, doi: 10.1088/1741-2552/abc902. Epub ahead of print. PMID: 33171452, 2020.

19. M. Bojarski et al., "End to end learning for self-driving cars," https://arxiv.org/abs/1604.07316, 2016.

20. Brahim Ait Skourt, Abdelhamid El Hassani, and Aicha Majda, Mixed-pooling-dropout for convolutional neural network regularization, Journal of King Saud University – Computer and Information Sciences, vol. 34, no. 8, part A, pp. 4756–4762, 2021.

21. G. Hinton et al., Deep neural networks for acoustic modeling in speech recognition: The shared views of four research groups, IEEE Signal Processing Magazine, vol. 29, pp. 82–97, 2012.

22. Kanchan M. Tarwani, and Swathi Edem, Survey on recurrent neural network in natural language processing, International Journal of Engineering Trends and Technology, vol. 48, pp. 301–304, doi: 10.14445/22315381/IJETT-V48P253, 2017.

23. Alex Sherstinsky, Fundamentals of recurrent neural network (RNN) and long short-term memory (LSTM) network, Physica D: Nonlinear Phenomena, vol. 404, Article 132306, 2020.

24. P. Nagabushanam, S. Thomas George, and Radha Sankararajan, EEG signal classification using LSTM and improved neural network algorithms, soft computing, vol. 24, doi: 10.1007/s00500-019-04515-0, 2020.

25. S. Kumar, A. Sharma, and T. Tsunoda, Brain wave classification using long short-term memory network based OPTICAL predictor, Scientific Reports, vol. 9, p. 9153, 2019.

26. B. Richhariya, and M. Tanveer, EEG signal classification using universum support vector machine, Expert Systems with Applications, vol. 106, pp. 169–182, ISSN 0957-4174, 2018.
27. H. Ines, Y. Slim, and E. Noureddine, "EEG Classification Using Support Vector Machine," 10th International Multi-Conferences on Systems, Signals & Devices 2013 (SSD13), pp. 1–4, doi: 10.1109/SSD.2013.6564011, 2013.
28. O. Aydemir, and T. Kayikcioglu, Decision tree structure based classification of EEG signals recorded during two dimensional cursor movement imagery, Journal of Neuroscience Methods, vol. 229, pp. 68–75, doi: 10.1016/j.jneumeth.2014.04.007. Epub 2014 Apr 19. PMID: 24751647, 2014.
29. Tianqi Chen, and Carlos Guestrin, "XGBoost: A Scalable Tree Boosting System," Proceedings of the 22nd ACM SIGKDD International Conference on Knowledge Discovery and Data Mining, arXiv:1603.02754, 2016.
30. S. Parui, A. K. Roshan Bajiya, D. Samanta, and N. Chakravorty, "Emotion Recognition from EEG Signal Using XGBoost Algorithm," 2019 IEEE 16th India Council International Conference (INDICON), pp. 1–4, doi: 10.1109/INDICON47234.2019.9028978, 2019.
31. T. Lv, J. Yan, and H. Xu, "An EEG emotion recognition method based on AdaBoost classifier," 2017 Chinese Automation Congress (CAC), pp. 6050–6054, doi: 10.1109/CAC.2017.8243867, 2017.
32. Annushree Bablani, Damodar Edla, and Shubham Dodia, Classification of EEG data using k-nearest neighbor approach for concealed information test, Procedia Computer Science, vol. 143, pp. 242–249, doi: 10.1016/j.procs.2018.10.392, 2018.
33. J. Machado, A. Balbinot, and A. Schuck, "A Study of the Naive Bayes Classifier for Analyzing Imaginary Movement EEG Signals Using the Periodogram as Spectral Estimator," 2013 ISSNIP Biosignals and Biorobotics Conference: Biosignals and Robotics for Better and Safer Living (BRC), pp. 1–4, doi: 10.1109/BRC.2013.6487514, 2013.
34. G. Xu et al., A deep transfer convolutional neural network framework for EEG signal classification, IEEE Access, vol. 7, pp. 112767–112776, 2019.
35. Ping Wang, Aimin Jiang, Xiaofeng Liu, Jing Shang, and Li Zhang, LSTM-based EEG classification in motor imagery tasks, IEEE Transactions on Neural Systems and Rehabilitation Engineering, pp. 1–1, doi: 10.1109/TNSRE.2018.2876129, 2018.

16 Effect of Age in Normal Women by Heart Rate Variability Analysis

Anjali C. Birajdar[1] and Vijaya R. Thool[2]
[1]Department of Electrical and Instrumentation Engineering,
MBE Society's College of Engineering, Ambajogai,
Maharashtra, India
[2]Department of Instrumentation Engineering,
SGGS Institute of Engineering and Technology,
Nanded, Maharashtra, India

CONTENTS

16.1 INTRODUCTION

In the past and in the present as well, women are the backbone of the family. A woman's health is her capital: the fit and healthier the woman, the happier the entire family is. Whether the woman is housewife or working professional, rich or poor, from rural area or urban, literate or illiterate, young or old, the basic need is to remain vigorous. Hence, this chapter has a forced focus to study the health conditions of women with respect to cardiovascular system and nervous system. The heart is the main organ of the human body, and its functioning plays a vital role in the survival of life. Diagnosing the status of the heart by electrocardiogram (ECG) is normal practice, but subtle morphological variations are hard to visualize and detect. Heart rate variability (HRV) is the extended version of analyzing the ECG signal. HRV is the beat-to-beat alteration in the heart rate of the ECG signal. HRV measures the healthiness of the status of the heart based on the variations available in heart rate. Bodily functions deteriorate as age increases, with the obvious changes in the skin, eyes, ears, and hair. As in external physiological systems, autonomic functions undergo similar modifications through the aging process as well.

An autonomic nervous system (ANS), which works in tandem to balance and regulate autonomic functions, has two subsystems, such as the sympathetic nervous

DOI: 10.1201/9781003324430-20

system (SNS) and the parasympathetic nervous system (PNS) [1]. The ANS, which belongs to the peripheral nervous system, senses the physiological status of the visceral body system through afferent pathways. Thus, feedback is to bring the body to homeostasis through the motor system via efferent pathways. The reflex arc passes through the medulla oblongata afferent neuron (which carries sensory information from the body viscera), one or more synapses (junctions between two neurons across which a nerve impulse is transmitted), and an efferent neuron (which performs regulatory action on target). Afferent neurons enter via dorsal roots, and efferent nerves leave via ventral roots in the spinal cord. The potential in sensory receptors is generated corresponding to the strength of the stimulus, and responses in the central system are graded in terms of excitatory postsynaptic potentials and inhibitory postsynaptic potentials at the synaptic junctions. The response reaches to the effectors, where it produces an action potential in the muscle. An ANS is divided into SNS and PNS, and these two systems work in opposition, where one system stimulates the organ and other one inhabits hence, both systems prepare the body for different situations. The SNS is generally activated in mentally or physically stressful circumstances, and to cope with such situations, it temporally enhances the physical performance of the body. It prepares the body for situations like alertness, fear, anger, excitement, or embarrassment; generally known as fight, fright, or flight. In such conditions of the SNS, cardiac muscles increase the heart rate by causing the dilation of lung bronchioles to increase the oxygen intake, which in turn causes the dilation of heart and skeletal muscles and blood vessels to increase the blood supply. PNS is the category of ANS that functions exactly in opposition with SNS, i.e., it slows down heart rate (HR), respiration rate, and blood pressure. It remains active in processes like digestion and rest. PNS stimulates the digestion process by stimulating digestive enzymes. An ANS functioning can be better understood by HR and HRV.

Various authors presented the linear methods of time domain (TD) and frequency domain (FD) for HRV analysis in different age groups [2–4] and also nonlinear methods [5, 6]. The heart rate variability is measured using time domain measures described with age, whereas the changes are measure dependent. Heart rate variability indices measured were less for the female gender, and these changes decreased with age [7]. This decrease in HRV parameters with increasing age was largely because of decreases observed in parasympathetic activity in HR [8]. Recent studies have also shown that standard ranges of HRV demonstrate influencing factors for healthy subjects that include age, gender, heredity, race, religion, diet, alcohol consumption, smoking, diseases, etc. [9–13]. Crone et al. [14] proposed and evaluated the HR and HRV analysis in three different age groups, from children to adolescents, beginning with 8-, 10-, and 12-year-olds, with a span of 2 years in each category, by observing the developmental change in feedback processing and rule shifting. Longin et al. [15] introduced an autonomic nervous system test battery to establish normative heart rate variability indices to find out the effect of autonomic nervous system tests on heart rate variability indices by comparing them with the baseline. Bricout et al. [16] experimented with the effect of sporting activity by the TD method of HRV analysis on a healthy soccer player at rest, training, and match conditions. Perseguini et al. [17] investigated heart rate autonomic modulation in older people, both in males and females, with respect to a change in the position of supine and standing posture using linear and nonlinear methods of HRV analysis. Vandeput et al. [18] presented features from nonlinear HRV analysis to provide the age and gender functioning in which features describe the information of autonomic HR modulation with complex behavior. Abhishekh et al. [19] described the changes occurring in the heart rate variability by analyzing it using TD and FD methods in normal healthy males and females with increases in the age stepwise. Poddar et al. [20] also described the declination in HRV with age by analyzing linear and nonlinear methods. Choi et al. [21] declared in respective study that aging affects the HRV parameters negatively. Silva et al. [22] carried out a meta-analysis to examine the changes that occurred because of fixed physical activity on healthy children using HRV analysis by time domain features. Voss et al. [23] analyzed the short-term HRV to observe the aging effect with gender in normal subjects by linear and nonlinear methods. This study explores heart rate variability analysis of normative females with four age groups of important stages of life span by linear and nonlinear methods.

The chapter is organized as follows: materials and methods, which include data and HRV analysis methods, are presented in Section 16.2. Results and discussion are presented in Section 16.3. The conclusion is presented in Section 16.4, followed by the reference list.

16.2   MATERIALS AND METHODS

16.2.1   DATA AND ITS RECORDING

Present-day research scenario is critical based on data and data recording as it has various aspects of maintaining the protocols. Basically, researchers wish to have a specific type of data for the research work to be carried out. Finding such subjects with the willingness to provide the data voluntarily is a hectic and tedious job. Subjects need to be convinced that such recorded data will be used for research and academic purposes only. Researchers also must maintain a phobia-free environment while recording the data within a certain bounded time frame. Ensuring the availability of specific subjects considered of interest is an equally challenging task. After recording the required data, it is necessary to make sure that the recorded data are fully noise free by observing a manual visualization of the entire data set.

After the various selection and omission criteria, the finally selected data for the analysis of HRV in normal healthy females were 194 in the overall age category of 18 and 75 years. The entire selected data have been stratified into groups as "a," "b," "c," and "d." Table 16.1 describes the details of stratified groups with age group categories and the total number of subjects considered. Determining the selection and exclusion criteria of data is tedious work for such an analysis, hence proper protocols have been strictly followed while choosing the subjects before recording. To avoid any kind of bias in the HRV analysis, the main exclusion protocols followed were the history of any disease, whether the subject is presently on any kind of medication, heredity-based diseases, any kind of mental stress the subject is going through, and the monthly menstrual cycle. The details of the data recording and its description with respect to recording setup, place of recording, initial recorded data, excluded data after recording, and final data for the analysis have been depicted in Figure 16.1.

TABLE 16.1
Description of Age Groups

Group	Age (Years)	No. of Subjects
A	18–30	85
B	31–45	53
C	46–60	32
D	61–75	24

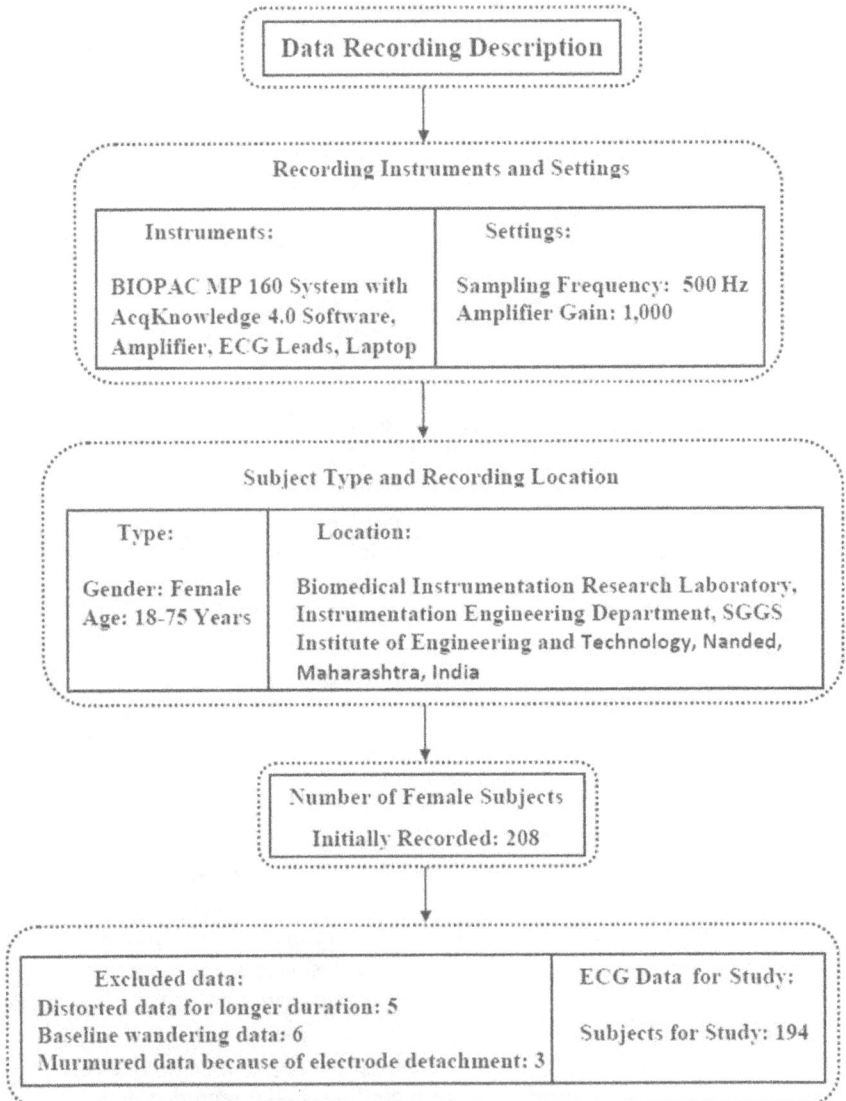

FIGURE 16.1   ECG data recording and its description diagram.

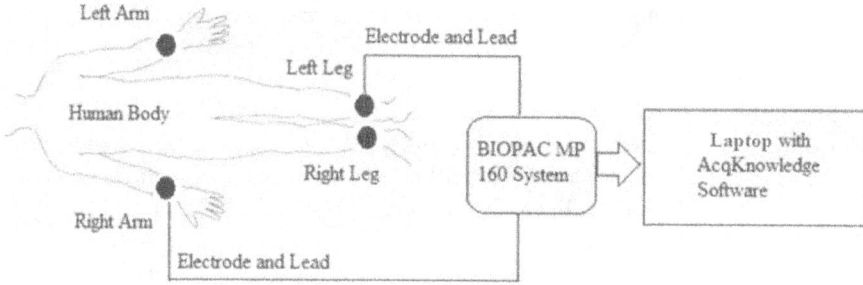

FIGURE 16.2 ECG recording setup with biopac system.

A 16-channel BIOPAC™ MP 160 system with AcqKnowledge software has been utilized to acquire the ECG signal in lead II combination for a minimum of 5 minutes of data. An entire set of data has been recorded at "Biomedical Instrumentation Research Laboratory of the Instrumentation Engineering Department, SGGS Institute of Engineering and Technology, Nanded, Maharashtra, India." Figure 16.2 depicts the ECG data acquisition system with essential hardware, which consists of the subject, ECG leads, MP160 system with amplifier, and the data monitoring and storing laptop. After recording the data, a manual observation was done on each recording from beginning to end to verify any kind of harmonics in the data and presence of ectopic beats. If there were fewer harmonics and countable ectopic beats in the recorded data, then these were eliminated, and if there were more harmonics and a high number of ectopic beats in recorded data, then such data are discarded to avoid its influence on further analysis. A simple flow of work carried out is shown in Figure 16.3. In this case, initially, recording of raw ECG data has been done, and thereafter the ECG data have been converted into RR interval HRV data by using AcqKnowledge software. Available HRV data have been further used for analysis purposes. In linear methods, features have been extracted by TD and FD. In FD of auto regressive (AR) modeling, Burg's method has been used to estimate the power spectral density (PSD) and the model order has been estimated using the final prediction error method [24–28]. AR modeling is a parametric method of analysis. The PSD plot with AR modeling is much smoother compared to the fast Fourier transform method. The details of all TD and FD features are shown in Table 16.2. The

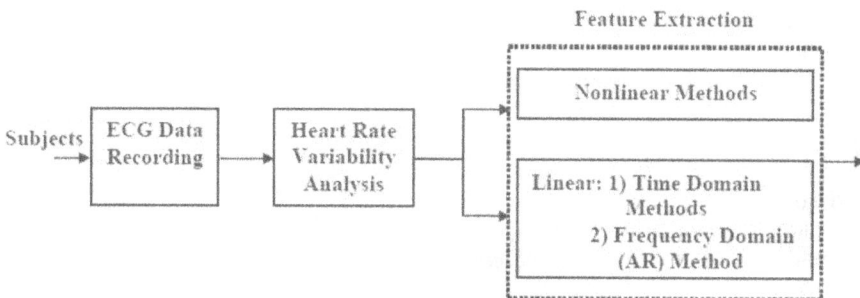

FIGURE 16.3 A proposed system with a simple schematic block diagram.

methodology calculates the mean NN intervals of entire data recorded and statistical values by considering data series as RR_i ($i = 0, 1... N$), i.e., $RR_1, RR_2, RR_3, ..., RR_N$ as RR_{Total}. Then time domain indices can be computed as per Table 16.2.

Similarly, in nonlinear methods, features have been extracted from Poincare plot (PP), approximate entropy (ApEn), and sample entropy (SampEn). Nonlinear techniques of HRV analysis can extract the inherent feature of biomedical signal like nonstationarity and nonlinear dynamics. Nonlinear methods like Poincare plot (SD1, SD2), ApEn of approximate entropy, and SampEn of sample entropy have been carried out. PP is the simple graphical portrayal of the current interval and its very next RR interval. It is a simple method to represent an RR interval change that compiles the functioning of the cardiovascular system. Let $RR_{Total} = (RR_1,$

TABLE 16.2
HRV Linear Parameters

Features	Description	Expressions
HR_{mean} (bpm)	Mean heart rate	$HR = \dfrac{60}{RR}$
Variance (ms²)	Variance	$Variance = \dfrac{1}{N}\sum\limits_{i=1}^{N}\left(RR_i - RR_{mean}\right)$ where $RRi, i = 1... N$ of data sample sequence as $RR1, RR2 ... RRN$. RR_{mean} = mean sample data sequence
SDNN (ms)	Standard deviation of the NN intervals	$SDNN = \sqrt{\dfrac{1}{N}\sum\limits_{i=1}^{N}\left(RR_i - RR_{mean}\right)^2}$
SDSD (ms)	Standard deviation of successive difference	$SDSD = \sqrt{\dfrac{1}{N}\sum\limits_{i=1}^{N}\left(dRR_i - dRR_{mean}\right)^2}$ where dRR_{mean} is the mean value of dRR_i $dRR_i = (RR_{(i+1)} - RR_i)$ RR_i is a sample point N is total number of dRR_i intervals.
RMSSD (ms)	Root mean square of successive difference	$RMSSD = \sqrt{\dfrac{1}{N-1}\sum\limits_{i=1}^{N-1}\left(RR_{i+1} - RR_i\right)^2}$
CV%	Coefficient of variance in percentage	$CV\% = \dfrac{SDNN}{RR_{mean}} * 100$
pNN50 (%)	Percentage of adjacent NN intervals differing by more than 50 ms	$pNN50 = \dfrac{\sum\limits_{i=1}^{N}\{|RR_{i+1} - RR_i| > 50\,\text{ms}\}}{N} * 100$
P-VLF (ms²)	Spectral power in very low frequency	0.0033–0.04 Hz
P-LF (ms²)	Spectral power in low frequency	0.04–0.15 Hz
P-HF (ms²)	Spectral power in high frequency	0.15–0.4 Hz
P-Total (ms²)	Spectral power in total frequency	0.0033–0.4 Hz

TABLE 16.3
HRV Nonlinear Parameters

Features	Description	Expressions
SD1 (ms²)	Short-term variability	
SD2 (ms²)	Long-term variability	$\begin{bmatrix} x_1 \\ x_2 \end{bmatrix} = \begin{bmatrix} \cos\dfrac{\pi}{4} & -\sin\dfrac{\pi}{4} \\ \sin\dfrac{\pi}{4} & \cos\dfrac{\pi}{4} \end{bmatrix}\begin{bmatrix} x \\ y \end{bmatrix}$
ApEn	Approximate entropy	$ApEn\,(m,r) = \Phi^m(r) - \Phi^{m+1}(r)$ where N = length of the data sequence (RR_1, RR_N) m = embedding dimension (2) r = tolerance (0.2 of SD)
SampEn	Sample entropy	$SampEn(m,r) = -ln\dfrac{\Phi(m+1,r)}{\Phi(m.r)}$ where m = embedding dimension (2) r = tolerance (0.2 of SD)

$RR_2, RR_3, \ldots, RR_N)$ be the total RR interval data series. It has been divided into the current RR interval series as $x = RR = (RR_1, RR_2, RR_3,\ldots, RR_{N-1})$ and the next RR interval series as $y = RR_{+1} = (RR_2, RR_3, RR_4,\ldots, RR_N)$.Then, x_1 and x_2 correspond to standard deviations SD_1 and SD_2, which are computed by the expression given in Table 16.3. ApEn is an index to calculate how complex or irregular the signal is. If a regular or highly predictable RR interval series is present, the value of the ApEn index will be lower; similarly, the more irregular or unpredictable the signal is, the higher the ApEn index value will be. Its mathematical expression is shown in Table 16.3. Sample entropy is a modified logarithm of an approximate entropy logarithm. SampEn is the negative natural logarithm of the conditional probability [12], and its equation is manifested in Table 16.3.

16.3   RESULTS AND DISCUSSION

In this section, comparative result analysis of all four age groups with respect to time domain, AR-based frequency domain, and nonlinear methods like PP, ApEn, and SampEn has been compiled and discussed. Table 16.4 summarizes all the parameters computed from the basic time domain and the spectral domain of linear and efficient parameters computed from nonlinear methods.

Although many other features have been computed in linear methods, clinically significant features are only considered for the analysis of HRV based on "p" values obtained from the student t-test. A comparative analysis of "p" values is demonstrated in Table 16.5 with all possible combinations of different age groups. The peculiar nature of behavior can be observed from the details of the "p" values. The "p" values are much higher when compared between age group "a" and

TABLE 16.4
Comparative Analysis of HRV Features of Normal Female Subjects with Different Age Groups

Features and Age Groups	a	b	c	d
HR$_{mean}$ (bpm)	78.67 ± 3.64	76.83 ± 5.21	73.73 ± 3.88	82.65 ± 4.75
Variance (ms²)	2756.9 ± 375.49	2277.85 ± 179.44	2053.99 ± 120.16	1871.25 ± 106.77
SDNN (ms)	54.36 ± 3.96	46.16 ± 2.93	40.43 ± 2.05	36.72 ± 1.07
SDSD (ms)	44.68 ± 4.31	38.19 ± 2.94	34.65 ± 1.944	21.04 ± 2.21
RMSSD (ms)	54.30 ± 5.65	36.75 ± 3.03	35.66 ± 1.88	20.79 ± 1.99
CV%	7.25 ± 1.38	6.21 ± 0.30	5.80 ± 0.49	5.04 ± 0.54
pNN50(%)	29.98 ± 2.74	16.95 ± 2.16	14.51 ± 1.209	6.64 ± 0.33
P-VLF (ms²)	407.29 ± 36.51	327.18 ± 30.60	257.42 ± 23.91	216.41 ± 19.67
P-LF (ms²)	371.81 ± 27.99	250.50 ± 37.64	159.42 ± 25.98	162.92 ± 24.39
P-HF (ms²)	323.39 ± 32.61	187.65 ± 28.04	128.23 ± 14.17	164.64 ± 16.54
P-Total (ms²)	1105.34 ± 83.71	765.70 ± 33.62	545.77 ± 34.31	543.98 ± 31.16
LF/HF	1.9552 ± 0.30	2.4888 ± 0.17	2.7276 ± 0.18	2.1754 ± 0.23
SD1 (ms²)	28.77 ± 2.82	20.59 ± 4.28	19.21 ± 3.39	17.21 ± 3.48
SD2 (ms²)	70.06 ± 8.57	60.82 ± 2.77	49.57 ± 5.17	46.63 ± 2.58
ApEn	1.1239 ± 0.0871	1.1498 ± 0.0801	1.0888 ± 0.0871	0.9380 ± 0.1798
SampEn	1.7181 ± 0.2694	1.5951 ± 0.2585	1.4417 ± 0.26	1.2811 ± 0.2135

TABLE 16.5
"p" Value Comparison Chart

Feature	a, b	a, c	a, d	b, c	b, d	c, d
HR$_{mean}$	0.0013	0.0406	0.0610	0.0906	0.6762	0.3674
Variance	3.1×10^{-7}	1.7×10^{-7}	0.0820	0.0599	0.0007	0.0002
SDNN	9.2×10^{-11}	1.5×10^{-12}	0.50173	0.0181	7.1×10^{-5}	1.1×10^{-6}
SDSD	6.4×10^{-10}	3.8×10^{-9}	6.2×10^{-5}	0.0525	0.4237	0.0257
RMSSD	6.3×10^{-10}	3.8×10^{-9}	6.2×10^{-5}	0.0525	0.4235	0.0257
CV%	2.4×10^{-12}	5.8×10^{-16}	0.0704	0.0034	8.8×10^{-6}	1.6×10^{-8}
pNN50	2.1×10^{-10}	1.4×10^{-9}	5.9×10^{-6}	0.0249	0.8800	0.0229
P-VLF	2.59×10^{-7}	1.8×10^{-6}	0.0002	0.0536	1.1×10^{-7}	1.3×10^{-5}
P-LF	0.0047	1.2×10^{-9}	0.0129	0.0463	0.7985	9.5×10^{-6}
P-HF	2.2×10^{-8}	3.3×10^{-8}	8.1×10^{-6}	0.0194	0.4322	0.0825
P-Total	3×10^{-8}	4×10^{-11}	0.0863	0.0162	0.0002	6.5×10^{-6}
LF/HF	4.5×10^{-9}	1.3×10^{-11}	5.1×10^{-16}	0.4213	0.0047	0.0559
SD1	7.2×10^{-10}	3.6×10^{-9}	6.6×10^{-5}	0.0661	0.4237	0.0308
SD2	2.1×10^{-10}	1.8×10^{-13}	0.7357	0.020	1.9×10^{-5}	3.2×10^{-7}
ApEn	0.0937	0.0621	2.8×10^{-10}	0.0021	1.2×10^{-9}	0.0001
SampEn	0.0095	5.9×10^{-6}	3.5×10^{-10}	0.0139	1.3×10^{-5}	0.0258

p > 0.05 = not significant, p < 0.05 = significant, p < 0.01 = very significant.

the remaining groups, "b," "c," and "d." Moreover, "p" values are moving toward higher to lower significant values as a comparison between higher age groups. A comparison of all TD parameters like HR_{mean}, variance, SDNN, SDSD, CV%, and pNN50 with consideration of all four age groups has been depicted with the help of boxplots in Figure 16.4. All the TD features were gradually diminishing linearly with increasing age. Moreover, HR_{mean} is declining gradually in the initial three age groups, but increased steeply in the elderly age group because of its advanced age, perhaps indicating the hectic mental stress caused by social and biological effects on the body. HR_{mean} has increased in the "d" age group, not the HRV, as it is diminishing linearly, which can be observed easily in Figure 16.4. The remaining

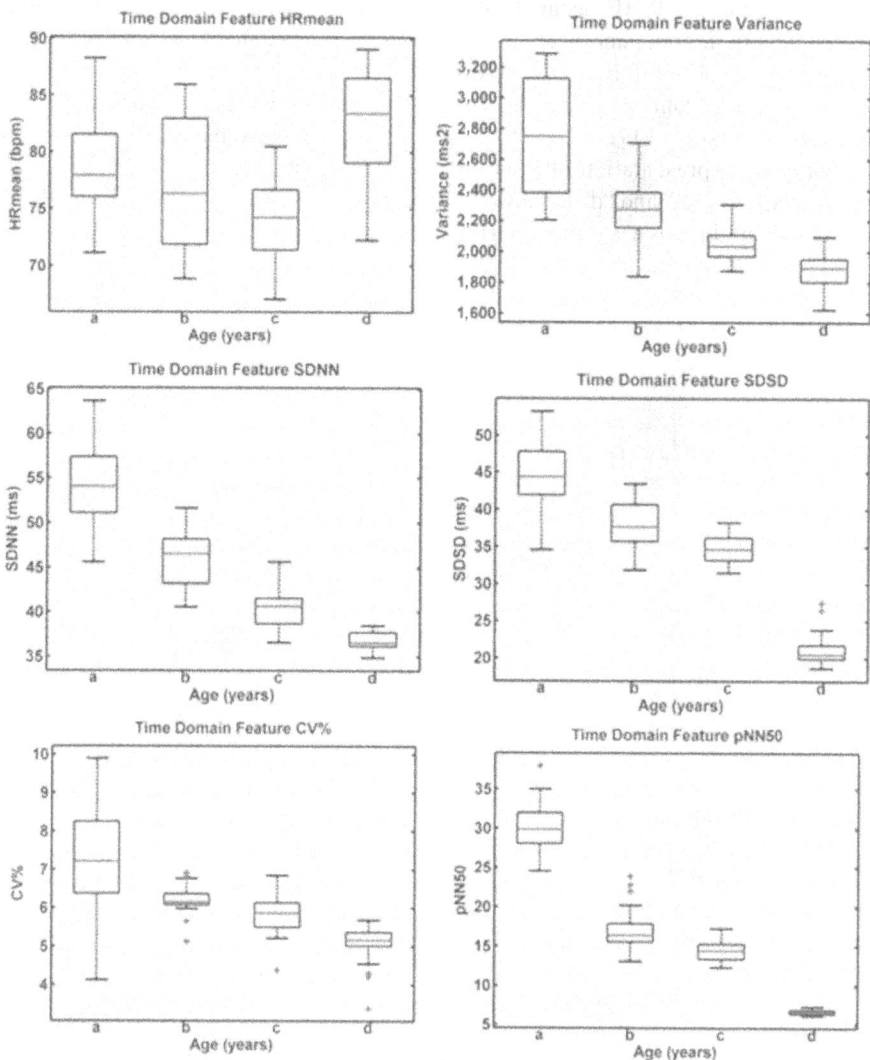

FIGURE 16.4   Boxplot of the HR_{mean}, variance, SDNN, SDSD, CV%, and pNN50 diagram.

TD features such as SDNN, SDSD, RMSSD, CV%, and pNN50 have linear decline from age group "a" to age group "b," from age group "b" to age group "c," from age group "c" to age group "d," and the same can be observed in Figure 16.4. It is evident from the declining trend of all TD features that sympathetic and parasympathetic activity of the ANS in the balancing act is in normal routine pattern. For AR-based spectral domain features like power in various frequency ranges, such as high, low, and very low, the entire range of frequency and LF/HF have been computed. A comparison of all FD parameters considering all four age groups is depicted with the help of boxplots in Figure 16.5. Feature P-VLF shows a gradual decline from the lower age group to the higher age groups. Features P-LF and P-HF have a steep decline in the age group from "a" to "b," and then a linear decline from "b" to "c," and in the last age group, "d," little positivity in P-LF and steep positivity in P-HF occur. Feature P-LF interrelates with sympathetic and parasympathetic tone, and whereas feature P-HF interrelates only with parasympathetic tone. LF/HF follows the similar pattern of P-LF and P-HF but in reverse, i.e., it escalates from age group "a" to "c" and then a down surge occurs in the last age group "d" since LF/HF corresponds to a sympathovagal balance.

A typical representation of PSD obtained from AR modeling in different age groups "a," "b," "c," and "d" is shown in Figures 16.6–16.9, respectively. From these figures, it can be observed that distribution of power occurs in different segments

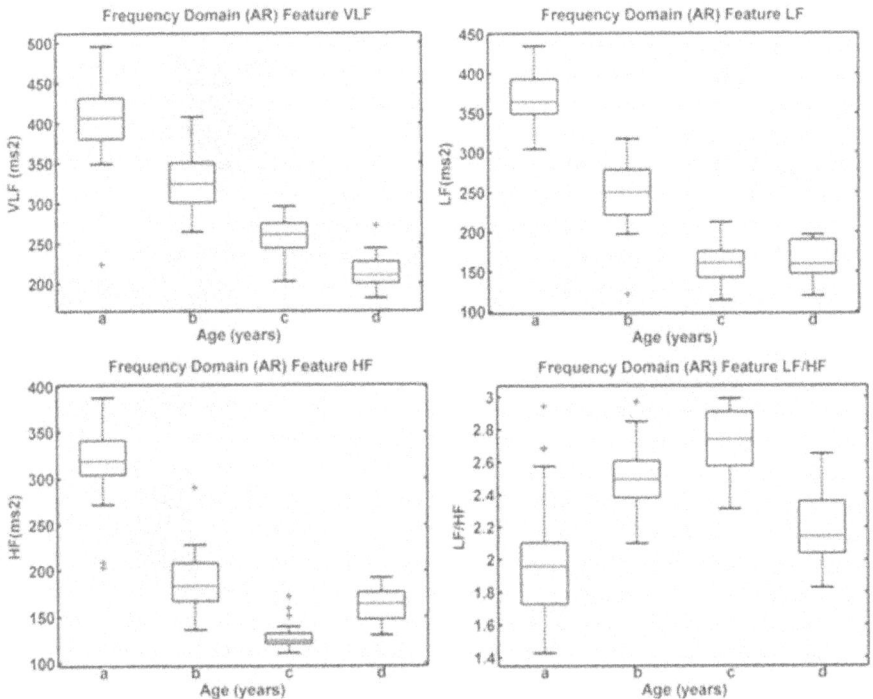

FIGURE 16.5   Boxplot of P-VLF, P-LF, P-HF, and P-LF/HF.

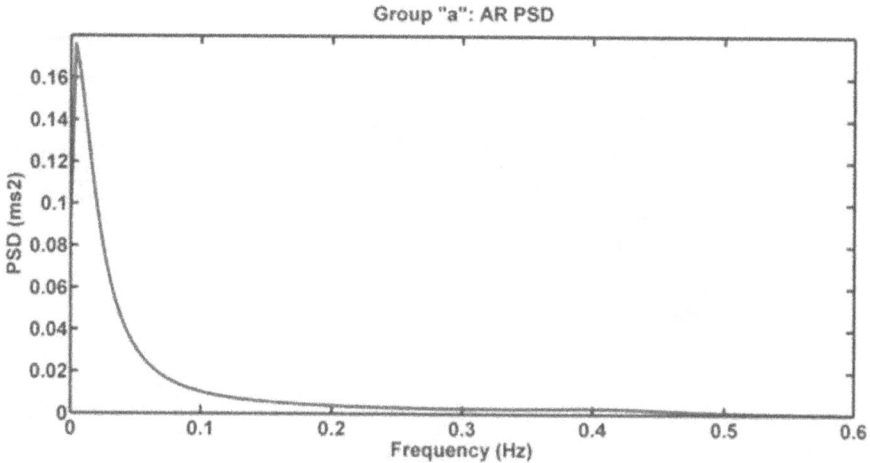

FIGURE 16.6 Sample representation of PSD by AR modeling in the age group "a."

of the frequency range like high, low, and very low, and variations occur in different age groups as well. Features from nonlinear HRV methods like SD1, SD2 of Poincare plot, ApEn of approximate entropy, and SampEn of sample entropy have been computed by considering all age groups. Nonlinear methods of HRV analysis can extract the inherent characteristics of biomedical signal like nonstationarity and nonlinear dynamics. All nonlinear indices exhibit a tapered-off nature of feature values with increasing age groups, which corresponds to the physiological and psychological aging of human organs. Both ApEn and SampEn, which describe the periodicity of the data for normal subjects, basically have a smaller overall

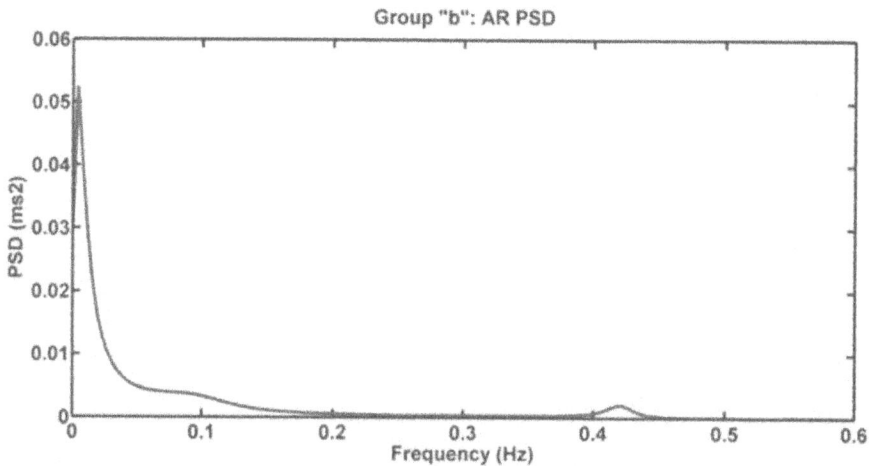

FIGURE 16.7 Sample representation of PSD by AR modeling in the age group "b."

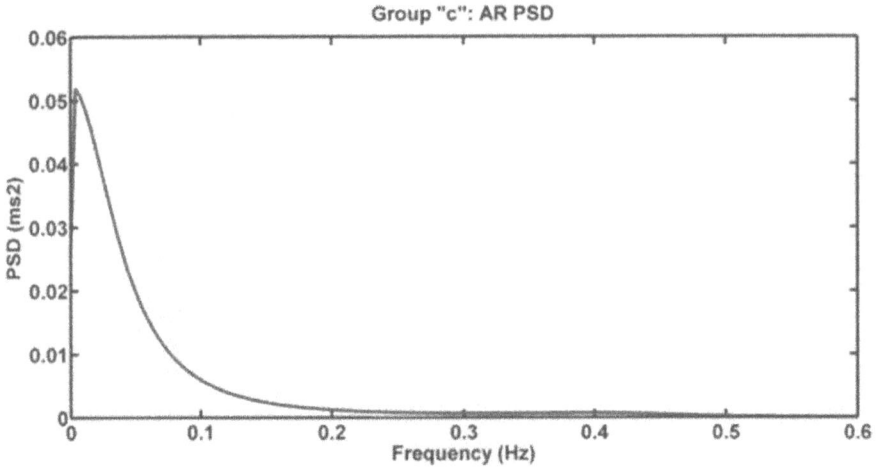

FIGURE 16.8   Sample representation of PSD by AR modeling in the age group "c."

range to express themselves but have slightly diminished values with increasing age groups. Figures 16.10 and 16.11 describe the Poincare plots age groups "a," "b," "c," and "d," respectively. From these figures, the spread of the data can be easily observed.

The data are more spread and away from the origin in the age group "a," and subsequently this spread of data is diminishing and moving toward the origin as age increases. For a comparative analysis of ApEn and SampEn, nonlinear parameters that consider all age groups have been depicted with the help of boxplots in Figure 16.12. Both the ApEn and SampEn indices have smaller ranges. In these smaller

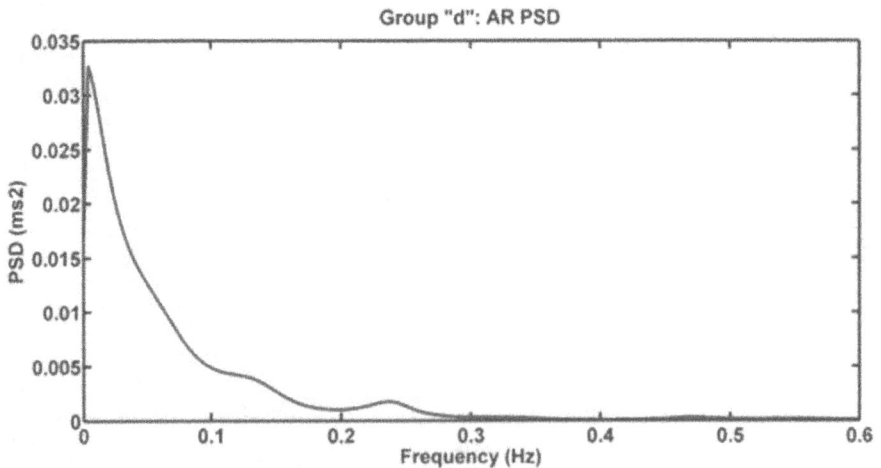

FIGURE 16.9   Sample representation of PSD by AR modeling in the age group "d."

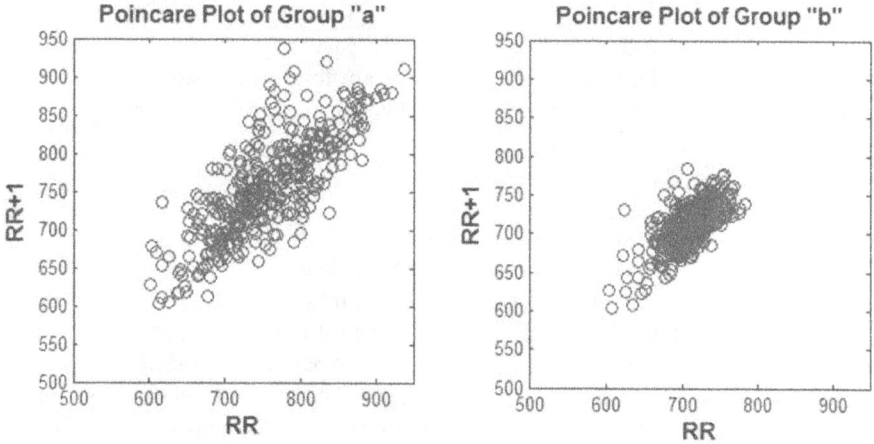

FIGURE 16.10   Sample representation of Poincare plots in the group "a" and group "b."

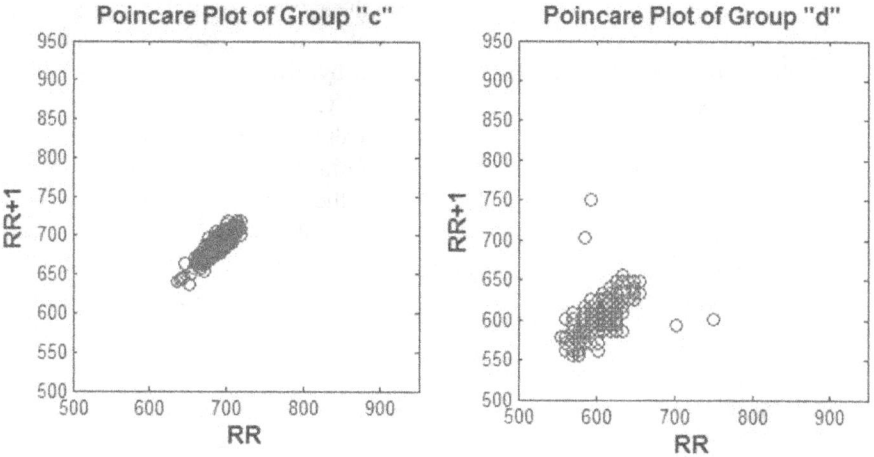

FIGURE 16.11   Sample representation of Poincare plots in the group "c" and group "d."

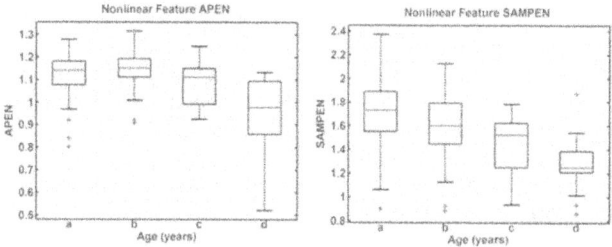

FIGURE 16.12   Boxplot of ApEn and SampEn.

ranges, it can be well observed that the values of indices diminish with progressive age groups though in the smaller quantities. In general, with the global scenario, all TD, AR-based FD, and nonlinear features are following a similar trend when compared with earlier research, although data acquisition has been carried out in the South Asian subcontinent region.

16.4 CONCLUSION

This study has attempted to analyze and diagnose heart rate variability by the features computed from the time domain, AR-based frequency domain, and nonlinear methods on normal healthy female subjects in four different age groups. The trend of variations in heart rate variability indices is measure based, but most of the heart rate variability indices decline with age. However, their normalized contribution toward autonomic control activity clearly shows the heart rate variability indices change with the aging process in women. Nonlinear methods of HRV analysis provide supportive significant information along with the time domain and frequency domain of linear methods, which are basic and yet effective measures to observe the discriminative idea of different age groups in normal healthy female subjects. This present study regarding HRV parameter variations with the aging of normal female subjects may help establish normal limits of HRV parameters in four psychosomatically different phases of total life span that are affected by different psychophysiological conditions of the body. There is a general saying: "Communities and countries and ultimately the world are only as strong as the health of their women." Hence, this methodology will provide a better tool to discriminate the normal healthy female subjects with different age groups and to establish the normal limits of HRV parameters in different phases of life span from young girl subjects to elderly women. This work enables us to compare HRV in different female age groups according to various HRV measures. These distinct HRV indices with female age will be helpful in preventing diseases related to ANS.

REFERENCES

1. Shimazu, T., N. Tamura, K. Shimazu. 2005. "Aging of the autonomic nervous system." *Nippon Rinsho*. **63**, no. 6: 973–977.
2. Acharya, U. R., N. Kannathal, O. W. Seng, L. Y. Ping, T. L. Chua. 2004. "Heart rate analysis in normal subjects of various age groups." *Biomedical Online Journal*. **3**: 24.
3. Lipsitz, L. A., J. Mietus, G. B. Moody, A. L. Goldberger. 1990. "Spectral characteristics of heart rate variability before and during postural tilt: Relations to aging and risk of syncope." *Circulation*. **81**: 1803–1810.
4. Malarvili, M. B., Mostefa Mesbah, Boualem Boashash. 2007. "Time-frequency analysis of heart rate variability for Neonatal Seizure detection." *Australasian Physical and Engineering Sciences in Medicine*. **29**: 1–10.
5. Faes, Luca, Ki H. Chon, Giandomenico Nollo. 2009. "A method for the time-varying nonlinear prediction of complex nonstationary biomedical signals." *IEEE Transactions on Biomedical Engineering*. **56**: 205–209.
6. Goya-Esteban, R., J. P. Marques de S, J. L. Rojo-Alvarez, O. Barquero-Perez. 2008. "Characterization of heart rate variability loss with aging and heart failure using sample entropy." In *Proceedings of the 2008 Computers in Cardiology*, Bologna, Italy: 41–44.

7. Umetani, K. U., D. H. Singer, R. McCraty, M. Atkinson. 1998. "Twenty-four hour time domain heart rate variability and heart rate: Relation to age and gender over nine decades." *Journal of American College of Cardiology.* **31**: 593–601.

8. Meersman, R. E. D., P. K. Stein. 2007. "Vagal modulation and aging." *Biomedical Psychology.* **74**: 165–173.

9. Task Force of European Society of Cardiology and the North American Society of Pacing and Electrophysiology. 1996. "Heart rate variability-standards of measurement, physiological interpretation and clinical interpretation and clinical use." *European Heart Journal.* **17**: 354–381.

10. Poddar, M. G., V. Kumar, Y. P. Sharma. 2013. "Linear-nonlinear heart rate variability analysis and SVM based classification of normal and hypertensive subjects." *Journal of Electrocardiology.* **46**: e25.

11. Poddar, M. G., V. Kumar, Y. P. Sharma. 2014. "Heart rate variability based classification of normal and hypertension cases by linear-nonlinear method." *Defence Science Journal.* **64**: 542–548.

12. Poddar, M. G., V. Kumar, Y. P. Sharma. 2015. "Automated diagnosis of coronary artery diseased patients by heart rate variability analysis using linear and non-linear methods." *Journal of Medical Engineering & Technology.* **39**: 331–341.

13. Poddar, M. G., Anjali C. Birajdar, Jitendra Virmani, et al. 2019. "Automated classification of hypertension and coronary artery disease patients by PNN, KNN, and SVM classifiers using hrv analysis." *Machine Learning in Bio-Signal Analysis and Diagnostic Imaging.* Amsterdam, the Netherlands: Elsevier, pp. 99–125.

14. Crone, Eveline A., Riek J. M. Somsen, Kiki Zanolie, Maurits W. Van der Molen. 2006. "A heart rate analysis of developmental change in feedback processing and rule shifting from childhood to early adulthood." *Journal of Experimental Child Psychology.* **95**: 99–116.

15. Longin, Elke, Carmen Dimitriadis, Samina Shazi, Thorsten Gerstner, Tamara Lenz, Stephan König. 2009. "Autonomic nervous system function in infants and adolescents: Impact of autonomic tests on heart rate variability." *Paediatric Cardiology.* **30**: 311–324.

16. Bricout, Véronique-Aurélie, Simon DeChenaud, Anne Favre-Juvin. 2010. "Analyses of heart rate variability in young soccer players: The effects of sport activity." *Autonomic Neuroscience.* **154**: 112–116.

17. Perseguini, N. M., A. C. M. Takahashi, J. R. Rebelatto, E. Silva, A. Borghi-Silva, A. Porta, N. Montano, A. M. Catai. 2011. "Spectral and symbolic analysis of the effect of gender and postural change on cardiac autonomic modulation in healthy elderly subjects." *Brazilian Journal of Medical and Biological Research.* **44**: 29–37.

18. Vandeput, Steven, Bart Verheyden, A. E. Aubert, Sabine Van Huffel. 2012. "Nonlinear heart rate dynamics: Circadian profile and influence of age and gender." *Medical Engineering and Physics.* **34**: 108–117.

19. Abhishekh, Hulegar A., Palgun Nisarga, Ravikiran Kisan, Adoor Meghana, Sajish Chandran, Trichur Raju, Talakad N. Sathyaprabha. 2013. "Influence of age and gender on autonomic regulation of heart." *Journal of Clinical Monitoring and Computing.* **27**: 259–264.

20. Poddar, M. G., V. Kumar, Y. P. Sharma. 2015. "Heart rate variability: Analysis and classification of healthy subjects for different age groups." In *Proceedings of IEEE International Conference on Computing for Sustainable Global Development*, New Delhi, India.

21. Choi, J., W. Cha, M. G. Park. 2020. "Declining trends of heart rate variability according to aging in healthy Asian adults." *Frontiers in Aging Neuroscience.* **12**: 610626.

22. Silva, Carla Cristiane, Ligia Maxwell Pereira, Jefferson Rosa Cardosa, Jonathan Patrick Moore, Fábio Yuzo Nakamura. 2014. "The effect of physical training on heart rate variability in healthy children: A systematic review with meta-analysis." *Pediatric Exercise Science.* **26**: 147–158.

23. Voss, A., R. Schroeder, A. Heitmann, A. Peters, S. Perz. 2015. "Short-term heart rate variability—Influence of gender and age in healthy subjects." *PLoS ONE*. **10**: e0118308.

24. Garavaglia, L., D. Gulich, M. M. Defeo, Mailland J. Thomas, I. M. Irurzun. 2021. "The effect of age on the heart rate variability of healthy subjects." *PLoS ONE*. **16**: e0255894.

25. Chung, E. K. 1989. *Principles of Cardiac Arrhythmias*. 4th edition, Baltimore, MD: Williams and Wilkins, 3–4.

26. Carvalho, J. L. A., A. F. Rocha, I. Dos Santos, C. Itoki, L. F. Junqueira, F. A. O. Nascimento. 2003. "Study on the optimal order for the auto-regressive time frequency analysis of heart rate variability." *IEEE EMBS 25th Annual International Conference*, September.

27. Aurelien, P., R. Manuel, A. J. Sophie, B. Claire de, D. Andre. 2006. "Spectral analysis of heart rate variability: Interchangeability between autoregressive analysis and fast Fourier transform." *Journal of Electrocardiology*. **39**: 31–37.

28. Poddar, M. G., V. Kumar, Y. P. Sharma. 2013. "Linear – nonlinear heart rate variability analysis and SVM based classification of normal and hypertensive subjects." *Proceedings of the 40th International Congress on Electrocardiology*, Glasgow, Scotland, 89–95.

17 EEG Signal Analysis Using Machine Learning and Artificial Intelligence for Identification of Brain Dysfunction

Rajeswari Aghoram[1] and S. B. Athira[2]
[1]Department of Neurology, Jawaharlal Institute of Postgraduate Medical Education and Research, Pondicherry, India
[2]Department of Physiology, Jawaharlal Institute of Postgraduate Medical Education and Research, Pondicherry, India

CONTENTS

DOI: 10.1201/9781003324430-21

17.1   INTRODUCTION

The neuron is an excitable electrical tissue that is polarized such that it receives input at the dendrites, provides output through its axons, and forms connections with other neurons called synapses. The brain is made of billions of such neurons connected in complex patterns to form neuronal networks. The cortical oscillations produced by these networked neurons are vital to the ability of the brain to process information. Sensors on the scalp measure the summated potential difference at a point on the scalp produced by the underlying oscillatory brain electrical activity. They record the extracellular current flow secondary to the synaptic activity. Other important contributors to scalp electrical signals include calcium spikes, intrinsic currents, after-hyperpolarizations, gap junctions, glial interactions, and ephatic effects [1]. The summation of all electrical activity within a volume of brain tissue at a given location in the extracellular medium can be measured in volts. A spatiotemporally smoothed record of such voltage changes using sensors on the scalp is called an electroencephalogram (EEG). The other methods of measuring the electrical activity are listed in Table 17.1.

In this chapter, we will restrict ourselves to scalp EEG. This is a simple noninvasive procedure that can be performed in outpatient settings. It is recorded using 17–32 electrodes placed on the scalp with standardized placements. When more than 64 electrodes are used, it is called high-density EEG. EEG can be looked upon as a multivariate discrete time series that carries a wealth of information about the underlying brain activity. EEG patterns vary with age, the mental state of the patient,

TABLE 17.1
Different Methods of Recording Brain Electrical Activity [1, 2]

Method	Description
Video EEG	EEG accompanied by time-locked video recording. Often used to record and classify events.
Ambulatory EEG	EEG recordings where patient is ambulatory. Uses wireless technology. Often fewer channels are used.
Amplitude averaged EEG	EEG records used in neonates; long-term recording using fewer channels where amplitude is averaged. Used for identifying neonatal seizures and monitoring hypoxic ischemic encephalopathy, etc.
ICU EEG	Continuous EEG with or without video; used in ICU settings for evaluation of disorders of consciousness and status epilepticus.
Invasive EEG	Using electrodes placed on the surface of the brain during surgery (electrocorticogram) or deep in the parenchyma (Stereo-EEG). They record the local field potentials and are often used prior to epilepsy surgery.
Magnetic encephalography	Studies the magnetic activity produced secondary to the electrical activity in the brain.
Voltage sensitive dye imaging	Optically image the voltage changes in genetically engineered neurons expressing voltage sensitive dyes.

drugs, etc. The duration, frequency, type of recording, and use of activation procedures also can influence the ability of EEG to predict underlying brain abnormalities. EEG records are currently read by an expert who visually inspects the EEG recordings for abnormalities. The abnormal patterns that are commonly obtained are in Table 17.2 [3].

Interpreting an EEG and recognizing abnormal patterns is a time-consuming exercise. Technicians and physicians who read EEGs undergo many years of training that is highly variable in its breadth and depth. Experience of the expert, inconsistency of reporting over time, unclear thresholding for flagging abnormalities, and subjectively defined frequency criteria may all contribute to further variability in EEG reporting. This means the interrater agreement for a given abnormality is only moderate [4] but improves when classification requires only grouping as normal or abnormal EEG [5]. Attempts have been made to standardize such reporting in the field of epilepsy and have been reasonably successful [6].

EEG signals have low signal-to-noise ratios [2]. Between the electrode on the scalp and the electrically active neural tissue, multiple capacitive layers including

TABLE 17.2
Abnormal EEG Patterns Commonly Encountered

Name	Frequency	Spatial Location	Common Pathologic Correlates
Focal polymorphic slow activity	Delta range (1–4 Hz) or theta range (4–7 Hz)	Localized to few leads	Underlying tumor, stroke, abscess, etc.
Generalized polymorphic slow activity	Delta or theta range	Generalized	Encephalopathies of metabolic, toxic, or infectious origin
Intermittent monomorphic slow activity	Delta or theta range	Focal, intermittent	Frontal localization in encephalopathy, lateralized focal involvement in deep (thalamic/periventricular) structural nature
Voltage attenuation	Variable, but reduction in amplitude	Focal or generalized	Focal-porencephaly or extra-axial hemorrhage, meningioma; generalized: anoxia, electrocerebral silence in brain death
Epileptiform discharges	Sharp waves & spikes: beta range, high amplitude, sometimes followed by slow wave	Focal or generalized Ictal or interictal discharges	Focal: focal cortical dysplasia and other focal epilepsy syndrome Generalized: absence epilepsy, juvenile myoclonic epilepsy, etc.

Others: Periodic complexes: generalized, bilateral, lateralized; stimulus-induced rhythmic, periodic, or ictal discharges.

bone and skin exist. These layers function as a low-frequency filter, reduce the amplitude of potential differences, and cause "smearing" of the electrical activity. This causes the activity measured by neighboring scalp electrodes to be highly spatially correlated [1, 2]. Such correlation presents difficulties with source localization, which is also called the inverse problem.

Further, the face and head area, where the electrodes are placed, have many muscles used for both voluntary and involuntary activities, like changing gaze, expressing emotion, articulation, eating, etc. Thus, there are multiple physiological events including muscle action and eye movement that contaminate the EEG and are called artifacts [1, 2]. Apart from these physiological artifacts, line noise and other electrical interference also affect EEG recordings. Individual skull shape and size are different. To accommodate these differences, standardized electrode placement methods using measurements of various circumferences of the head are used. Such externally marked placements are limited in their ability to correspond to specific brain areas. For instance, F8/F9 are frontal electrodes, but they mostly measure activity from the temporal poles [6]. Other technical factors like impedance and electrode contact also affect the quality of recordings.

The advent of the second disruption has opened new avenues for EEG processing. Machine learning can rapidly sift through, analyze, and classify data, and is a promising new tool for EEG analysis. The high dimensionality of EEG coupled with the difficulties in obtaining sufficient expertise makes it ideal problem to be tackled by automation [6]. Machine learning using EEG can function as early alarm mechanisms and screening tools, particularly in resource-poor areas. They can also provide standardized reporting that can be translated across settings and compared directly. Further, they can function as signal decoders for brain computer interfaces. They can also be used for artifact removal, data augmentation, and multimodal integration. The advantages and problems associated with using machine learning in EEG are summarized in Table 17.3.

A review of all the literature in signal processing and artificial intelligence in EEG is beyond the scope of the current chapter due to the sheer volume of information.

TABLE 17.3

Using Machine Learning in EEG Analysis: Advantages and Problems

Advantages	Problems
Current methods of interpretation are time consuming	Low signal-to-noise ratio in EEG
Expertise requires years of training and often is inconsistent	High spatial correlation between electrodes
Resource-poor settings are left out	Inverse problem
High-dimensional time-variant data	"Black box learning" in unsupervised machine learning may not be appropriate for clinical decision making
Excellent temporal resolution	Data availability in public domain is limited
Standardized reporting	High intersubject and intrasubject variability

Therefore, in this chapter, we restrict ourselves to the various machine learning methods that have been used in literature to process routine scalp EEGs to manage various brain pathologies.

17.2 METHODOLOGY

We performed a literature search using keywords and the medical subheading (Mesh) terminology for machine learning, artificial intelligence, and electroencephalography in PubMed using appropriate Boolean operators. The relevant study abstracts were included after screening. We also searched the references of chosen articles and used Google search using keywords for salient articles. The results are presented qualitatively. We then filtered the results for original articles in the previous year. We used the title and abstract to identify the themes in the research presented. The results of this analysis are presented graphically and using text.

17.3 RESULTS AND DISCUSSION

The PubMed search was last conducted on September 23, 2021. It identified 3,281 individual articles, including 140 reviews. Most (2,235; 68.1%) were published in the last 10 years. Two hundred and seventy original research articles that were published in the preceding year were analyzed thematically. The focus of these articles showed over 31 individual areas where machine learning approaches have been used to analyze scalp EEG (Figure 17.1). Brain computer interfaces, cognitive processes, epilepsy, and sleep staging were the domains most often studied.

In the following sections, we review the various methodologies associated with processing EEGs and discuss the current state-of-the-art applications of ML/DL with EEG in some individual neurological disorders.

17.3.1 Machine Learning Pipelines for EEG

Machine learning leverages computing technology and statistics to model large amounts of data to classify or make predictions. With the advent of parallel computing and the graphic processing units, the field of machine learning has expanded to include artificial neural networks and deep learning algorithms. Though ML has been used to process EEG since the 1990s, the last decade has seen an exponential growth in the literature. EEG processing using ML pipelines is shown in Figure 17.2.

17.3.1.1 Preprocessing of EEG

EEG, particularly scalp EEG, has a low signal-to-noise ratio and hence, preprocessing steps are important in EEG analysis. The methodological variations across studies in this step result in problems with the ability to replicate results [7]. During EEG preprocessing, the researcher identifies the time window to be used; the frequency band of interest and appropriate filtering procedures; electrodes to be studied depending upon the nature of the experiment and the quality of recording; the reference to be used; rejection of extraneous artifacts; and exclusion of outliers. To standardize these procedures, ML pipelines have been proposed. Different pipelines

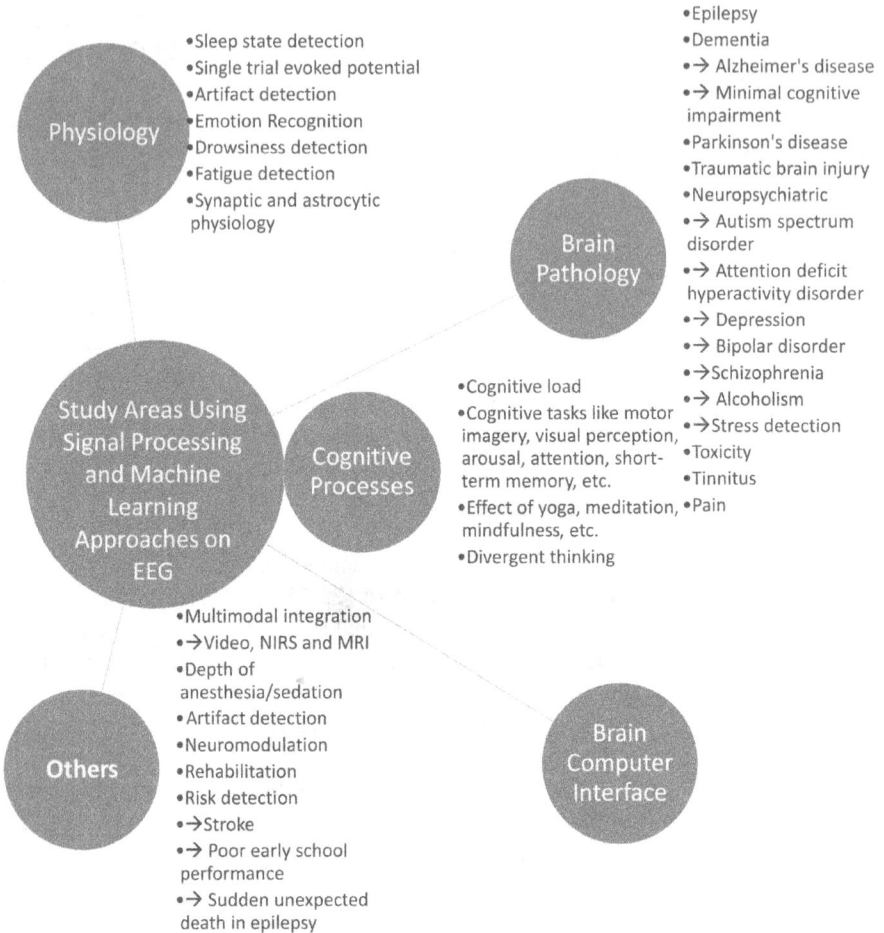

FIGURE 17.1 Domain areas of papers using the machine learning approach EEG.

offer variable functionalities and may be suitable for different studies. For instance, the PREP pipeline removes line noise and performs an average referencing and can be used generically, while HAPPE from Harvard corrects artifacts but cannot be used for evoked response EEG studies. EEG processing open-source scripts (EPOS) is the latest addition to these preprocessing pipelines and can be applied in all types of EEG studies [7]. EEG raw signal has also been used with success as input in some deep learning algorithms.

17.3.1.2 Architecture

Supervised, unsupervised, and neural networks have all been employed in the evaluation of EEG. Of late, there is a trend toward greater use of neural networks [8]. The advantage of neural networks and deep learning algorithms is that they can be used for end-to-end processing without need for feature engineering and much preprocessing. There is also some evidence to suggest that deep learning algorithms may be

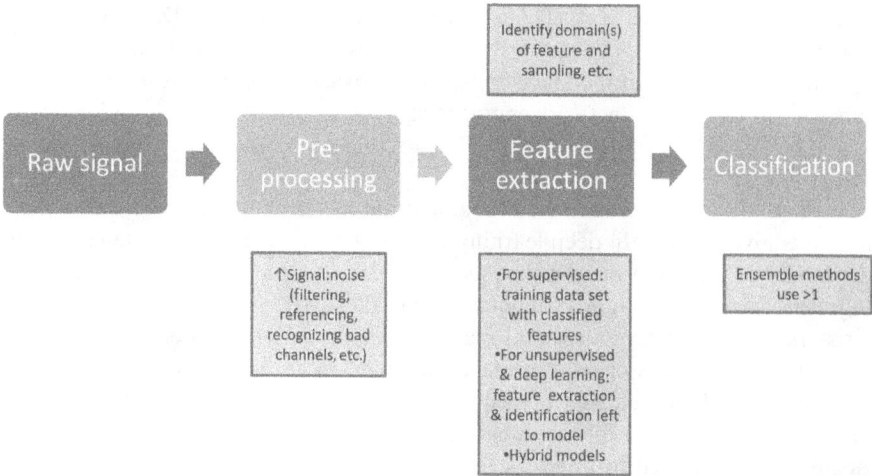

FIGURE 17.2   Process flow diagram for ML/DL in EEG.

more accurate than other supervised machine learning methods [8]. Of the various neural network architectures, convoluted neural networks (CNNs) are the most used in EEG studies [8]. This may be the result of their remarkable success in image and natural language processing and also because CNNs allow hierarchical processing while enabling dimensionality reduction. Due to the time-variant nature of EEG, recurrent neural networks have also been used, particularly long short-term memory (LSTM). Shallower architectures seem to provide better accuracy than deeper architectures in EEG studies [8].

17.3.1.3   Feature Extraction

EEG is time-variant, spatially correlated multidimensional data. Feature extraction for EEG is thus a time-consuming activity. It can be done manually (supervised) or using automation (unsupervised) [9]. Input to ML can be calculated features, images, or raw signals [10]. Calculated features can belong to the frequency domain, time domain, spatial features, connectivity measures, complexity measures, or a combination of these. These can be simple, like power spectral density, or more complex, like fractal components. Input for ML can also be created by mapping features to generate images. This approach has been particularly successful for convoluted neural networks. As EEG signals are nonstationary, it may be difficult to understand signal dynamics solely based on observed patterns in the time series [11]. Some approaches to deal with this include use of wavelet transform and time-variant autoregressive models. More than one feature can also be used. The features can be selected manually based on the task at hand, such as power spectral density in studies of sensorimotor rhythms or event-related synchronization and desynchronization in brain computer interface applications [12]. This needs considerable domain expertise. Automated approaches to feature selection include independent and principal component analysis, but these again are constrained by the features selected as input to these models [8, 10]. In deep learning algorithms, the feature selection is left entirely to the network. The nature of features identified by DL algorithms is not obvious and is difficult to reconstruct. As networks may have to be engineered to optimize the function of the algorithms, some experts argue that DL replaces "feature engineering" with "network engineering."

17.3.1.4   Training

The extracted feature is then classified, and the labels compared to a training set in an iterative process. In deep learning algorithms, these errors are often added to the model as a penalty or cost that should be minimized [8]. Unsupervised training using back-propagation techniques often takes a very long time, and there is a risk of getting stuck in local minima of the cost function. This can be overcome by pretraining models or using transfer learning. Deep belief networks restricted Boltzmann machines, etc., have been used to provide an appropriate representation of the EEG input signal for the target task classification as part of pretraining [11]. Regularization is used to impose certain constraints on the neural network while training so that the results are more generalizable [8]. In EEG studies, weight decay, early stopping, dropout, and label smoothing have all been utilized for regularization, though weight decay appears to be the most common method. Optimizers are used to maintain the balance between training error and test error by updating parameters. The most used optimizer is Adam, as it well suited for nonstationary and noisy data like EEG [8]. Hyperparameter searching is another important step in training. Grid search, manual, and Bayesian optimization have all been used to find the best hyperparameter set. Most studies that reported on the methods used to find the optimum hyperparameter have reported using grid or manual search [8].

17.3.1.5   Decoding

The final step for all ML algorithms is some sort of classification or labeling. The result of such ML output is reported most often as accuracy of classification. The accuracy is evaluated using test data. Test data, also called the test set, is kept separate from the training and validation set [10]. Sometimes cross-validation using a "leave one out cross-validation" approach or a combination of cross-validation and test set are used in EEG studies. The results of such classification can also be compared across algorithms. In EEG studies, it has been criticized that the performance of the DL algorithm is often compared some very simple ML models such as SVM. However, there is some evidence that in EEG research, simple classification models may perform as well as state-of-the-art research [13]. Apart from accuracy, in EEG studies, it is also important to consider inter- and intrasubject variability and how the algorithm handles this [10]. ML algorithms perform well with intrasubject variability, and more recently DL algorithms have shown reasonable success in handling intersubject variability also.

17.3.1.6   Other Considerations

Most machine learning algorithms are data hungry and perform better with more data. There is limited EEG data that are available in the public domain, and by nature EEG is high dimensional. These two factors together contribute to the so-called "curse of dimensionality problem." As with all machine learning algorithms, there is the added risk of generalization, and over- or underfitting of data [12]. Reproducibility of the study results remains an issue with ML. The reasons are the availability of code and data, both of which are limited in the public domain. The reporting of these studies is also not uniform. Further, the algorithms are trained against labeling by experts. Expert opinion is often inconsistent, leading to reduced replicability [10]. Establishment of publicly available EEG data corpus like the TUH database and an ongoing effort to standardize reporting procedures of ML studies may improve things in the near future [8].

17.3.2   ML Applications Using EEG in Brain Pathology

17.3.2.1   Stroke

Stroke is an emergency characterized by a sudden onset a focal neurological deficit due to ischemia or hemorrhage in an area of central nervous system. Visual EEG changes that can be seen in stroke include focal slow wave activity, periodic lateralized epileptiform discharges, and voltage attenuation. The use of EEG in acute stroke has been limited principally by time required for acquisition and interpretation. With the advent of dry electrodes and machine learning, there is now increasing interest in the utility of EEG in stroke. The pathological processes causing tissue destruction and recovery processes including neuroplasticity can result in EEG changes. This accentuates the preexisting inter- and intrasubject variability of EEG and is another challenge in using ML for stroke EEG [14]. The ability of DL to handle such differences has made it the preferred approach in stroke studies.

DL models have been employed for diagnosis and prognosis of stroke. A model using a deep learning approach with EEG and clinical characteristics was shown to perform better (area under curve of receiver operating characteristic [ROC] curve 87.8) than clinical characteristics alone (area under the curve [AUC]: 62.3) in identifying patients experiencing stroke or transient ischemic attack and for identifying large vessel occlusion (AUC 86.4 vs. 80.4) [15]. Similar accuracy rates have been reported with deep learning of EEG signals in elderly stroke patients [16]. Machine learning methods trained on 19 channel EEG in combination with a baseline scale to measure severity of stroke (National Institutes of Health Stroke Severity Scale) performed better than the stroke severity scale alone in predicting 6-month outcomes (AUC 0.8 vs. 0.7 $p<0.05$) [17]. Discrimination of poststroke dementia from normal controls and mild cognitive impairment was shown to improve with machine learning. The authors used a hybrid preprocessing approach for artifact removal, extracted three entropy features (spectral, permutation, and Tsallis), and used two classification schemes with fuzzy neighborhood preserving analysis and QR decomposition. They found that this approach provides classification accuracy for vascular dementia of 90.4% [18].

By far, the largest amount of work in machine learning with EEG in stroke is on brain–computer interfaces (BCI) [19]. BCI have been used in the rehabilitation of both motor and nonmotor deficits following stroke. This can take the approach of augmenting using an external device or facilitating recovery by enhancing neuroplasticity [20]. It can also be used to track the changes in brain activity during recovery [14] and rehabilitation [21]. The use of motor imagery–related signals in stroke patients to control external devices like a wheelchair or neuro-prosthesis was first demonstrated in 2008 [22]. A magnetoencephalography (MEG)-based system was used in this study to pick up brain electrical activity. EEG, being easier and less expensive to record, has since replaced MEG, and various machine learning algorithms have been successfully used to extract motor imagery–related features. Another approach uses BCI to reward attempted movement and promote neuroplasticity with the aim of facilitating motor recovery [14]. Machine learning algorithms to facilitate neurofeedback using EEG signals, to enhance emotional and cognitive recovery, have also been studied [20].

17.3.2.2 Neuropsychiatric Disorders

The management of neuropsychiatric disorders is increasingly moving away from a diagnosis-based management to a more personalized approach using patterns of behavior and psychopathology [23]. Such pattern recognition can be done as well or better by ML. ML techniques used include SVM, KNN, and random forest apart from DL. Advanced imaging data and EEG are the most common type of data used [24]. EEG, being cheaper and noninvasive, is increasingly explored in the areas of psychobiology. EEG studies using ML or DL algorithms are most common for depression, schizophrenia, autism spectrum disorder, and attention deficit hyperactivity disorder [23]. A recent systematic review of studies using DL techniques showed that resting EEG was most often used for diagnosis of the neuropsychiatric condition. A few studies have used DL/ML on EEG to explore response to therapy or progression of disease. For depression, the hemispheric asymmetry is the most often studied feature for identification of depression [25]. The CNN with a variable number of hidden layers is the most used architecture [23]. The most common features were time domain features, though often with filtering at specific frequencies. The studies in this review reported accuracies of ML for the various tasks to be between 69–99% [23].

17.3.2.3 Epilepsy

Epilepsy is characterized by seizures, and seizures are defined as an abnormal synchronous excitation of a neuronal population [26]. The EEG records the brain's electrical activity and is an important tool for diagnosis, monitoring, and managing epilepsy. EEG changes in epilepsy can vary depending on whether the EEG is recorded during a seizure (ictal), just before a seizure (preictal) or long after a seizure (interictal). Interictal changes include focal or generalized spikes and sharp waves apart from focal slow wave activity. Preictal records usually show a change in background with a buildup that culminates in the seizure. This is variable in morphology and tempo. Ictal records often have spikes and are contaminated by movement artifacts. Thus, invasive EEG with fewer artifacts is better for studying ictal EEG changes. A large body of work exists on the use of ML in epilepsy as follows:

  I. Seizure detection
     Seizure detection and classification are necessary for appropriate management of the patient. However, EEG signatures of seizures differ between patients and between seizures in the same patient. Support vector machines,

Naive Bayes, random forest classification, RNN, and CNN have all been studied for seizure detection [27, 28]. These methods have shown accuracy of >80% using both single features and multiple features [27]. There is some suggestion that using a feature-based decoding framework can achieve accuracies similar to DL for seizure detection [28]. "Line length" is a time-frequency domain feature that is sensitive to frequency and amplitude while also serving as a measure of complexity. This has been particularly successful in classifying seizure and nonseizure [29]. Seizure type classification has also been done using scalp EEG with good success [30].

II. Seizure prediction

Prediction of seizure is an important clinical outcome, particularly if done with adequate lead time. This can allow early alarm systems that can enable patient safety measures and possibly abortive therapy [31, 32]. The challenge here is to identify the preictal EEG. Apart from the inter- and intrasubject variability, another problem with seizure prediction using ML is that the training data set is likely to be imbalanced due to the unpredictable and episodic nature of seizures [29]. Further, data processing should be real-time for the process to be meaningful. The nonstationarity of EEG data becomes more important for this task than in others like evoked responses [11]. Investigators have also integrated EEG with other clinical or physiological measures features for prediction tasks. Algorithms that have been studied include SVM, Gaussian mixture models, CNN, and RNN. DL algorithms are increasingly preferred due to their ability to use raw EEG, which makes real-time processing easy. Hybrid DL architectures such as deep belief networks followed by CNN or CNN in combination with RNN are also common. The reported sensitivities are 70.5–92.8%, specificities are 61–90.6%, and lead times are 1–45 minutes [33].

III. Seizure localization

EEG channels exhibit high spatial correlation, and scalp EEG has blind zones where neural activity is not reflected in surface recording, such as medial aspects of the cortex or depths of sulci. Thus, scalp EEG alone is often not used for localization [31].

IV. Others

Epileptic networks in the brain can be modeled in silico, and such models can be used to make predictions about surgical margins, drug response, response to neuromodulatory techniques, etc. [30]. This requires multimodal integration of EEG data along with imaging, clinical, and possibly genetic data. Such integration has been done using ML. Such multimodal integration including EEG data has been used to localize seizure onset zone and deliver personalized epilepsy medicine [32].

17.3.2.4 Continuous EEG Monitoring

This type of EEG monitoring is done in the critical care units for detecting seizure activity, dosing sedation, and monitoring encephalopathy. Seizure detection ML in ICU settings are commercially available (RiskSLIM, Neurotrend), though their accuracy is not very good [34]. For monitoring encephalopathy, SVMs have been traditionally used. More recently, researchers have used CNN and LSTM together and have shown that such a hybrid algorithm has an AUC of 0.8 for detecting delirium and can predict level of consciousness with an accuracy of 70% compared to nurse-technician agreement of 59% to detect change in level by one on the Richmond Agitation Sedation Scale for level of consciousness [35]. By extension, continuous EEG can also be used to monitor depth of anesthesia and titrate sedation. Using a hybrid of LSTM and sparse denoising autoencoder on multiple features extracted from EEG, Li et al. [36] demonstrated a predictive probability for depth of anesthesia of 0.8556.

17.3.2.5 Dementia

Of the various causes for dementia, Alzheimer's disease is the most common neurodegenerative condition. EEG changes in neurodegenerative dementias may result from direct neuronal dysfunction and/or the changes in connectivity [37]. Lower alpha power and higher delta power in Alzheimer's disease has been reported by many authors. SVM and KNN have been commonly used to identify Alzheimer's disease. Some studies also sought to correlate EEG changes to progression of cognitive decline [38]. Most studies have used resting state EEG as task EEG is often more difficult to interpret. Apart from power spectral density, other features like entropy to measure complexity and phase lag index to measure coherence have also been used. Deep learning methods like CNN have also been studied for this task.

Apart from the preceding discussed brain pathologies, machine learning algorithms for EEG have been developed in areas of estimation of cognitive load associated with stress and anxiety, other types of dementia like Cruetzfeldt Jakob disease, traumatic brain injury, and neuro infections.

17.4   IMPACT OF ML/DL

Potential applications of ML/DL technology in the field of EEG are many. In routine patient care, these technologies can provide predictive platforms using EEG to accomplish diagnosis. As discussed previously, this is an area where a lot of research is ongoing. ML/DL can also be used to screen EEG for common abnormal patterns and provide more standardized reporting. This is of particular benefit in resource-poor settings where the availability of domain expertise is often limited. EEG can also be potentially leveraged to provide functional maps of the networks of the brain similar to other functional imaging modalities like functional magnetic resonance imaging. Considering the sheer volume of data that need to be analyzed for such mapping, it can only be done with use of artificial intelligence. Such maps can be superimposed on structural imaging, again with the help of similar technology, to provide guidance for neurosurgical and neuromodulatory procedures. Real-time processing of EEG using AI can be used to feed into brain–computer interfaces that can perform tasks ranging from simple ones such as turning on lights to complex tasks like surgeries using robots. Such processing power can also be leveraged to provide therapeutic alternatives such as responsive neurostimulation for conditions like epilepsy. Finally, the hope of personalized or precision medicine for a whole range of neurological and neuropsychiatric conditions can be realized using AI technology by integrating EEG with other modalities. Thus, disruptive technology using EEG can enable faster, more reliable, and more equitable care pathways for patients.

17.5   LIMITATIONS

This is a qualitative summary of the work done using machine learning on EEG for evaluation of brain pathologies. The list of pathologies is long, and it would not be possible to summarize all the work done in every field. Here we have concentrated on the most common conditions that are encountered in routine clinical practice. For any given brain pathology, one can create algorithms for diagnosis, therapeutic classification and prognosis. Most studies on ML with EEG have so far focused only on diagnosis. Exploration of this technique for other uses has only been done in the field of epilepsy. Another important aspect not covered in this review is multimodal integration with imaging such as MRI or with video or other physiological signals like electromyogram. Such integration is possible with ML. This type of integration often combines complementary information that can improve performance of the algorithm, though it makes it more complex. Finally, one should bear in mind that ML and DL fields are rapidly evolving, and knowledge is accruing at a rapid pace. Hence reviews only provide an indication of the nature and amount of work done; more details can be obtained only by going back to the literature.

17.6   CONCLUSION

EEG is a noninvasive measure of brain function that has been around for over 70 years. It is high-dimensional, time-variant data that are reflective of the complexity of the underlying brain activity. Machine learning and deep learning methods are uncovering faster and newer methods to leverage this information to enable better clinical management. Data paucity is an important bottleneck. This can be overcome by using pretraining or innovative ML to generate EEG and augment data. Similarly, the low signal-to-noise ratio can be handled using preprocessing ML pipelines. However, the black box nature of unsupervised learning hampers its integration into routine clinical decision-making pathways. This calls for innovative approaches to untangle the learning processes and reduce the complexity. Using a standardized approach to ML and DL research and reporting will also help improve confidence in these techniques by increasing replicability. Considering its success in natural language processing and image processing, it won't be long before ML and DL techniques are integrated in EEG processing pipelines for various conditions.

ACKNOWLEDGMENT

I would like to acknowledge Ila Nishad for her help in preparing the images.

ABBREVIATIONS

CNN   Convoluted neural network
DL   Deep learning
EEG   Electroencephalograph
KNN   K-nearest neighbor
LSTM   Long short-term memory
ML   Machine learning
MRI   Magnetic resonance imaging
RNN   Recurrent neural network
SVM   Support vector machines

REFERENCES

1. Buzsaki G, Anstassiou A, Koch C, The Origin of Extracellular Fields and Currents—EEG, ECoG, LFP and Spikes. Nature Reviews Neuroscience. 2012; 13: 407–420. ISSN 1471–0048.
2. Jackson AF, Bolger DJ, The Neurophysiological Bases of EEG and EEG Measurement: A Review for the Rest of Us. Psychophysiology. 2014; 51: 1061–1071. doi: 10.1111/psyp.12283.
3. Hahn CD, Emerson RG. Electroencephalography and Evoked Potentials. In Daroff RB, Jankovic J, Mazziotta JC, Pomeroy SL. Bradley's Neurology in Clinical Practice. 7 ed. China: Elsevier; 2016, 348–352.
4. Grant AC, Abdel-Baki SG, Weedon J, Arnedo V, Chari G, Koziorynska E et al., EEG Interpretation Reliability and Interpreter Confidence: A Large Single Centre Study. Epilepsy & Behavior. 2014; 32: 102–107.
5. Jing J, Herlopian A, Karakis I, Ng M, Halford JJ, Lam A, Maus D, Chan F et al., Interrater Reliability of Experts in Identifying Interictal Epileptiform Discharges in Electroencephalograms. JAMA Neurology. 2020; 77(1): 49–57. doi: 10.1001/jamaneurol.2019.3531.
6. Tatum WO, Rubboli G, Kaplan PW, Mirsatari SM, Radhakrishnan K, Gloss D, Caboclo LO, Drislane FW et al., Clinical Utility of EEG in Diagnosing and Monitoring in Adults. Clinical Neurophysiology. 2018; 129(5): 1056–1082. doi: https://doi.org/10.1016/j.clinph.2018.01.019.
7. Rodrigues J, Weib W, Hewig J, Allen JJB, EPOS: EEG Processing Open Source Scripts. Frontiers in Neuroscience. 2021; 15: 660449. doi: 10.3389/fnins.2021.660449.
8. Roy Y, Banville H, Albuquerque I, Gramfort A, Falk TH, Faubert J, Deep Learning-Based Electroencephalograph Analysis: A Systematic Review. Journal of Neural Engineering. 2019; 16: 051001. doi: 10.1088/1741-2552/ab260c.
9. Udousoro IC, Machine Learning: A Review. Semiconductor Science and Information Devices. 2020; 2(2): 5–15. doi: 10.30564/ssid.v2i2.1931.
10. Craik A, He Y, Contreras-Vidal JL, Deep Learning for Electroencephalography Classification Tasks: A Review. Journal of Neural Engineering. 2019; 16: 031001. doi: 10.1088/1741-2552/ab0ab5.
11. Movahedi F, Coyle JL, Sejdic E, Deep Belief Networks for Electroencephalography: A Review of Recent Contributions and Future Outlooks. IEEE Journal of Biomedical and Health Informatics. 2018; 22(3): 642–652. doi 10.1109/JBHI.2017.2727218.
12. Cao Z, A Review of Artificial Intelligence for EEG Based Brain Computer Interfaces and Applications. Brain Science Advances. 2020; 6(3): 162–170. doi: 10.26599/BSA.2020.9050017.

13. Mortaga M, Brenner A, Kutafina E, Towards Interpretable Machine Learning in EEG Analysis. German Medical Data Sciences. 2021. doi: 10.3233/SHTI210538.

14. Leamy DJ, Kocijan J, Domijan K, Duffin J, Roche RAP, Commins S, Collins Ward TE, An Exploration of EEG Features During Recovery Following Stroke—Implications for BCI Mediated Neurorehabilitation Therapy. Journal of Neuro Engineering and Rehabilitation. 2014; 11: 9. doi: 10.1186/1743-0003-11-9.

15. Erani F, Zolotova N, Vanderschelden B, Khoshab N, Sarian H, Nazarzai L, Wu J, Chakravarthy B, Hoonpongismanont W et al., Electroencephalography Might Improve Diagnosis of Acute Stroke and Large Vessel Occlusion. Stroke. 2020; 51: 3361–3365. doi: 10.1161/STROKEAHA.120.030150.

16. Choi YA, Park SJ, Jun JA, Pyo CS, Cho KH, Lee HS, Yu JH, Deep Learning Based Stroke Disease Prediction System Using Real-Time Bio Signals. Sensor. 2021; 21: 4629. doi: 10.3390/s21134269.

17. Chiareli AM, Croce P, Assenza G, Merla A, Granata G, Giannantoni NM, Pizzella V, Tecchio F, Zappasodi F, Electroencephalography-Derived Prognosis of Functional Recovery in Acute Stroke through Machine Learning Approaches. International Journal of Neural Systems. 2020; 30(12): 2050067. doi: 10.1142/S0129065720500677.

18. Al-Qazzaz NK, Ali S, Ahmad SA, Escudero J, Classification Enhancement of Post-Stroke Dementia Using Fuzzu Neighbourhood Preserving Analysis with QR Decomposition. Annual International Conference of the IEEE Engineering in Medicine and Biology Society. 2017; 3174–3177. doi: 10.1109/EMBC.2017.8037531.

19. Hosseini MP, Hemiingway C, Madamba J, McKee A, Ploof N, Schuman J, Voss E, Review of Machine Algorithm for Brain Stroke Diagnosis and Prognosis by EEG Analysis. Electrical Engineering and System Science. 2020. arXiv:2008:08118.

20. Mane R, Chouhan T, Guan C, BCI for Stroke Rehabilitation: Motor and Beyond. Journal of Neural Engineering. 2020; 17: 041001. doi: 10.1088/1741-2552/aba162.

21. Monge-Pereira E, Molina-Rueda F, Rivas-Montero FM, Ibanez J, Serrano JI, Alguacil-Diego IM, Miangolarra-Page JC, Electroencephalography as a Post Stroke Assessment Method: An Updated Review. Neurologia. 2017; 32(1): 40–49. doi: 10.1016/j.nrleng.2014.07.004.

22. Buch E, Weberr C, Cohen LG, Braun C, Dimyan MA, Ard T, Mellinger J et al., Think to Move: A Neuromagnetic Brain Computer Interface System for Chronic Stroke. Stroke. 2008; 39(3): 91–97. doi: 10.1161/STROKEAHA.107.505313.

23. de Bardeci M, Ip CT, Olbrich S, Deep Learning Applied to Electroencephalogram Data in Mental Disorders: A Systematic Review. Biological Psychology. 2021; 162: 108117. doi: 10.1016/j.biopsycho.2021.108117.

24. Shatte ABR, Hutchinson DM, Teague SJ, Machine Learning in Mental Health: A Scoping Review of Emthods and Applications. Psychological Medicine. 2019: 1–23. doi: 10.1017/S0033291719000151.

25. Su C, Xu Z, Pathak J, Wang F, Deep Learning in Mental Health Outcomes Research: A Scoping Review. Translational Psychiatry. 2020; 10: 116. doi: 10.1016/j.neuroimage.2020.117021.

26. Scharfman HE, The Neurobiology of Epilepsy. Current Neurology and Neuroscience Reports. 2007; 7(4): 348–354. doi: 10.1007/s11910-007-0053-z.

27. Usman SM, Khalid S, Aslam MH, Epileptic Seizures Prediction Using Deep Learning Techniques. IEEE Access. 2020; 8: 39998. doi: 10.1109/ACCESS.2020.2976866.

28. Gemein LAW, Schirmeister RT, Chrabaszcz P, Wilson D, Boedecker J, Schulze-Bonhage A, Hutter F, Ball T, Machine Learning Based Diagnostics of EEG Pathology. Neuro Image. 2020; 220: 117021. doi: 10.1016/j.neuroimage.2020.117021.

29. Siddiqui MK, Morales-Menendez R, Huang X, Hussain N, A Review of Epileptic Seizure Detection Using Machine Learning Classifiers. Brain Informatics. 2020; 7: 5. doi: 10.1186/s40708-020-00105-1.

30. An S, Kang C, Lee HW, Artificial Intelligence and Computational Approaches for Epilepsy. Journal of Epilepsy Research. 2020; 10: 8–17.
31. Si Y, Machine Learning Applications for Electroencephalograph Signals in Epilepsy: A Quick Review. Acta Epileptologica. 2020: 2–5. doi: 10.1186/s42494-020-00014-0.
32. Abbasi B, Goldenholz DM, Machine Learning Applications in Epilepsy. Epilepsia. 2019; 60: 2038. doi: 10.1111/epi.16333.
33. Usman SM, Khalid S, Aslam MH, Epileptic Seizure Prediction Using Deep Learning Techniques. IEEE Access. 2020; 8: 39998–40008.
34. Chaudhry F, Hunt RJ, Hariharan P, Anand SK, Sanjay S, Kjoller EE, Bartlett CM et al., Machine Learning Application in the Neuro ICU: A Solution to Big Data Mayhem? Frontiers in Neurology. 2020; 11: 554633. doi: 10.3389/fneur.2020.554633.
35. Sun H, Kimchi E, Akeju O et al., Automated Tracking of Level of Consciousness and Delirium in Critical Illness Using Deep Learning. NPJ Digital Medicine. 2019; 2: 89. doi: 10.1038/s41746-019-0167-0.
36. Li R, Wu Q, Liu J, Wu Q, Li C, Zhao Q, Monitoring Depth of Anesthesia Based on Hybrid Features and Recurrent Neural Network. Frontiers in Neuroscience. 2020; 14: 00026. doi: 10.3389/fnins.2020.00026.
37. Bailey NW, Hoy KE, The Promise of Artificial Neural Networks, EEG and MRI for Alzheimer's Disease. Clinical Neurophysiology. 2021; 132: 207–209. doi: 10.1016/j.clinph.2020.10.009.
38. Perez-Valero E, Lopez-Gordo MA, Morillas C, Pelayo F, Vaqureo-Blasco MA, A Review of Automated Techniques for Assisting the Early Detection of Alzheimer's Disease with a Focus on EEG. Journal of Alzheimer's Disease. 2021; 80: 1363–1376.

Part V

Recent Trends in Biomedical Applications

18 Cervical Cancer Screening Methods

Comprehensive Survey

Swati Shinde, Madhura Kalbhor, and Aditya Shinde
Pimpri Chinchwad College of Engineering, Pune,
Maharashtra, India

CONTENTS

18.1 INTRODUCTION

Cancer is becoming a greater health hazard in developing countries and underdeveloped countries, where health infrastructure is poor. There is no part of the world that is immune to cancer. While China and the United States are the leading countries for cases of cancer, India ranks at number 3. Approximately 1 million new cases of cancer are reported in the country every year. Of this number, about 70% of the patients are women [1]. Breast cancer, cervical cancer, and oral cancer are often seen in women. Cervical cancer is a disease that can be found in the cervix. The cancerous cells are formed by the cells on the tissue of the cervix present inside the vagina. Cervical cancer is the leading cause of death among women in low- and middle-income countries. Breast cancer is one of the leading cancers among women, and oral cancer is a common cancer among men and women. But cervical cancer, which affects women, is the least discussed. About 29% of the total fatalities among women cancer patients are due to cervical cancer. Also, treatment of cervical cancer is very expensive [2].

To reduce the burden of cervical cancer, early detection and treatment is crucial. Cervical cancer develops slowly over a period, hence testing for it has to be done in regular intervals of two, three, or five years if the human papillomavirus

DOI: 10.1201/9781003324430-23

(HPV) vaccine is taken [3]. Testing of cervical cancer requires the patient to come to the clinic or hospital and lay on the testing bed; the doctor or examiner then inserts a metallic speculum inside the vagina for a view of the cervix. The process thus becomes a hindrance for women to come to testing centers. Many women feel uncomfortable to get examined in this way by another person. Thus it becomes very important to make patients comfortable before testing.

18.2 SCREENING METHODS

To identify cervical cancer, three methods are used. One of the ways is to identify cancerous cells on the cervix by taking sample cells from the cervix from the transformation zone where the cancer starts. This process is known as pap smear testing [4] (see Figure 18.1). In a pap smear test, the patient is asked to lay on the testing bed and a speculum is inserted into the vagina to displace vaginal walls and a brush or spatula is used to collect a sample. The sample is then sent to the pathology lab for further processing, which includes staining and viewing the sample under a microscope [5]. Pap smear tests are time consuming because of the distance the sample must travel to reach the pathology lab and since each sample must be seen under the microscope, making it a cumbersome task.

Another way of identifying cancer in the cervix is by colposcopy test (see Figure 18.2), which should be done by an expert or medical practitioner [6]. A colposcopy test requires the patient to lay on the testing bed, and a speculum is then used to widen vaginal walls, similar to the way that the pap smear test is conducted. But in a colposcopy, the test cervix is viewed by the expert, and hence a clear view of the entire cervix is important. A colposcopy test requires illumination for a clear view, and if vernacular patterns are not visible by the naked eye, acetic acid is applied on the cervix. If the

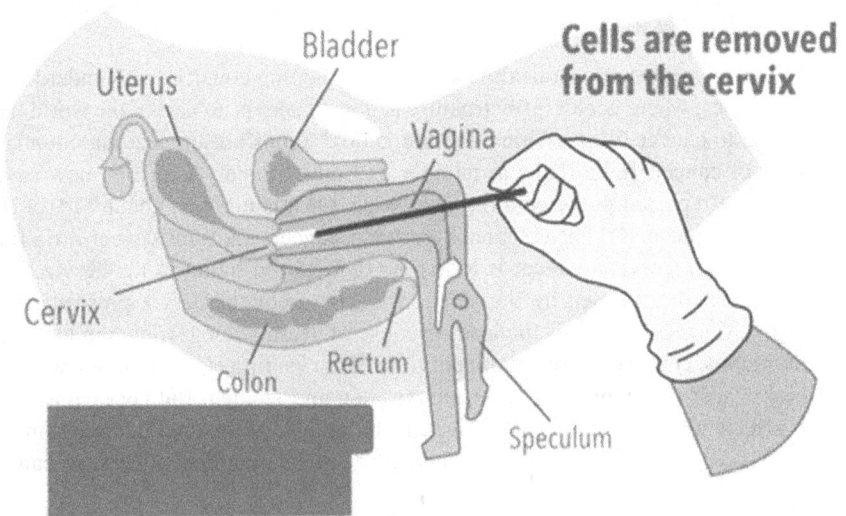

FIGURE 18.1 Pap smear for cervical cancer screening. A healthcare worker collecting sample.

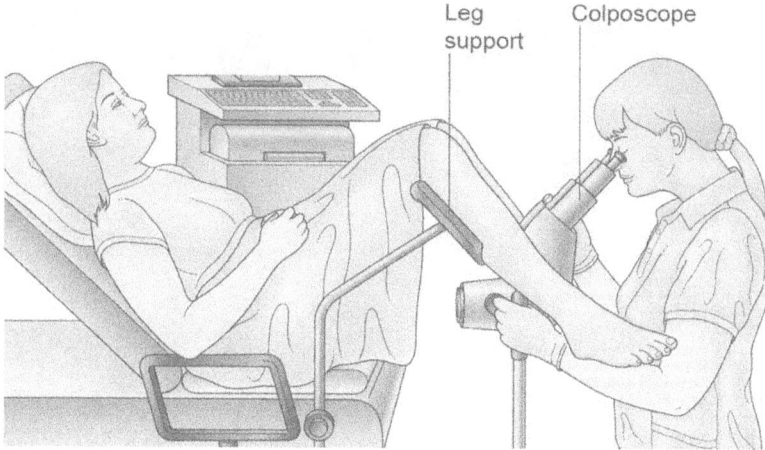

FIGURE 18.2 Colposcopy for cervical cancer screening. The doctor is examining the cervix of the patient.

cervical epithelium has an abnormal load of cellular proteins, the acetic acid causes the proteins to coagulate, giving the affected region an opaque and white appearance. When compared to normal epithelium, a precancerous lesion has a greater protein concentration. This leads to formation of acetowhite, which is an indication of the presence of cancerous cells. This method is known as visual inspection using acetic acid (VIA). Another visual inspection is done by applying Lugol's iodine. It turns cancerous lesions into yellow, and the normal epithelium turns black. This method is known as visual inspection using Lugol iodine (VILI) [7]. If a pap smear or colposcopy test confirms the presence of cancerous lesions, biopsy is done to identify the damage done by the cancer. In the biopsy, a small piece of tissue from the cervix is removed and viewed under a microscope. Due to high diagnosing cost and time consumption in biopsy, VIA makes the process easier and less expensive in low resource setting which is the need of the hour for low- and middle-income countries [8].

18.3 COLPOSCOPY SCREENING DEVICES

Conventional colposcopy screening devices available in the market include conventional speculums like Graves, Pederson, or Cusco speculums [9]. Such speculums are used to separate the vaginal wall and hold it for the duration of visual inspection. Conventional colposcopy like Wallach Tristar uses a halogen light source, is heavy, and has a working length of around 30–50 cm from the subject. Some of the conventional colposcopes are mounted with single-lens reflex (SLR) digital cameras [10]. The magnification factor for the conventional type of colposcope has limitations depending upon the camera type mounted in it. If the mounted camera is digital, then its magnification will limit until the camera's limit. Some conventional colposcopies also have binoculars mounted in them (see Figure 18.3a). Depending on the magnification factor, binoculars have a better view, but the image cannot be stored digitally, so they require an additional device for storage of the image. Binoculars and

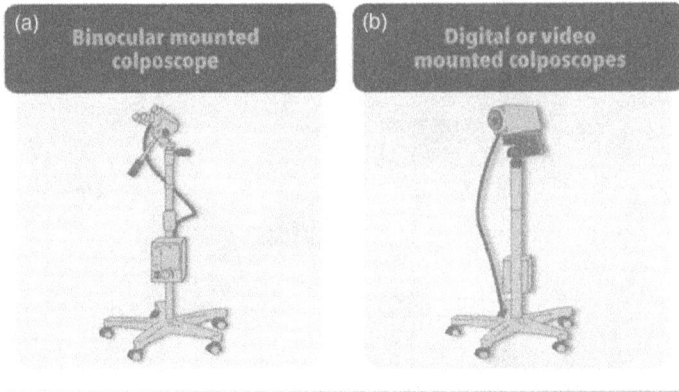

FIGURE 18.3 (a) Binocular mounted colposcope; (b) colposcope with a digital camera or mobile phone mounted.

cameras need to have a high magnification factor due to its working distance, which is long. Many modifications are done to conventional colposcopes depending upon the requirements and availability of equipment. There have been instances of mobile cameras being used to capture cervix images. Also, Canon and Olympus cameras have been used along with binoculars to capture images digitally (see Figure 18.3b). Due to the increasing number of devices mounted for a single purpose, the cost of these devices rises and is unaffordable to low- and middle-income countries. Their cost can range from 2,000 to 24,000 US dollars. Also, they require a separate software setup for digitally transferring images in clinical settings and remote access of clinical images [11]. Ad hoc setup of colposcope equipment may help view the cervix and do the colposcope test, but most of the time such a setup is inconclusive for the diagnosis. Depending on the factors mentioned, like cost, weight, and outcome, there is a need for an alternative colposcope device for better testing of cervical cancer.

To overcome the drawbacks and disadvantages in the conventional colposcope, Duke University developed a device that they named the pocket colposcope. There are two variants of the pocket colposcope developed by Duke University: the 2.0 MP pocket colposcope, and the 5.0 MP pocket colposcope [12]. The pocket colposcope is a novel and low-cost digital colposcope. It is a tampon-sized device that can be inserted and that enables viewing the cervix from the working distance of 30 mm. It is also mounted with illuminating led lights for clear images along with high optics and a high-resolution camera on 2.0 MP and 5.0 MP. The colposcope is connected to mobile device using the OTG USB communication protocol for seamless transfer of images from the healthcare center to medical doctors for diagnosis and testing. Along with a 2.0 MP camera, Duke University's pocket colposcope provides a tampon-sized introducer, which is an alternative to the speculum used in conventional colposcope testing. This introducer helps in widening vaginal walls and helps to get a clear view of the cervix. The introducer and 2.0 MP camera pocket colposcope are useful for healthcare workers to test in low-resource settings and in low- and middle-income countries. Claims of inventor of the tampon-sized introducer, named *callascope*, are that it reduces the discomfort that occurs with a metal

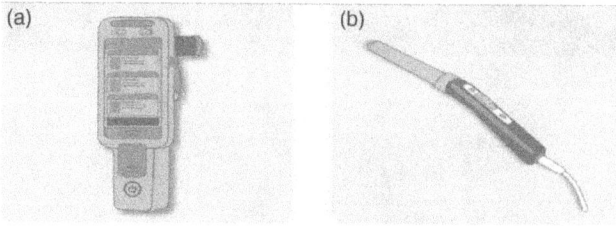

FIGURE 18.4 (a) Mobile ODT portable colposcope; (b) pocket colposcope by Duke University of 5.0 MP.

speculum [13]. The 5.0 MP variant of the pocket colposcope can be used for self-testing by the patient. The ergonomics of the 5.0 MP colposcope are such that it is easily inserted into the vagina and can reach close to the cervix are to capture cervix images. Due to higher resolution, the camera takes good-quality images.

Another colposcope device on the market is Mobile ODT, which is created by EVA Visual Check AI in conjunction with the National Cancer Institute (NCI) (see Figure 18.4a). The service includes a cervical cancer screening site that may be used as a baseline for developing screening tools [14]. It uses artificial intelligence for image analysis and prediction before sending it to experts for opinion. Mobile ODT is portable device with illumination lights and a mobile-size display device mounted on a hand-held instrument specifically designed for doing colposcope examination [15]. It operates at a working distance of 25–30 cm. The device requires use of a speculum for widening of vaginal walls for clear visibility. Mobile ODT is backed by AI, which helps in better and speedy decisions required for testing. Images captured by it are shared with experts on the portal, where they can decide further action. Mobile ODT uses a 12 MP or 16 MP camera along with a 1.6 GHz octa-core powerful processor. The mobile display device in Mobile ODT includes Wi-Fi, Bluetooth, and 4G LTE connectivity. It has an illuminating light of 3 W LED with a polarizer for glare reduction. Mobile ODT weighs around 600 grams and has dimensions around 25 cm × 8 cm × 11 cm. Due to AI, portal and good camera quality mobile ODT gained popularity and is used by as many as 27 countries around the world.

One low-resource setting and cheap alternative for the colposcope device is developed by the India-based company Periwinkle. The Periwinkle model CX1.0 device is similar to the Duke 5.0 MP pocket colposcope but small in size and can be used by health workers for examination (see Figure 18.4b). It is portable and has a disposable sheath cover. The model is 18 cm long and has a diameter of 12 mm in a tube-like structure. It is connected to the application for storage and image processing [16].

18.4 INSTRUMENTS USED

18.4.1 SPECULUM

The use of speculums discourages women to undergo cervical cancer screening. The main reasons behind this resistance are anxiety, fear, discomfort, pain, and embarrassment during the procedure [17]. A study done in Tanzania revealed that concerns for patients are embarrassment and fear of pain due to the speculum during

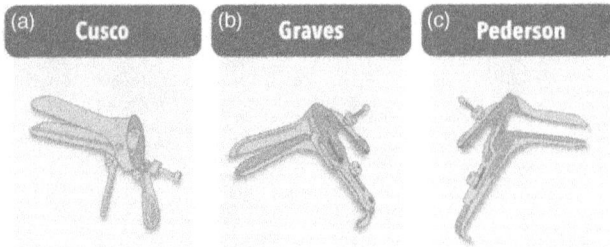

FIGURE 18.5   (a) Cusco speculum invented in 1870; (b) Graves speculum invented in 1878; (c) Pederson speculum with modification in previous designs.

the screening. Similar results were obtained by the study done in Australia and the United States, where the access to healthcare and compliance rate for cervical cancer screening is high. Due to changes in the vagina and skin around it, less painful and invasive speculums are needed.

The father of gynecology, J. Marion, developed the first prototype of the modern speculum from a bent spoon. Later in 1870, the Cusco speculum was designed, and in 1878 the Graves speculum was invented (see Figure 18.5). These were made of metal and were cold. Later some modification on this design was done, and the duck-billed speculum came into existence. But these speculums were for external users, and self-insertion was not possible with these speculums. Also, due to the difficulty in viewing the cervix in case of bigger body sizes, these speculums were extended too much, causing discomfort and pain. Other instruments and devices used now for testing mainly include brush, microscope slide, microscope, cotton ball for acetic acid application, colposcopy camera, and illumination for the colposcope. Of all of these, the metallic speculum is the one that is most uncomfortable for the patient. It is due to their reusable property that these speculums are popular among the medical fraternity. Another reason for their popularity is the ability to increase and decrease its opening with the help of a mechanism present in the speculum. Speculum design has not changed for many years due to these points. But considering from the patient's point of view, it is important to make speculum design comfortable. Many startups and designers have worked over the years to improve the design. Some of them have succeeded, but others failed to gather praise from medical practitioners.

Some of the creative and successful designs are the callascope by Duke University, which is a tampon-sized speculum [13]. The developer of his callascope did a thorough study of different designs similar to the tampon-size speculum depending on the material and opening diameter. A mechanical billed expander, silicone expander, and probe inserter are different potential replacements for the speculum that were studied by Duke University. A mechanically built expander is a minispeculum at the tip of the probe. It is inserted and then opened when close to the cervix. The expander helps widen around 1 inch of the vaginal walls. Another contender is a silicone expander with a stem made of medical-grade plastic and mounted with a silicone menstrual cup. During insertion, the menstrual cup is folded and inserted into the vagina. It opens inside the vagina and is further pushed with the help of a stem. A third model was a simple insertion and removal model with a funneled outtip of a smaller opening compared to the menstrual cup model of around 2.5 cm [17]. In the study and testing done by Duke University, the percent visualization area of the billed expander was much smaller compared to another model for a tilted cervix. The probe inserter and silicone expander performed very well, but due to complexity of insertion and removal, the silicone expander was not studied further. The alternative selected for the conventional metallic speculum for cervical cancer screening was a probe inserter with a smaller diameter than a menstrual cup with a modified design introducing a curved tip for adjustment of the cervix and a separate spray channel with syringe for acetic acid application.

Another alternate for metal speculum is the Yona Care speculum [18]. It is developed by group of engineers that included mechanical engineers and both men and women. They removed screws and mechanisms that used to look scary and increase patients' fear. With smooth design and less need for wider opening, it became a good alternative for metal speculums. Another attempt for giving an alternative for speculums was offered by FemSpec which can be inflated to expand vaginal walls, but medical practitioners did not embrace it and it didn't gain popularity. The Vedascope is another all-encompassing speculum/colposcopy device created in Australia that dilates the vaginal canal with air input and is connected to a camera and light for a colposcopy [19]. But the device is heavy, costly, and needs to be placed by a doctor. It also carries the danger of an air embolism, which can be deadly. Due to various complications that could arise due to its use, many speculum designs were dropped and failed to gather momentum in the medical fraternity.

18.4.2 AGENTS USED FOR VISUAL INSPECTION

In colposcope screening after insertion of a speculum or speculum-like device, agents like acetic acid or Lugol's iodine are applied on the cervix. This helps in better understanding of cancerous lesions and tissue on the endocervix. Acetic acid with 3–4% concentration is applied on the cervix; if acetowhite is formed, then it is inferred that cancerous lesions are present. Acetic acid reacts with a high quantity of protein present on a cancerous cervix to form acetowhite. If glycogen is present in the cervix, Lugol iodine reacts with glycogen to form brown or black coloration if not cancerous, while it turns yellow if cancerous lesions are present. These techniques are known as visual inspection with acetic acid (VIA) and visual inspection using Lugol's iodine (VILI), respectively [20].

18.4.3 BRUSH

In the pap smear testing method, after widening of vaginal walls, a cytology brush is used to collect samples, which are then sent to pathology lab for staining and viewing under the microscope. Collection of samples is also an important task since patients did not need to be called again and again for sample collection. Thus, brush design needs to be taken into consideration for better sample collection. Conventionally, a spatula and cytology brush that is used to take samples

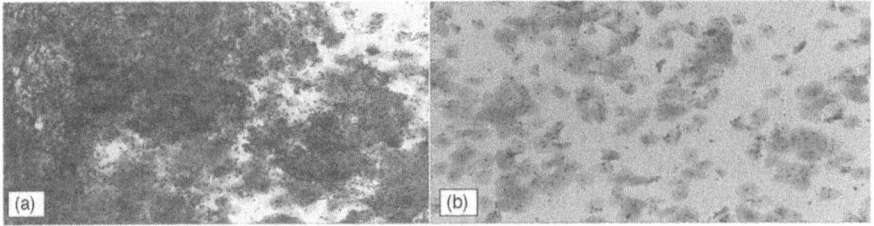

FIGURE 18.6 (a) Pap smear sample under a microscope with the conventional process of staining and viewing under the microscope; (b) pap smear sample under a microscope with LBC preprocessing performed on it.

from the endocervix region are used. Design changes in the brush have also taken place, and brushes with broom-like bristles have been designed. Modern cytology brushes use this broom type of brush as it causes less discomfort, and the area and quantity of samples are greater compared to the other two types of sample collection equipment, spatulas and endocervix brushes [21]. Once the sample is collected from the transformation zone of the cervix, it is transferred on a microscope slide, and the fixation solution is spread on it to avoid decaying of the sample, then it is sent to pathology for further processing.

18.4.4 CYTOLOGY PROCESS

Once samples reach the pathology laboratory, they can be studied in two ways, conventional cytology and liquid-based cytology (LBC). In conventional cytology, the slide is stained and viewed under a microscope (see Figure 18.6a). In LBC, before staining it is processed with lubricants and glacial acetic acid for removal of impurities and mucus from the sample collected (see Figure 18.6b). This is done with the help of a centrifuge machine for cytology testing. After preprocessing, it is stained and looked at under a microscope. LBC helps in accurately identifying cancerous cells as other impurities are removed [22].

18.5 CONCLUSION

From the existing screening methods, we can infer that pap smear cytology screening is costly and requires time as a sample is collected and sent to pathology labs for processing, while for low- and middle-income countries, the colposcope screening method has turned out to be an alternative that is fast and requires less infrastructure or processing to test cervical cancer. Different equipment used in cervical cancer includes speculum, brush, and agents used in cytology. Different pathology processes on pap smear samples were reviewed, and new modern alternatives were studied. Depending upon the accuracy, cost, and speed of getting results, different methods are used. Many develop countries rely on pap smear screening where healthcare infrastructure is good, while many low-income countries rely on colposcopy screening methods to test women for cervical cancer.

REFERENCES

1. https://kauveryhospital.com/blog/cancer/the-three-most-common-cancers-in-india/
2. Singh, M. P., Chauhan, A. S., Rai, B., Ghoshal, S., & Prinja, S. (2020). Cost of Treatment for Cervical Cancer in India. *Asian Pacific Journal of Cancer Prevention: APJCP, 21* (9), 2639–2646. doi: 10.31557/APJCP.2020.21.9.2639
3. Wang, Renjie, Pan, Wei, Jin, Lei, Huang, Weiming, Li, Yuehan, Wu, Di, Gao, Chun, Ma, Ding, & Liao, Shujie. (2020). Human Papillomavirus Vaccine Against Cervical Cancer: Opportunity and Challenge. *Cancer Letters, 471*, 88–102. ISSN 0304–3835.
4. Tan, S. Y., & Tatsumura, Y. (2015). George Papanicolaou (1883–1962): Discoverer of the Pap Smear. *Singapore Medical Journal, 56*, 586–587.
5. Gupta, Ruchika, Sardana, Sarita, Sharda, Akhileshwar, Kumar, Dinesh, Verma, Chandresh Pragya, & Gupta, Sanjay. (2020). Impact of Introduction of Endocervical Brush on Cytologic Detection of Cervical Epithelial Cell Abnormalities: A Clinical Audit of 13-years' Experience at a Cancer Research Centre. *European Journal of Obstetrics & Gynecology and Reproductive Biology, 250*, 126–129. ISSN 0301–2115.
6. Yu, Yao, Ma, Jie, Zhao, Weidong, Li, Zhenmin, & Ding, Shuai. (2021). MSCI: A Multistate Dataset for Colposcopy Image Classification of Cervical Cancer Screening. *International Journal of Medical Informatics, 146*, 104352. ISSN 1386–5056.
7. Keerthana, M. (2020). *Visual Inspection of Cervix of Lugol's Iodine and Acetic Acid for Early Detection of Premalignant and Malignant Lesions of Cervix with Colposcopy and HPE Correlation.* Master's thesis, Tirunelveli Medical College, Tirunelveli.
8. Tassang, A., Ekane, G. E. H.-, Nembulefack, D., Orock, G. E.-, Cho, F. N., Ewane, T., Tassang, T., Ebong, C. E., Orock, A. E. E.-, Folefac, L., Ndakason, W., Ncham, G., & Fru, P. N. (2020). Cervical Cancer Screening in a Low-Resource Setting: Buea-Cameroon. *International Research Journal of Oncology, 3* (2), 138–146. Retrieved from https://journalirjo.com/index.php/IRJO/article/view/60
9. World Health Organization. (2020). WHO technical guidance and specifications of medical devices for screening and treatment of precancerous lesions in the prevention of cervical cancer.
10. Lam, C. T., Krieger, M. S., Gallagher, J. E., Asma, B., Muasher, L. C., Schmitt, J. W., & Ramanujam, N. (2015). Design of a Novel Low Cost Point of Care Tampon (POCkeT) Colposcope for Use in Resource Limited Settings. *PLoS One, 10* (9), e0135869. doi: 10.1371/journal.pone.0135869
11. Søfteland, S., Sebitloane, M. H., Taylor, M., Roald, B. B., Holmen, S., Galappaththi-Arachchige, H. N., Gundersen, S. G., & Kjetland, E. F. (2021). A Systematic Review of Handheld Tools in Lieu of Colposcopy for Cervical Neoplasia and Female Genital Schistosomiasis. *International Journal of Gynecology and Obstetrics, 153* (2), 190–199. doi: 10.1002/ijgo.13538
12. Lam, C. T. (2018). *The Pocket Colposcope, a Novel Low Cost Digital Colposcope, to Improve Access to Cervical Screening in Resource Limited Settings* (Doctoral dissertation, Duke University).
13. Asiedu, Mercy, Agudogo, Júlia, Dotson, Mary, Skerrett, Erica, Krieger, Marlee, Lam, Christopher, Agyei, Doris, Amewu, Juliet, Asah-Opoku, Kwaku, Huchko, Megan, Schmitt, John, Ali, Samba, Srofenyoh, Emmanuel, & Ramanujam, Nirmala. (2020). A Novel Speculum-Free Imaging Strategy for Visualization of the Internal Female Lower Reproductive System. *Scientific Reports, 10*, 16570. doi: 10.1038/s41598-020-72219-9
14. https://www.mobileodt.com/products/eva-colpo/
15. Mink, Jonah, & Peterson, Curtis. (2016). MobileODT: A Case Study of a Novel Approach to an MHealth-Based Model of Sustainable Impact. *MHealth, 2*, 12–12. doi: 10.21037/mhealth.2016.03.10

16. Rahatgaonkar, V., Uchale, P., & Oka, G. (2020). Comparative Study of Smart Scope® Visual Screening Test with Naked Eye Visual Screening and Pap Test. *Asian Pacific Journal of Cancer Prevention: APJCP, 21* (12), 3509–3515. doi: 10.31557/APJCP.2020.21.12.3509

17. Asiedu, M. N., Agudogo, J., Krieger, M. S., Miros, R., Proeschold-Bell, R. J., Schmitt, J. W., & Ramanujam, N. (2017). Design and Preliminary Analysis of a Vaginal Inserter for Speculum-Free Cervical Cancer Screening. *PLoS One, 12* (5), e0177782. doi: 10.1371/journal.pone.0177782

18. https://yonacare.com/Speculum

19. Wong, K., & Lawton, V. (2021). The Vaginal Speculum: A Review of Literature Focusing on Specula Redesigns and Improvements to the Pelvic Exam. *Columbia Undergraduate Research Journal, 5* (1). doi: 10.52214/curj.v5i1.8084

20. Benski, Anne-Caroline, Viviano, Manuela, Jinoro, Jéromine, Alec, Milena, Catarino, Rosa, Herniainasolo, Joséa, Vassilakos, Pierre, & Petignat, Patrick. (2019). HPV Self-Testing for Primary Cervical Cancer Screening in Madagascar: VIA/VILI Triage Compliance in HPV-Positive Women. *PLoS One, 14* (8), e0220632.

21. Zou, Y., Tuo, X., Wu, L., Liu, Y., Feng, X., Zhao, L., Han, L., Wang, L., Wang, Y., Hou, H., Shi, G., & Li, Q. (2020). Comparison of Cervical Cytopathological Diagnosis Using Innovative Qi Brush and Traditional Cervex-Brush® Combi. *Frontiers in Medicine, 7,* 369. doi: 10.3389/fmed.2020.00369

22. de Oliveira, A., Domingues, A., Neufeld, F., Fleury, M., & Nogueira Neto, M. J. F. (2020). Comparison between Conventional Cytology and Liquid-Based Cytology in the Tertiary Brazilian Navy Hospital in Rio de Janeiro. *Acta Cytologica, 64,* 539–546. doi: 10.1159/000508018

19 Understanding Assessment Methods and Sensors for ADHD Hyperactive-Impulsive Type among Children

Thulasi Kumar and M. B. Malarvili
Universiti Teknologi Malaysia, Johor Bahru, Johor, Malaysia

CONTENTS

19.1 ADHD

Attention deficit/hyperactivity disorder (ADHD) is a childhood-onset neurodevelopmental disorder in primary care settings [CPG, 2008; DSM-5, 2013]. ADHD is categorized into three subtypes, namely inattention also known as ADHD-I,

TABLE 19.1
ADHD Subtypes and Its Characteristics

ADHD Subtype	Characteristics
Inattention	Fails to give close attention to details or makes careless mistakes, difficulty sustaining attention in tasks or play activities, not seem to listen when spoken to directly, not follow through on instructions and fails to finish the given task, lack of organization, reluctant to engage in a task that requires mental effort, loses stuff, and forgetful.
Hyperactive-impulsive	Hyperactive: often fidgets with hands or feet or squirms in seat, unable to seat at one place, runs about or climbs excessively in situations in which it is inappropriate, has difficulty playing or engaging in leisure activities quietly, acts as if "driven by a motor" and often talks excessively.
	Impulsive: often blurts out answers before questions have been completed, has difficulty awaiting turn and often interrupts or intrudes on others (e.g., butts into conversations or games).
Combined	The combination symptoms of inattentive and hyperactivity-impulsivity subtypes.

Source: Adapted and modified from Kaufmann et al. (2000) and SAMHSA (2016).

hyperactivity impulsivity, or ADHD-H, and combined, ADHD-C (a fusion with features of ADHD-H and ADHD-I), which are developmentally inconsistent with the age of the child [CPG, 2008; DSM-5, 2013; Hall et al., 2016; Zentall, 2006]. Table 19.1 indicates the characteristics of ADHD subtypes.

19.2   SCOPE OF ADHD STUDIES

The worldwide research revolving around ADHD can be divided into different scopes of studies or fields, such as cause or etiology, prevalence, and case studies, policies and reviews, assessments and rating scales, treatment or aid, and diagnosis or detection. An overview of the scope of ADHD studies is shown in Figure 19.1.

19.2.1   ETIOLOGY OF ADHD

Since ADHD inclined more toward subjective concern and only could be identified through abnormal repetitive behaviors over time, the exact etiology of ADHD in a general concept for a population is still unknown [Zentall, 2006]. Many researchers conclude two main potential etiologies of ADHD: genetic and environmental aspects of a child being born and raised [Amado-Caballero et al., 2020; Cecil and Nigg, 2022; Zentall, 2006].

The genetic study of ADHD is the study of the inborn abnormalities in the structure or chemistry of the brain or the inheritance of abilities or temperament [Zentall, 2006]. In this study, it was mentioned that more than 80% of the differences in activities between ADHD and non-ADHD children could be explained by genetic assessments. It was a known genetic factor for the boys to have relatively higher rates of apparent ADHD symptoms compared to the girls. Genetically, it proved for

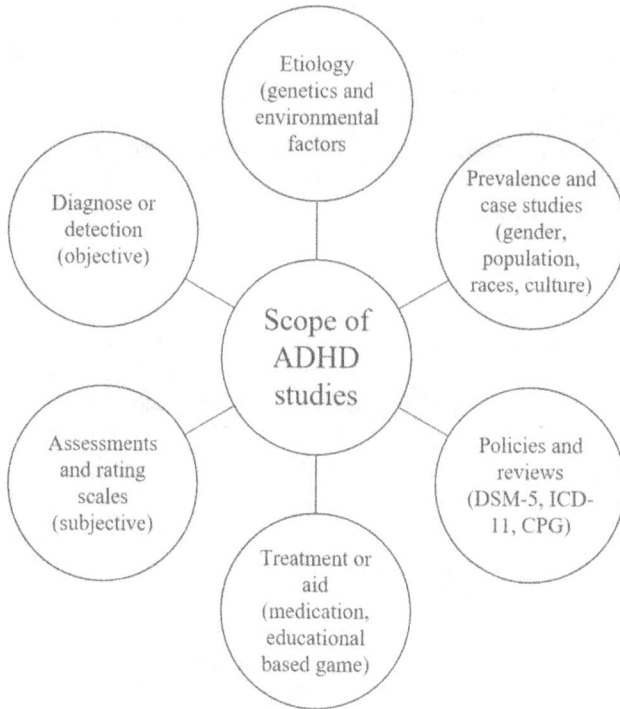

FIGURE 19.1   An overview scope of ADHD studies.

individuals with ADHD to have a longer than normal D4 gene, making the nerve cells less sensitive toward dopamine neurotransmitters, whereby the conveying of signals from one neuron to another neuron takes more times or lapsing in between [Jensen, 2001; Zentall, 2006]. As artificial intelligence (AI) being main part of influences, Loh et al. (2022) reported a few AI studies using machine learning (ML) and the deep learning (DL) models incorporating genetic data to identify ADHD genetic variants.

Apart from genetic factor, the study of environmental factors are to analyze the changes occurring in the biological functions of a child such as disease, trauma, and other health conditions [Zentall, 2006]. The tests used to study the influences of the environmental factors are usually neurofeedback tests such as electroencephalogram (EEG), electrocardiogram (ECG), and functional magnetic resonance imaging (fMRI) associated with subjective assessments [Ghiassian et al., 2016; Loh et al., 2022; Paloyelis et al., 2007].

19.2.2   PREVALENCE AND CASE STUDIES OF ADHD

Some ADHD studies focus on the case studies or prevalence rates in small communities within a country, and these are to understand the distribution of ADHD in the specified population. In the United States, boys aged from four to nine years old are most likely to be diagnosed, and the ADHD disorder is found in all the communities, although variation is present in the prevalence figures across races, cultures, and living style, and the research documenting the statistics is still ongoing across the regions [Chadd.org, 2020; IMH.org, 2020; Lerner and Lerner, 2008; Loh et al., 2022; NIMH, 2006; Zentall, 2006]. The common tests used to report case studies and/or prevalence values are the gold standard ADHD assessments and rating-scale interviews with teachers and parents.

19.2.3 POLICIES AND REVIEWS OF ADHD

By decades, ADHD definition and its associative information like ages and related behaviors change over time based on the respective years of research contribute to the policies and reviews of ADHD being revised and updated.

The common approved published policies are *Diagnostic and Statistical Manual of Mental Disorders*, fifth edition (DSM-5), the eleventh revision of International Classification of Diseases (ICD-11), and Clinical Practice Guidelines (CPG) in each country to update any changes in the terminology and the defined characteristics of ADHD subtypes. The latest global revaluation of these policies, including guidelines for clinical tests and public use, are lastly reviewed on 2013 for DSM-5 and 2019 for ICD-11 [DSM-5, 2013; ICD-11, 2019]. A new text revision of DSM-5 known as DSM-5-TR is published in year 2022 to include a new diagnosis, prolonged grief disorder, and new symptom codes. The DSM components in this book comprise the diagnostic classification of diagnostic codes of ICD-10-clinical modification (CM), the diagnostic criteria sets, and the descriptive text of each illness. In the same year of 2022, the policy of ICD-11-CM is being officially in effect for the national and international recording and reporting of causes of illness, death, and many more with more than 120 000 digital term codes are being used online [WHO, 2022]. The ADHD term code is digitally reported as 6A05 according to International Classification of Diseases for Mortality and Morbidity Statistics, 11th Revision, v2023-01 [Find-A-Code, 2023]. On this website page, the subscription and newsletter of ADHD are available officially.

Besides the policies, there are review studies that document all the published articles to get a good grasp of the emerging researchers elsewhere in the world, centralizing the topic of ADHD [De Crescenzo et al., 2016; Hall et al., 2016; Loh et al., 2022]. They and many more other reviewers collected a bulk of ADHD published journal papers elsewhere in the previous years and classified them into a several point of views, and thus their work has become a crucial reference point for researchers.

19.2.4 TREATMENT OR AID OF ADHD

After understanding the factors influencing ADHD among children and its serious consequences for children's cognitive and gross and fine motor development [James et al., 2022], the researchers experimented with various treatment or aid to help the children to overcome some of the ADHD symptoms so they can focus better, respond appropriately, and perform daily tasks without any hindrance. The rapidly developing research on treatment of ADHD advocates stimulant medications such as methylphenidate and amphetamine or other types of stimulant and nonstimulant medications that need to be taken for a longer term [Hall et al., 2016; Halperin et al., 1992; Konrad et al., 2005].

Medications alone could not overcome repetitive occurrence of ADHD symptoms. Hence aids needed to help children, for example special education, differential approach in the mainstream classroom, educational-based games, and neurofeedback training (NFT) [Wang, 2017; Ye et al., 2019]. These types of aid programs can assist ADHD children to have a normal life like typical children and slowly overcome the signs of ADHD symptoms. The unity efforts of various professionals from different fields could help ADHD children to recognize their abilities and temperament changes and lessen the effects of ADHD on their daily life [IMH.org, 2020; Zentall, 2006].

19.2.5 Assessments and Rating Scales of ADHD

When looking into the factors that cause ADHD among children, prevalences, individual case studies, related policies in defining ADHD, and reviews of previous research, those analyses need tools to assess ADHD prototypically prior to initiating any treatment.

The improvised assessments over years, particularly the subjective assessments of various tests and checklist items used to diagnose ADHD among children, are the continuous performance tasks (CPT), Conner's tests for parents and teachers, the Child Behavior Checklist (CBCL), DSM-IV, or DSM-5-TR, the Schedule for Affective Disorder and Schizophrenia for School-Age Children (K-SADS), Das–Naglieri Cognitive Assessment System (DN: CAS), *Wechsler Intelligence Scale for Children*, fourth edition (WISC-IV), and many other tools [De Crescenzo et al., 2016; Hall et al., 2016; Loh et al., 2022]. The selected assessment tools are tabulated in Table 19.2.

19.2.6 Diagnosis or Detection

Although there are many established assessment tools to identify ADHD among children, the negligence still happens, and because no diagnosis of ADHD takes place, thus delaying treatment, many ADHD children experience the symptoms into adulthood, experiencing low self-esteem, lack of confidence, and depression, besides having problems with school, work, and relationships [Ginsberg et al., 2014]. Diagnosis has never been an easy task, as the ADHD tests involved are usually subjective assessments that begin with the self-reporting from parents or teachers to medical practitioners first [IMH.org, 2020; Loh et al., 2022; Pierangelo and Giuliani, 2007; Zentall, 2006]. Further analysis would lead to the clinical examination such as subjective assessments to be conducted in inclusive settings, interviews, camera recording of the child's movement during assessments, and also fMRI and other neurodevelopmental scans to verify the disorder and also to identify the subtypes of ADHD prior prescribing medication [Hall et al., 2016; Halperin et al., 1993; Konrad et al., 2005; Myhealth.gov.my, 2020]. To date, there is no lab test available for ADHD [Lewin, 2003; Soref, 2019].

Therefore, further discussion in the next sections concentrate on objective methods used in detection of ADHD subtypes, and the topic will narrow down into the ADHD-HI subtype.

TABLE 19.2
Selected ADHD Assessment Tools for Children Aged Group

Assessment	Feature	Explanation
CPT, Conner's CPT, and other CPT tasks	ADHD-C	Is a continuous performance test of computer-based program, which involves rapid presentation of visual or auditory stimuli. Participants are asked to respond when a given target occurs but to withhold the response to nontargets.
Sleep quality	Sleeping efficiency	Assessing sleeping efficiency, high in ADHD comorbidities.
Kiddie-SADS PL/E, K-SADS	Psychopathology	Schedule for Affective schizophrenia interview tests comorbidities including ADHD.
SRS	ADHD	Social responsiveness scale measure social ability of children (4–18 years old) to differentiate ADHD individuals from patient with autistic spectrum disorder (ASD).
IVA-CPT	ADHD-I	Evaluate visual and auditory attention using computerized continuous performance tests.
WISC-R	ADHD-I	Wechsler Intelligence Scale-Revised measure intelligence by assess 10 abilities
NPESY	Use as class determinants	Neurophysiological functioning and severity assess five domains: Attention/Executive functioning, Language, Visuospatial, Sensorimotor, and Memory.
Kiddie CPT, CPT, MFFT	ADHD-I	Computerized continuous performance tests, neurophysiological test to assess severity of ADHD, and matching familiar figures test is part of CPT.
Go-No-Go task, memory task	Assess inhibitory control	Participants responding by pressing the key/ withhold response to measure implicit social cognition.
Rating-scale, teacher rating	Parents/teachers	Score student's behavior through observation and understanding by someone close to children.
BASC-2	Assess emotion and behavior	Behavior Assessment System for Children is a multidimensional assessment system evaluates clinical and adaptive aspects of behavior and emotional/personality functioning. Done by teacher/parents and including personality self-report, structured developmental history, and student observation system.
CSI-IV	ADHD-C	Child symptom inventory 4; refer to DSM-5 to assess emotional and behavioral system.
CBCL	Diagnostic screener	Child behavior checklist is a questionnaire used by caregiver to identify behavior problem in child.
BRIEF-P	ADHD-HI	Behavior rating inventory of executive function in preschool for parents and teachers.
Movement-ABC-2 / MVPA (Taiwan)	Protocols approved by Taiwan government	Movement-ABC-2 is motor competence assessment battery for children and MVPA is moderate-to-vigorous physical activity assessment which measurement involves actigraph.
Episodic buffer	Working memory component	Preclinical behavioral studies used to fractionate the multicomponent working memory system. Episodic buffer is part of working memory component apart from phonological and visuospatial.

Source: Adapted and modified from the previous selected studies of Amado-Caballero et al. (2020), Chu et al. (2020), De Crescenzo et al. (2016), Duda et al. (2017), Faedda et al. (2016), Gilbert et al. (2016), Hall et al. (2016), Kofler et al. (2017), Loh et al. (2022), Oztekin et al. (2021), and Yu et al., (2019).

19.3 OBJECTIVE DETECTION METHODS OF ADHD SUBTYPES

This section discusses the emerging studies on the objective detection methods of ADHD children. Based on previous studies, since the subjective assessments are taking longer and need observation reports from the guardians of a child as a first step, the objective assessments are getting more distinguished for different subtypes of ADHD. These developing objective assessments are helpful in assisting during the subjective assessments, and they further find ADHD occurrence in children especially in medical aspects. For initial diagnosis of ADHD symptoms among children, the research is still developing, and many researchers have proposed various engineered-based research drafts or solutions that could be used to identify ADHD. The classification and features of these objective methods for three subtypes of ADHD are summarized in the following subsections.

19.3.1 COMBINED SUBTYPE (ADHD-C) AND OTHERS

Let us look at the availability of the objective detection method for the combined subtype of ADHD and others before we get to know the objective methods used to diagnose ADHD-I and ADHD-HI subtypes.

The combined subtype of ADHD-C uses sensors and a clinical system together because of the ADHD-HI subtype's recognized movements, such as fidgeting, while the ADHD-I subtype is about cognitive aspects. Thus, the current developed objective methods in clinical settings to detect the ADHD-C subtype are electrophysiological alterations such as handcrafted feature of electroencephalogram (EEG), electrooculogram (EOG) aided with EEG, and heart rate variability (HRV) analysis by using electrocardiogram (ECG) and EEG tools [Ahmadi et al., 2021; Altınkaynak et al., 2020; Griffiths et al., 2017; Hall et al., 2016; Tanko et al., 2022]. There are also researches done by using acceleration and angular velocity sensors for arm movement (pronation and supination) during ADHD-I assessments, auxiliary diagnosis by using sensors during clinical setting assessments such as the study of wearable sensors for body posture, and measurement of physiological conditions via HRV using skin electrical sensors at the same time during task completion [Griffiths et al., 2017; Hall et al., 2016].

Besides these, recently an AI-related gaming of virtual reality (VR) in a classroom proved to be able to differentiate ADHD from non-ADHD children by using ML model incorporating task performance and neurobehavior aspect [Yeh et al., 2020]. Wiguna and others used DL model, a subset of ML model to develop ADHD-VR digital game aimed to diagnose ADHD among children [Wiguna et al., 2020]. There are a few game-related ADHD assessments, and one of them can be traced back to Heller et al. (2013), which used rapid adoption of tangible user interface devices collaborated with popular interactive video games of "Groundskeeper." In this game assessments, ADHD indicative feature variables converted mathematically into machine learning algorithms, and diagnostic models were developed to aid psychiatric clinical assessments of ADHD. A study in 2022 used brain-computer interface (BCI) in EEG-BCI application game to test ADHD and non-ADHD children [Serrano-Barroso et al., 2021].

Besides the three subtypes of ADHD, there is another category that the previous studies of ADHD focused on as well, which is known as comorbid ADHD. It means there are other disease(s) or disorder(s) coexisting with ADHD disorder, and this condition is called ADHD comorbidity(ies). To detect comorbid ADHD, one of the studies used the gold standard method of CPT to identify two or more disorders in measuring anxiety disorders and bipolar disorder and differentiating them with ADHD symptoms or physiological parameters by using both subjective and objective assessments for detection such as using nonwearable sensor during the assessments [Faedda et al., 2016; Hall et al., 2016].

19.3.2 INATTENTIVE SUBTYPE (ADHD-I)

The ADHD-I subtype, which shows symptoms such as failing to give attention to details, not engaging, and being forgetful, has inspired the development of attentive objective tests. One of the well-established objective tests is EEG, which is usually used by medical practitioners to validate after the confirmation of ADHD-I subtype via subjective assessments. The experimental classifiers and features used for EEG is theta/beta ratio (TBR) [Marcano et al., 2017]. Another medically approved objective test is assessment of neurodevelopmental delay using functional magnetic resonance imaging (fMRI), and one can find online the analysis of the collection of fMRI clinical and imaging data from the ADHD-200 data set [Ghiassian et al., 2016]. Another EEG study used additional tool of functional near-infrared spectroscopy (fNIRS) to identify the changes in the concentration of oxy-Hb during a task [Guven et al., 2020].

Aside from these, researchers from gaming and educational fields have amalgamated the educational games with AI by using software such as the Contextualized and Objective System (COSA), FOCUS (a serious EEG-based game), the Cambridge Neuropsychological Test Automated Battery (CANTAB), and machine learning [Adamis et al., 2017; Alchalabi et al., 2018; Ye et al., 2019]. There are also combination testing of EEG and eye-movement during assessments using software [Adamis et al., 2017; Alchalabi et al., 2018]. Another article covers research on the pupillary light reflex to measure the emotion dysregulation among ADHD children during the assessment [Hamrakova et al., 2019]. The uncontrollable eye movement in ADHD patients can be a potential biomarker for diagnosis of ADHD [Das and Khanna, 2021; Varela et al., 2019].

19.3.3 HYPERACTIVE-IMPULSIVE SUBTYPE (ADHD-HI)

ADHD-HI subtype symptoms inclined more toward movements, thus the data collected objectively were activities quantified through using wearable and nonwearable sensors. One of the wearable sensors is an actigraph device such as Motionlogger Micro, GENEActiv, ActiGraph, Ambulatory Monitoring, and others that can be worn on the wrist, ankle, and waist of the subjects [De Crescenzo et al., 2016; Hall et al., 2016]. Besides actigraphs, other articles have covered different types of the wearable sensors to study the movement activities of a subject, such as accelerometers (worn on the ankle and wrist), inertial measurement unit (IMU, consists of a gyroscope and an accelerometer) and pedometers [Hall et al., 2016; Jiang et al., 2020; Muñoz-Organero et al., 2018; O'Mahony et al., 2014]. The nonwearable sensors used to detect ADHD-HI are infrared motion analysis and impulse radio ultrawideband

(IR-UWB) radar sensor [Gunther et al., 2012; Hall et al., 2016; Yim et al., 2019]. An example of infrared motion analysis is to track the location of a reflective marker worn on a cap worn by the participant before collecting and recording movement during subjective assessments such as Qbtest which is a part of CPT assessment tool [Gunther et al., 2012; Hall et al., 2016; Teicher, 1995]. IR-UWB radar sensors are usually used to calculate the movement of a subject by measuring the vital signs such as respiration and heart rates in a clinical setting based on the positioning and tracking system in the laboratory room [Yim et al., 2019].

19.4   OBJECTIVE ASSESSMENT OF ADHD-HI SUBTYPE DETECTION

After the analysis of various fields of ADHD scopes, the focus is narrowed down into the less studied area of objective detection methods compared to the numerous available subjective assessments to diagnose ADHD. However, there is no suitable subjective detection method for ADHD-HI subtype because the scaling method of behavioral assessments is using descriptive language and lacking quantitative standard, and for the EEG application which affects emotional tension among ADHD-HI children and gives rise to inaccurate evaluation results, requiring more tests or tools for analysis [Jiang et al., 2020]. Figure 19.2 represents overall information about objective detection methods for ADHD subtypes. Among these objective methods, the less studied ADHD-HI subtype is the focus of the current study, as there are many features that could be used for future improvements in this field.

There are two types of sensors used in the detection of the ADHD-HI subtype, namely wearable and nonwearable. The wearable sensors are actigraph, IMUs,

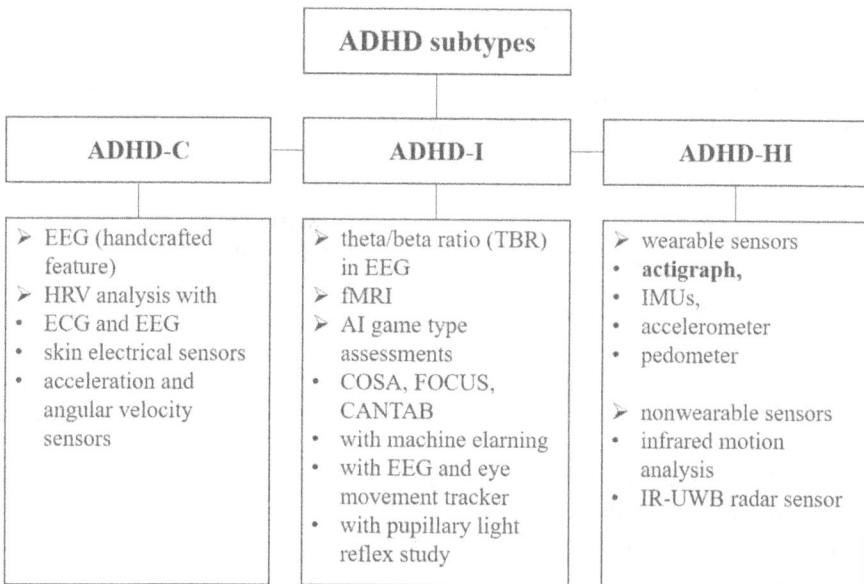

ADHD subtypes		
ADHD-C	**ADHD-I**	**ADHD-HI**
➢ EEG (handcrafted feature) ➢ HRV analysis with • ECG and EEG • skin electrical sensors • acceleration and angular velocity sensors	➢ theta/beta ratio (TBR) in EEG ➢ fMRI ➢ AI game type assessments • COSA, FOCUS, CANTAB • with machine elarning • with EEG and eye movement tracker • with pupillary light reflex study	➢ wearable sensors • **actigraph,** • IMUs, • accelerometer • pedometer ➢ nonwearable sensors • infrared motion analysis • IR-UWB radar sensor

FIGURE 19.2   Summarized objective detection methods for ADHD subtypes.

accelerometers, and pedometers, while the nonwearable sensors are infrared motion analysis and radio ultrawideband radar sensors. Actigraph, also known as actometer or actimeter, is a proportional device. Examples of actigraph devices are Motionlogger or a solid-state device that uses pizoelectric sensors, accelerometers, light/position sensors, and IMUs within it. This is different compared to other wearable sensors, such as IMUs that consists only of triaxial accelerometers and triaxial gyroscopes, accelerometers that have single and triaxial acceleration position, and pedometers that are binary devices. A detailed information of input, feature, classifier, output, and limitation of these sensors' application in the studies were tabulated in Table 19.3.

Among the wearable and nonwearable sensors to measure activities of a subject's movement, a wearable sensor is most suitable, as it can be used in a flexible condition either indoors, outdoors, or in an open flexible setting environment without hindering the subjects from behaving as they normally do as they carry out their daily activities [Hall et al., 2016; Muñoz-Organero et al., 2018; Yim et al., 2019]. Otherwise, the aforementioned infrared cameras, other fixed cameras, or IR-UWBs, which measure the breathing movements as part of nonwearable sensors, are only suitable to be used in a clinical setting whereby other assessments are being carried out at the same time [Jiang et al., 2020; Loh et al., 2022]. Also, such cameras are inflexible and expensive to use in other settings apart from the fixed testing clinical room [Amado-Caballero et al., 2020; Faedda et al., 2016; Hall et al., 2016; Yim et al., 2019].

19.5   EXPERIMENTAL FEATURES OF THE ADHI-HI SUBTYPE WEARABLE SENSOR OF THE ACTIGRAPH DEVICE

A few articles have been selected from years 2015 to 2022 to study their experimental setup as shown in Table 19.4.

The first benchmark study is a systematic review of 16 published articles from 1980 to 2015 using the actigraph device during CPT tests and other assessments [Hall et al., 2016]. The experimental feature of time domain is for both diurnal and nocturnal activities with the calculations of epochs of time to measure the intensity of the movement and gravitational acceleration. The subjects wore wearable sensors on different parts of their bodies, such as the wrist, ankle, waist, and/or leg. The collected frequency levels of the actigraph signals for these studies vary from slow or fast, very low, low, moderate, high, to very high. The main calculations used in the experiments are receiver operating characteristics (ROC) curve analysis, commission and omission errors, and/or mean motor activities to analyze the big picture through the correlated factors (using the Cholesky model), logistic regression, and/or confidential intervals (CI) and more to measure the accuracy, sensitivity, and specificity and identify the positive and negative predictive values (true positive vs false positive). A study within this meta-analysis identified that the magnitude of movements yielded an area under the curve (AUC) of up to 0.8 to differentiate ADHD from control, and this value has been used as reference value or threshold value for other studies' aftermath [Wood et al., 2009].

Another meta-analysis article discussed the role of actigraphy as an objective tool for the ambulatory monitoring of sleep and activity in ADHD, collecting 19 articles

TABLE 19.3
Wearable and Nonwearable Sensors of ADHD-HI

Sensor	Input (Ref.)	Feature	Classifier	Output
Wearable	Actigraph [Hall et al., 2016]	Body movements (ankle, wrist, and waist) including sleeping for a certain time period + sleep logs, use CPT/DSM-5 to define measurement characteristics	Direct assessment using commercial software and/or further analysis using MATLAB[a], re-modelling/modified algorithm	Hyperactive children have higher activity levels compared to control group
	IMUs [O'Mahony et al., 2014]	Measure total inertia force (inclination angle/motion of pose) and angular velocity (rotational characteristics of the movement)	Commercial sensor module of APDM[b] Opal sensor provides data to be saved directly to an on-board memory for post-processing @ SVM[c] tool	High sensitivity and specificity in par with TOVA test (~ 95%)
	Accelerometer [Muñoz-Organero et al., 2018]	24 hours movement of wrist and ankle, + daily logs	Processed algorithm, 2D[d] analysis, CNN[e] via MATLAB[a]	Higher deviations (high-intensity movements) compared to control group (insensitive to non-locomotor move)
	Pedometer [Gapin et al., 2009]	Assessing activities levels, activated by the impact of foot and ground (step counts) in a fixed environment	Direct observation of activity / counts on pedometer watch	Higher counts of steps / speeds in ADHD children vs control (insensitive to non-locomotor move)
Non-wearable	Infrared motion analysis (exclude Qbtest-infrared camera) [Hall et al., 2016]	Recorded abnormality movement patterns in seated condition + CPT	Analysis of tracked position of four markers 50 times per second to a resolution of 0.04 mm	Frequent fidgety and larger amplitude movements of ADHD seated children
	Impulse radio ultra-wideband radar sensor, IR-UWB [Yim et al., 2019]	Detecting movements (able to detect breathing) in testing room + CAT[f]	Quantity calculation of spatial (vector change) and sedentary (magnitude change) of body movement via MATLAB[a] (signal processing algorithm)	Big $M_{sedentary}$[f] value and high significant difference for $M_{spatial}$[g] is expected for ADHD children during the test if active movement happen

a MATLAB: MATrix LABoratory.
b APDM: ambulatory Parkinson's disease monitoring.
c SVM: support vector machine.
d 2D: 2-dimensional.
e CNN: convolutional neural network.
f CAT: clinical assessment of attention deficit.
g M: movement.

TABLE 19.4
Significant Experimental Setting and Limitation/Recommendation of Selected Published Articles from Year 2015 to 2022

Ref.	Significant Experimental Setting (Ref.)
Hall et al. (2016)	1. Actigraph used during CPT test or other assessments (all 16 articles) 2. All age groups are 6–12, 6–13, 6–18, 7–11, 7–12, 8–12, 9 or 9.6 (mean) except 3–4 of preschoolers [Rajendran et al., 2015] 3. ADHD-C [Hall et al., 1997] 4. 24 hours observational of a subject [De Crescenzo et al., 2014 Porrino et al., 1983] 5. Inclusive/indoor setting [Alderson et al., 2012; Dane et al., 2000; Inoue et al., 1998; Marks et al., 1999; Wood et al., 2009] 6. School vs test situation [Konrad et al., 2005] 7. Inclusive medications/treatment [Borcherding et al., 1989; Donnelly et al., 1989; Halperin et al., 1993, 1992; Konrad et al., 2005; Porrino et al., 1983; Rapoport et al., 1980] 8. **Limitation:** did not perform quality assessment of the papers and their findings and samples are clinic-referred and community-based samples, which may have influenced the clinical utility of the CPT.
De Crescenzo et al. (2016)	1. 24 hours observational of a subject 2. Structured experimental sessions 3. Estimating heterogeneity (CI) among various studies (low CI, high ADHD) 4. 3–4, 9 (mean), 14.1–15.1 (mean) years old children and adolescents 5. **Limitation:** differs in sample size and time domain may overpower certain results and usage of different actigraphic devices influence the variability actigraph signals.
Faedda et al. (2016)	1. 24 hours observational of a subject 2. Differentiating pediatric bipolar disorder from ADHD 3. 5–18 years old 4. **Recommendation:** further studies needed to confirm the usage of actigraph as part of laboratory test to identify early onset BD.
Gilbert et al. (2016)	1. Actigraph used during CPT test 2. Inclusive/indoor setting 3. Diurnal activity 4. 6–11 years old 5. **Limitation:** lack of clinical comparison may lead to spectrum bias, test accuracy could differ between subgroups of patients with different characteristics (including presence and severe), age and race limit, needed replication studies using cross-cultural samples.
Kofler et al. (2017)	1. Actigraph used during assessment 2. Inclusive/indoor setting 3. Diurnal activity 4. Ages 8–13 years old 5. **Limitation:** more limitation are mentioned on the probability occurrence of deficits in other experiment settings and assessments task used (phonological, visuospatial, buffer) and the differences could have influenced results and more future studies needed in this area.

(Continued)

TABLE 19.4 *(Continued)*
Significant Experimental Setting and Limitation/Recommendation
of Selected Published Articles from Year 2015 to 2022

Ref.	Significant Experimental Setting (Ref.)
Yu et al. (2019)	1. Actigraph and EEG used during assessment 2. Inclusive/indoor setting 3. Diurnal activity 4. 7–12 years old 5. **Limitation:** very small sample size, this cross-sectional design employed precludes causal inferences, participants who were with high level of MVPA should be further examined due to different time domain and limited on explicitly assessing all MC components due to fewer measurement items, especially fine motor competence relative to other measurement.
Chu et al. (2020)	1. Actigraph and EEG used during CPT test 2. Inclusive/indoor setting 3. Diurnal activity 4. 6–12 years old (hospital's outpatient department and elementary school) 5. **Limitation:** small sample size, non-match group of ADHD vs control age and some experiment parts not under control.
Amado-Caballero et al. (2020)	1. 24 hours observational of a subject; period separated by activity term (day/night) 2. Inclusive/indoor and outdoor; setting separated by activity term (24 hours/ sleeping quality assessment/performing task) 3. 6–15 years old 4. **Limitation:** children study group; limited to heterogamous sample and large age span. 5. **Recommendation:** future study on each activity term/ windows (different time domain) as different methodologies to identify homogeneous sample based on specific pathology, age and gender.
Loh et al. (2022)	1. Actigraphy: the experimental settings are from the previous studies which are in discussion in Tables 19.2 and 19.3 [Amado-Caballero et al., 2020; Faedda et al., 2016; Muñoz-Organero et al., 2018; and O'Mahony et al., 2014] 2. **Recommendation:** future direction of AI in diagnosis ADHD by using cloud computing to combine and analyze data of genetic, MRI, EEG, questionnaires and neurophysical tests, wearable devices and from smartphones.

from years 1992–2014 inclusive of eight studies assessing activity mean and 11 studies assessing sleep patterns. The study shows evidence that a higher mean activity is present in ADHD children during structured sessions, a similar sleep duration, and a moderately altered sleep pattern (De Crescenzo et al., 2016). The time domain used in the experiment feature are from 0.25 to 1 minute epochs to calculate the movements from the wrist, arm, waist, leg, and ankle with the frequency of low, moderate, and high. The involved calculations are SD and 95% CI for activity mean, wake after sleep onset and sleep duration, latency, and efficiency. The big picture of meta-analysis statistics is to measure standardized mean difference (SMD) effect sizes for each comparison with confidence intervals (95%), determining an overall effect size and estimating heterogeneity (95% CI).

Faedda et al. (2016) focused on both diurnal (D) and nocturnal (N) activities with 1 minute epochs via a belt-worn actigraph, and the monitoring activities for these two sessions were done by parents. The researchers then used the collected data to measure activity levels of both D and N sessions as well as the rhythms and fluctuations of circadian variances and amplitudes. The parameters used to calculate the activity levels are active hours (at most ten and at least five), percentages of activity proportions (very low, low, moderate, high, and very high), D skew, time-dependent coefficient of variation (TD-COV), and oscillator model calculations such as Mesor 3 Oscillator Model. These calculations including sleep and circadian measurements make use of machine learning algorithms such as support vector machine (SVM) and artificial neural networks (ANN).

The study by Gilbert et al. (2016) is similar to the articles chosen in Hall et al. (2016) whereby the experimental setup is focused on the measurement of motion sensors during CPT testing. However, the study used *Kcal* unit [per min and body mass (kg)] to measure activities collected from the wrist and ankle with the frequency of light, moderate, and vigorous. The statistics used are normality, skewness, analysis of variance (ANOVA), Levene and Welch statistics, and Bonferroni and discriminant function analyses (DFA) for coefficient and cross-validation.

Another study used four actigraphs in one subject worn at the nondominant wrist, both ankles, and at the back of four-caster swivel chair during assessments [Kofler et al., 2017]. The frequencies measured are low, intermediate, and high movement intensity at 16 times per second (16 Hz) at 1 minute epochs and gross motor movement calculation from the back of the chair. The analysis involved is total movement level (TML) and an episodic buffer (part of the working memory component) functions by using Bayesian model statistics for power analyses, single-modality performance, and Bayesian mixed-model ANOVA.

Other than those studies previously mentioned, a study finding the occurrence of the relationship between TBR of EEG during the resting state and motor competence (MC) during physical activities while conducting the assessments to study the cortical functioning [Yu et al., 2019]. The time domain used in the experiment setting is 60 second epochs with an actigraph worn at the waist for seven hours for seven days to analyze the frequency signals of sedentary (lying and sitting) with < 100 counts per minute, moderate (brisk walking) with > 2,295 and ≤ 4,011 counts per minute, and vigorous with ≥ 4,012 counts/minutes. The calculations used are means and standard deviation (SD) in an effort to analyze the statistics data via significant covariates, Pearson correlations for demographic variables, age, severity of the aggression/anxiety-depression/attention Child Behavior Checklist (CBCL-AAA) profile using T-scores (sum of the CBCL-AAA scales), body mass index (BMI), socioeconomic status (SES), moderate–to-vigorous physical activity (MVPA), MC, and TBR.

In conjunction to the aforementioned study, there is another similar study using EEG (attention and meditation) and actigraph (activity) to identify the potential indicators of CPT [Chu et al., 2020]. No information is mentioned on the signal analysis of the actigraph and on which side it was worn. The calculation used was correlation analysis, repeated measures ANOVA, and regression analysis to investigate which indicators can be used for ADHD diagnosis. The results summarized that high activity amounts indicates high impulsive behavior of the participants and high omissions target in the CPT. However, it concluded that the actigraph outperforms the EEG in

$$\|(x,y,z)\| = \overset{f_s = 1Hz}{\sqrt{\left(x^2 + y^2 + z^2\right)}}$$

FIGURE 19.3 Formula used to calculate movement signal of a subject. (Adapted from Amado-Caballero et al., 2020.)

screening of ADHD because CI was identified to be the most important indicator to diagnose ADHD that was not related to the brain waves.

The second last chosen study proposes an end-to-end methodology for automatic diagnosis of ADHD-C [Amado-Caballero et al., 2020]. An actigraph device is worn on the dominant wrist of the subject with time domain of 1 minute epochs for 24 hours, and an aggregate signal r-value is calculated as input using the formula (Figure 19.3) as one identification (ID) equivalent to one signal for one subject, and the calculation is about movement counting.

The analysis is recorded as the split signal in the windows with the same size using convolutional neural networks (CNN) architecture to classify the spectrograms of activity windows. The windows are separated as activity of short, medium, and long term with differences in time domain. A power input signal from these three groups are set up to 0.022 as minimum to avoid bias from the network or inefficient training during assessments. The spectrogram creation has features such as correct visualization with signal frequency peak, and the input images are same size regardless of window size and period. Binary classification is used for each window with SVM classifier support and 10-fold repetitive process for performance evaluation.

The last reviewed article discussed about the types of ADHD diagnostic tools utilized to develop AI models in a few tools such as MRI, physiological signals, questionnaires or rating scales data, game simulation and performance tests, and motion data [Loh et al., 2022]. In motion data section of actigraphy and accelerometers, the experimental settings of the selected four articles from 2018 to 2020 have been discussed elsewhere in this study and Loh and others highlighted the features and models used such as 28 metrices, end-to-end, IMUs, and acceleration image features and ML (CNN) and DL (SVM) models [Amado-Caballero et al., 2020; Faedda et al., 2016; Muñoz-Organero et al., 2018; O'Mahony et al., 2014].

19.6   SELECTED DOMAINS FROM EXPERIMENTAL FEATURES

The accumulated selected domains from the experimental features of various studies are time domain, actigraph signal frequency, and type of assessments conducted. In the time domain, there are variations of study involved and research is being conducted continuously on this aspect, such as differences in epochs time (0.25–1 minute/Hz), period of study (diurnal and/or nocturnal), the location of actigraph influence time domain (wrist, arm, waist, leg, or ankle), and the primary calculations of these signals obtained from the time domain based on the frequency measurements (i.e., Kcal unit, movement counts, intensity movement, gravitational acceleration, gross motor movement, and motor competence). However, the goal is finding significant differences among the parameters being tested.

Another domain that influences the study is the demographic status of the participants, such as age group, experiment groups (ADHD and control; inpatient, outpatient, or healthy groups), gender, cross-culture or specific community-based, and other almost negligible parameters such as weight, height, and BMI, which are probably insignificant for the objective of these studies. Yet there are no other studies that are being compared on this area as well for further arguments.

Besides these, the environment of the experiment setting varies between studies, such as indoors (during assessments either in the classroom or clinical setting, sleeping or resting stage in the clinical setting or in the subjects' houses, and free activity within the clinical setting) or outdoor assessments (free activity in school or outside the school compounds and house). Few previous studies have been done in outdoor or external environments without any indoor experimental setting in an outdoor environment as to control certain parameters to study a specific feature without hindrance and also to reduce unforeseeable errors that might affect the results.

Depending on the experiment settings, the signal frequency from an actigraph is varied and relies on the study context, such as slow or fast, very low, low, moderate, high, or very high (some only use three from these five signal peaks), and sedentary, moderate, or vigorous. The aggregation or cumulative values to categorize the signals into these peaks differ from one study to another.

The last selected domain is the assessments used in each study, and these assessments are described and explained in Table 19.3.

19.7   SELECTION OF ACTIGRAPH DEVICE TO BE USED IN THIS STUDY

All of the selected commercial actigraph devices are commonly used for physical activities (exercises) and sleeping measurement. Narrowing down to the objective detection of ADHD, particularly the ADHD-HI subtype, and excluding research involving sleeping activities (circadian measurement) while neglecting the involvement of medication and other aspects in the identification of the ADHD-HI subtype, only a few articles have been retrieved to match the requirement for this study. Among those selected actigraph-related articles, a few of commercial actigraph devices are listed in Table 19.5.

Among these articles, in terms of available open-source software to analyze and extract raw data, GENEActiv Original or also known as GENEActiv: Raw Data Accelerometry proved to be more affordable compared to other commercial actigraphs that are associated with a must-buy software package. This technical design offers 0.5 GB of optimal raw data collection in an open-source analysis format and comes as fully waterproof with two months of battery life and can be worn 24 hours a day [ActiveInsights, 2022]. For the vast majority of applications, GENEActiv Original is the most suitable device to be used to measure movement activities among school children [ActiveInsights, 2022]. The general properties of GENEActiv Original are included in Appendix 19.1.

An example of an obtained data set after performed movement activities by using the GeneActiv wristwatch with its free software is included in Appendix 19.2. This actigraph data set is about a 10-year-old subject who wore the wristwatch in the classroom for two hours. The spreadsheet collected information of x, y, and z axes movement position of the wristwatch.

TABLE 19.5
List of Selected Revised Actigraph Devices

Feature	Actigraph Corp	Active-Insights	Phillips	Ambulatory Monitoring	CamNtech
Actigraph	ActiGraph LEAP™, GT3X, GT9X CentrePoint® Insight watch	GENEActiv, Activinsights Band	Actiwatch, Actiwatch Spectrum	Micro Motionlogger® Watch, Sleep Watch® 2.0	MotionWatch 8, MotionWatch Rugged
Supplier	Florida	UK	US, Malaysia	New York	UK
Publication	>200[a]	>850	>400[b]	> 400	>600
ADHD publication	2[c]	1[d]	0	4[e]	2[f]
Movement detection	√	√	No (only sleeping)[g]	√	√
Software	√ Paid	√ Open-source	√ Open-source	√ Paid	√ Paid
Extract raw data	√	√	√	√	√

[a] 119 found exclude sleeping in 2020 and only about 50 plus articles being posted in the updated website for evidence in April 2023.

[b] Others > 400 related to newsletters or outside scientific papers.

[c] Gilbert et al. (2016) (GT3X) and Wood et al., 2009.

[d] Furrer et al. (2019).

[e] Kofler et al. (2018), Alderson et al. (2012), Dane et al. (1996), and Halperin et al. (1993).

[f] Chu et al. (2020) and Konrad et al. (2005) (+medication).

[g] Sleep/wake history reliably tracks sleep and two types of the actigraphs has added quantifiable physical activity data.

19.8   CONCLUSION

This chapter gives an insight of an overall research fields of ADHD, differential assessment of ADHD-HI subtype detection, and the experimental trends of the objective detection method of the ADHD-HI subtype. The published studies support that objective assessment to detect the ADHD-HI subtype is possible, and the actigraph device was found to be a promising experimental tool for the future. However, these publications mentioned limitations that need to be addressed in the future and more tests needed to refine the detection features toward a betterment of objective assessment. Adding an objective measure of activity to detect movements allows research to measure certain ADHD-HI subtype symptoms in closed or open experiment settings, and this may improve the clinical utility of wearable and nonwearable sensors. These sensors are more accessible and flexible and could aid subjective assessments to identify activity movement of children during experiments. The selection of sensors are includes either of single, or double wears or more depends on the research objectives, experimental settings, the field, and scope of the study.

Although this study chose the actigraph device to present its features, further investigation is needed to establish an objective tool to identify ADHD-HI subtype symptoms among children, which can facilitate faster, high sensitivity diagnosis, affordable marketing price, and the ability to detect early the disorder early.

APPENDIX

	GENEActiv
Sensor outputs	Acceleration, light, and temperature data at up to 100 Hz
Connectivity	Setup through USB cradle on PC or Android and download to PC
Data format	High resolution, raw SI unit data in an open format
Data storage	Sovereign data store or use of Activinsights' cloud store
Data analytics	Raw data analytics using proprietary, customised or open-source data analytics tools (e.g. R)
Battery life	1 week to 1 month
Data capacity	0.5 Gb
Waterproof	Yes
Body locations	Wrist, upper arm, chest, waist, thigh, ankle
Approvals	FDA 510(k) exempt, European Class 1 medical device
Size and weight	40 mm wide x 13 mm deep 27 G (16 G without strap)
Operating temperature	$5 - 40°C$
Warranty	1 year

APPENDIX 19.1 Types of Properties of GENEActiv (Adapted and modified from Activinsights, 2012; 2022; 2023)

Timestamp	x axis (g)	y axis (g)	z axis (g)	Light level (lux)	button (1/0)	Temperature (?)	Sum of vector magnitudes	SD of x axis	SD of y axis	SD of z axis	Peak lux
Timestamp of epoch end	Mean x axis	Mean y axis	Mean z axis	Mean lux	Sum button	Mean temperature (?)					
2020-10-09 16:00:46:000	-0.7888	-0.0597	-0.5616	794	0	27.1	156.24	0.1235	0.1523	0.1295	600
2020-10-09 16:01:46:000	-0.7801	-0.0386	-0.6915	293	0	27.4	149.02	0.1462	0.1462	0.32	580
2020-10-09 16:02:46:000	-0.9404	-0.1519	-0.6605	206	0	27.4	85.34	0.0794	0.1773	0.1499	420
2020-10-09 16:03:46:000	-0.9624	-0.0134	-0.1061	196	0	27.4	76.98	0.1009	0.1383	0.1982	300
2020-10-09 16:04:46:000	-0.9655	0.0172	-0.1899	259	0	27.7	56.89	0.0653	0.0463	0.1182	540
2020-10-09 16:05:46:000	-0.9895	0.023	-0.1106	244	0	27.7	29.84	0.0131	0.0137	0.0358	300
2020-10-09 16:08:46:000	-0.9904	-0.0250	-0.0737	217	0	27.7	43.54	0.0338	0.0468	0.071	300
2020-10-09 16:07:46:000	-0.9052	-0.034	-0.0925	200	0	27.7	134.92	0.3517	0.2596	0.2121	520
2020-10-09 16:08:46:000	-0.9542	-0.1304	-0.0295	300	0	27.7	167.41	0.1113	0.2009	0.1446	300
2020-10-09 16:09:46:000	-0.934	-0.1307	-0.0295	186	0	27.7	235.62	0.2017	0.2401	0.226	500
2020-10-09 16:10:46:000	-0.8186	0.0543	-0.1457	171	0	27.7	90.47	0.388	0.2853	0.2713	380
2020-10-09 16:11:46:000	-0.7813	0.1147	-0.1728	210	0	27.8	123.45	0.4416	0.3185	0.2342	400
2020-10-09 16:12:46:000	-0.9046	-0.1549	-0.2275	258	0	27.8	136.76	0.0907	0.1394	0.151	440
2020-10-09 16:13:46:000	-0.957	-0.1501	-0.1061	228	0	27.7	184.11	0.1191	0.1662	0.1231	320
2020-10-09 16:14:46:000	-0.9519	0.0021	-0.191	223	0	27.7	113.77	0.064	0.1168	0.1331	380
2020-10-09 16:15:46:000	-0.9389	-0.1018	-0.0281	225	0	27.8	110.88	0.5435	0.1863	0.1705	440
2020-10-09 16:16:46:000	-0.9735	-0.0721	-0.0483	204	0	27.8	134.43	0.0936	0.1594	0.1319	320
2020-10-09 16:17:46:000	-0.957	-0.0678	-0.1526	211	0	27.9	145.14	0.0944	0.1678	0.1069	360
2020-10-09 16:18:46:000	-0.9497	-0.1598	-0.1277	213	0	27.9	164.79	0.1055	0.1826	0.1298	340
2020-10-09 16:19:46:000	-0.2799	-0.3365	0.3517	239	0	27.9	197.86	0.5398	0.3196	0.5704	560
2020-10-09 16:20:46:000	-0.9757	-0.0803	-0.0436	217	0	27.9	191.78	0.1594	0.171	0.15	320
2020-10-09 16:21:46:000	-0.9672	-0.0689	-0.1412	237	0	28	106.57	0.0713	0.1367	0.1116	420
2020-10-09 16:22:46:000	-0.8462	-0.0672	-0.5185	230	0	28.1	181.7	0.7083	0.3104	0.2859	580
2020-10-09 16:23:46:000	-0.9552	-0.0479	-0.1491	98	0	28.2	145.23	0.1383	0.1758	0.1714	380
2020-10-09 16:24:46:000	-0.765	0.1585	0.1151	82	0	28.4	286.33	0.798	0.4104	0.4647	580
2020-10-09 16:25:46:000	0.7501	0.2359	0.582	25	0	28.5	318.43	0.2	0.2888	0.5712	100
2020-10-09 16:26:46:000	0.7097	0.1181	0.5835	21	0	28.7	236.6	0.1275	0.2243	0.1639	120
2020-10-09 16:27:46:000	0.6982	-0.0633	0.6577	22	0	29	126.05	0.1887	0.2021	0.1481	140
2020-10-09 16:28:46:000	0.5816	-0.2283	-0.0335	109	0	29.1	304.7	0.2587	0.3225	0.8965	600
2020-10-09 16:29:46:000	0.417	-0.0776	-0.8532	361	0	29.1	138.02	0.1652	0.1896	0.1155	620
2020-10-09 16:30:46:000	0.1623	-0.1145	-0.5354	232	0	29.2	258.59	0.8123	0.4174	0.4071	660
2020-10-09 16:31:46:000	0.7947	-0.1421	-0.4953	387	0	29	155.15	0.1395	0.2128	0.1966	560
2020-10-09 16:32:46:000	0.8886	-0.0164	-0.4062	260	0	29.8	103.29	0.0797	0.1255	0.1238	420
2020-10-09 16:33:46:000	0.8474	-0.0736	-0.2507	248	0	28.6	214.46	0.2611	0.1673	0.3918	400
2020-10-09 16:34:46:000	0.8907	-0.2469	-0.2541	249	0	28.5	178.96	0.1131	0.2217	0.1508	380
2020-10-09 16:35:46:000	-0.3521	-0.0668	-0.2709	245	0	28.4	142.3	0.164	0.1793	0.2607	520
2020-10-09 16:36:46:000	-0.9039	0.3154	0.0713	224	0	28.2	157.31	0.1148	0.1936	0.1936	320
2020-10-09 16:37:46:000	0.9233	-0.2301	0.0118	211	0	28	198.21	0.1498	0.215	0.2241	300
2020-10-09 16:38:46:000	0.6746	0.1525	0.321	150	0	27.9	318.26	0.411	0.52	0.3222	320
2020-10-09 16:39:46:000	-0.0873	0.1391	-0.2078	216	0	27.9	332.68	0.4108	0.4437	0.8215	680
2020-10-09 16:40:46:000	0.3972	-0.0388	-0.8689	427	0	27.9	142.7	0.1981	0.1695	0.1279	640
2020-10-09 16:41:46:000	-0.4931	0.0073	-0.8499	422	0	27.8	64.11	0.677	0.0653	0.0628	600
2020-10-09 16:42:46:000	0.5403	0.0704	-0.8037	413	0	27.7	71.1	0.1369	0.0987	0.0715	630
2020-10-09 16:43:46:000	-0.506	-0.0351	-0.7578	378	0	27.6	132.06	0.14	0.1513	0.1361	560
2020-10-09 16:44:46:000	-0.7948	-0.0295	-0.5475	396	0	27.4	205.9	0.1451	0.1589	0.1597	520
2020-10-09 16:45:46:000	-0.9129	-0.0155	0.5504	202	0	27.4	68.1	0.0799	0.0847	0.1425	460
2020-10-09 16:46:46:000	0.5894	-0.1073	0.1398	164	0	27.4	213.68	0.6312	0.4025	0.8537	480
2020-10-09 16:47:46:000	0.6897	0.2843	0.2543	80	0	27.4	157.81	0.4601	0.5448	0.1973	260
2020-10-09 16:48:46:000	0.9386	0.0564	-0.2367	137	0	27.4	66.19	0.1301	0.1691	0.146	700
2020-10-09 16:49:46:000	0.9424	0.0315	-0.2866	187	0	27.5	47.1	0.0541	0.0932	0.1064	200
2020-10-09 16:50:46:000	0.9763	0.056	-0.3268	119	0	27.6	47.82	0.0651	0.0818	0.1163	220
2020-10-09 16:51:46:000	-0.8797	-0.1008	-0.3851	131	0	27.7	111.5	0.108	0.1668	0.1853	320
2020-10-09 16:52:46:000	-0.883	-0.0636	-0.4149	141	0	27.7	136.09	0.2048	0.1317	0.163	320
2020-10-09 16:53:46:000	-0.7814	0.0237	-0.5951	191	0	27.7	47.76	0.0659	0.0495	0.1037	260
2020-10-09 16:54:46:000	-0.8403	0.023	-0.5134	131	0	27.5	50.22	0.5966	0.0514	0.0549	180
2020-10-09 16:55:46:000	0.9145	-0.0213	-0.9481	153	0	27.5	65.55	0.0746	0.0641	0.142	480
2020-10-09 16:56:46:000	-0.8373	-0.0527	0.5193	182	0	27.4	57.76	0.040	0.0499	0.0653	300
2020-10-09 16:57:46:000	0.9103	-0.0667	-0.5204	181	0	27.5	111.45	0.1294	0.1519	0.1496	540
2020-10-09 16:58:46:000	0.9051	0.075	-0.2763	184	0	27.5	101.99	0.1818	0.1277	0.2686	560
2020-10-09 16:59:46:000	-0.9155	-0.1384	-0.5983	143	0	27.7	142.02	0.7515	0.1854	0.2306	340
2020-10-09 17:00:46:000	0.8834	-0.0691	0.8158	131	0	27.7	164.82	0.2085	0.1603	0.2669	320
2020-10-09 17:01:46:000	-0.901	-0.0907	0.1735	147	0	27.7	236.44	0.209	0.2432	0.2766	540
2020-10-09 17:02:46:000	-0.9636	-0.1137	-0.0786	147	0	27.7	152.55	0.1398	0.1473	0.1548	300
2020-10-09 17:03:46:000	-0.939	-0.0243	-0.2999	130	0	27.7	104.89	0.1295	0.1163	0.1228	220
2020-10-09 17:04:46:000	-0.9988	0.025	-0.2399	148	0	27.7	77.41	0.072	0.0641	0.1559	340
2020-10-09 17:05:46:000	-0.9297	0.0053	-0.2619	208	0	27.7	119.05	0.0952	0.1515	0.1867	520
2020-10-09 17:06:46:000	-0.9303	0.0295	-0.2432	172	0	27.7	88.17	0.2179	0.1465	0.2041	460
2020-10-09 17:07:46:000	-0.974	0.0237	-0.197	115	0	27.7	42.22	0.0358	0.0257	0.0641	160
2020-10-09 17:08:46:000	-0.9727	-0.0315	-0.1958	115	0	27.8	154.83	0.7027	0.2157	0.2056	720
2020-10-09 17:09:46:000	-0.957	0.0019	-0.276	119	0	27.9	41.94	0.019	0.0313	0.0804	160
2020-10-09 17:10:46:000	0.9404	-0.056	-0.2062	121	0	27.8	44.42	0.0377	0.0424	0.0848	180
2020-10-09 17:11:46:000	-0.9558	-0.1173	-0.0707	124	0	27.9	71.63	0.059	0.1172	0.1097	240
2020-10-09 17:12:46:000	0.5089	0.2115	-0.803	160	0	27.8	197.02	0.5214	0.2601	0.415	780
2020-10-09 17:13:46:000	0.3706	0.0845	-0.7538	269	0	27.9	161.3	0.8812	0.2262	0.3208	560
2020-10-09 17:14:46:000	-0.5112	-0.2119	-0.5906	183	0	27.9	137.08	0.4826	0.2778	0.2197	520
2020-10-09 17:15:46:000	-0.4132	-0.2631	-0.2566	178	0	27.8	217.96	0.6578	0.354	0.4275	600
2020-10-09 17:16:46:000	-0.8942	0.075	-0.3038	151	0	27.8	162.97	0.1166	0.1291	0.2052	600
2020-10-09 17:17:46:000	-0.9273	-0.0678	-0.2213	142	0	27.8	152.86	0.1339	0.2159	0.183	300
2020-10-09 17:18:46:000	-0.4518	0.3051	0.4401	35	0	27.7	398.33	0.8731	0.508	0.4753	300
2020-10-09 17:19:46:000	-0.6183	0.0302	-0.0146	150	0	27.7	368.14	0.411	0.4103	0.6013	980
2020-10-09 17:20:46:000	-0.5844	0.2044	-0.1589	167	0	27.5	339.98	0.343	0.4759	0.5807	520
2020-10-09 17:21:46:000	-0.9512	-0.0001	-0.3777	25	0	27.4	149.37	0.2907	0.6985	0.1147	720
2020-10-09 17:22:46:000	-0.8577	0.0118	-0.3063	136	0	27.4	213.36	0.1577	0.1613	0.3672	520
2020-10-09 17:23:46:000	0.4669	0.1143	0.6534	47	0	27.5	205.98	0.6766	0.3307	0.3402	440
2020-10-09 17:24:46:000	-0.7967	0.0532	0.3181	86	0	27.7	168.52	0.3499	0.11	0.3915	260
2020-10-09 17:25:46:000	-0.7915	-0.0758	0.569	77	0	27.9	153.56	0.1553	0.1476	0.1693	180
2020-10-09 17:26:46:000	-0.7429	0.1009	0.4127	97	0	27.9	146.34	0.3595	0.4176	0.3026	260
2020-10-09 17:27:46:000	-0.4589	0.3761	0.2624	83	0	27.9	102.66	0.4895	0.5201	0.1723	480
2020-10-09 17:28:46:000	-0.6036	0.3322	0.323	110	0	27.8	223.22	0.5673	0.5295	0.4931	680
2020-10-09 17:29:46:000	-0.9475	0.0356	0.1796	132	0	27.7	73.54	0.1358	0.1592	0.1964	520
2020-10-09 17:30:46:000	-0.6963	-0.1117	0.1748	139	0	27.7	153.46	0.23	0.2523	0.249	520
2020-10-09 17:31:46:000	-0.8668	-0.0555	0.283	187	0	27.3	155.44	0.2007	0.2184	0.2936	540
2020-10-09 17:32:46:000	-0.9605	0.0035	0.7055	85	0	27.7	216.3	0.134	0.23	0.193	440
2020-10-09 17:33:46:000	-0.8662	-0.0663	0.2544	111	0	27.7	199.37	0.7925	0.347	0.3073	420
2020-10-09 17:34:46:000	-0.8509	0.1545	0.4407	110	0	27.7	292.38	0.1409	0.1956	0.196	360
2020-10-09 17:35:46:000	-0.6653	0.2311	0.4675	82	0	27.6	241.38	0.3589	0.3707	0.2993	380
2020-10-09 17:36:46:000	-0.4949	0.3549	0.2315	91	0	27.3	377.98	0.4884	0.9054	0.4734	1420
2020-10-09 17:37:46:000	-0.2197	0.0446	0.6879	116	0	27.3	190.45	0.2806	0.2801	0.5276	560
2020-10-09 17:38:46:000	-0.4341	-0.0815	0.6754	364	0	27.3	107.87	0.1134	0.1191	0.0814	500
2020-10-09 17:39:46:000	-0.5781	-0.049	-0.7626	338	0	27	131.27	0.1288	0.1227	0.1039	540
2020-10-09 17:40:46:000	-0.622	-0.0543	-0.4452	230	0	26.9	178.06	0.2148	0.1469	0.2866	600
2020-10-09 17:41:46:000	-0.9674	0.1114	-0.0658	171	0	26.9	129.9	0.0958	0.1403	0.1405	320
2020-10-09 17:42:46:000	-0.7709	0.2032	0.0454	155	0	26.9	215.17	0.3493	0.4062	0.382	360
2020-10-09 17:43:46:000	-0.7281	0.2778	0.1336	147	0	26.9	377.26	0.344	0.4453	0.3977	500
2020-10-09 17:44:46:000	-0.814	-0.2462	-0.0395	190	0	26.9	135.05	0.3242	0.3208	0.2667	480
2020-10-09 17:45:46:000	-0.7018	-0.7816	-0.7674	239	0	26.9	104.44	0.4031	0.3575	0.3222	540
2020-10-09 17:46:46:000	-0.9383	0.0596	0.28	151	0	27.3	68.99	0.1046	0.1171	0.1573	540
2020-10-09 17:47:46:000	-0.9311	0.0261	0.3254	137	0	27.5	54.92	0.0573	0.0959	0.1114	200
2020-10-09 17:48:46:000	-0.9614	0.0127	0.2466	142	0	27.2	140.1	0.1998	0.0994	0.1853	760
2020-10-09 17:49:46:000	-0.914	-0.0191	0.3672	117	0	27.4	56.74	0.0811	0.0986	0.1361	200
2020-10-09 17:50:46:000	0.8459	0.0425	0.3976	142	0	27.4	196.21	0.2317	0.2511	0.5047	580
2020-10-09 17:51:46:000	0.7495	-0.3977	0.4345	64	0	27.4	280.19	0.2281	0.299	0.2119	840
2020-10-09 17:52:46:000	-0.8647	-0.4931	-0.12	75	0	27.5	90.11	0.1562	0.2621	0.5891	400
2020-10-09 17:53:46:000	-0.3870	-0.5671	-0.4917	164	0	27.2	306.15	0.4271	0.2053	0.2843	1000
2020-10-09 17:54:46:000	-0.0002	0.6983	0.5232	228	0	27.6	506.16	0.6284	0.5564	0.4952	1000
2020-10-09 17:55:46:000	-0.6009	-0.4127	0.2901	75	0	27.6	209.18	0.3966	0.3593	0.369	1400
2020-10-09 17:56:46:000	-0.8304	-0.4539	0.1521	73	0	27.4	130.68	0.1894	0.232	0.1731	420
2020-10-09 17:57:46:000	-0.5784	-0.4168	0.212	53	0	27.4	212.98	0.2607	0.6031	0.2305	220
2020-10-09 17:58:46:000	-0.8413	-0.3743	0.1951	50	0	27.4	348.11	0.2463	0.7668	0.2599	480
2020-10-09 17:59:46:000	-0.8737	-0.178	0.2562	55	0	27.6	131.99	0.0989	0.1262	0.1133	380
2020-10-09 18:00:46:000	-0.863	0.4179	0.1497	50	0	27.7	130.11	0.1075	0.2178	0.1908	180

APPENDIX 19.2 Actigraph Dataset of a 10 Years Old Subject Wearing GeneActiv Wristwatch

REFERENCES

Activinsights; GENEActiv instructions. (2012). Online version downloaded from Activinsights Ltd. website on 15th Oct 2020 from https://www.activinsights.com/resources-support/geneactiv/downloads-software/

Activinsights; GENEActiv instructions. (2022). Online version downloaded from Activinsights Ltd. website on 10th May 2022 from https://activinsights.com/wp-content/uploads/2022/06/Product-Comparison-Sheet.pdf

Activinsights; GENEActiv Raw Data Accelerometry and Activinsights Band: Advanced Actigraphy. (2023). Online version revised from Activinsights Ltd. website on 25th Apr 2023 from https://activinsights.com/technology/

Ahmadi, A., Kashefi, M., Shahrokhi, H., & Nazari, M. A. (2021). Computer aided diagnosis system using deep convolutional neural networks for ADHD subtypes. *Biomedical Signal Processing and Control, 63*, 102227.

Altınkaynak, M., Dolu, N., Güven, A., Pektaş, F., Özmen, S., Demirci, E., & İzzetoğlu, M. (2020). Diagnosis of Attention Deficit Hyperactivity Disorder with combined time and frequency features. *Biocybernetics and Biomedical Engineering, 40*(3), 927–937.

Adamis, D., Unal, M., & O'Mahony, E. (2017). Use of eye-tracker device to detect attention deficits in adults with ADHD. *European Psychiatry, 41*(S1), S764–S764.

Alchalabi, A. E., Shirmohammadi, S., Eddin, A. N., & Elsharnouby, M. (2018). Focus: Detecting ADHD patients by an EEG-based serious game. *IEEE Transactions on Instrumentation and Measurement, 67*(7), 1512–1520.

Alderson, R. M., Rapport, M. D., Kasper, L. J., Sarver, D. E., & Kofler, M. J. (2012). Hyperactivity in boys with attention deficit/hyperactivity disorder (ADHD): The association between deficient behavioral inhibition, attentional processes, and objectively measured activity. *Child Neuropsychology, 18*, 487–505.

Amado-Caballero, P., Casaseca-de-la-Higuera, P., Alberola-Lopez, S., Andres-de-Llano, J. M., Lopez-Villalobos, J. A., Garmendia-Leiza, J. R., & Alberola-Lopez, C. (2020). Objective ADHD diagnosis using convolutional neural networks over daily-life activity records. *IEEE Journal of Biomedical and Health Informatics, 24*(9), 2690–2700.

Borcherding, B. G., Keysor, C. S., Cooper, T. B., & Rapoport, J. L. (1989). Differential effects of methylphenidate and dextroamphetamine on the motor activity level of hyperactive children. *Neuropsychopharmacology, 2*, 255–263.

Cecil, C.A.M., Nigg, J.T. (2022). Epigenetics and ADHD: Reflections on Current Knowledge, Research Priorities and Translational Potential. *Mol Diagn Ther, 26*, 581–606. https://doi.org/10.1007/s40291-022-00609-y

Chadd.org. Children and Adults with Attention-Deficit/Hyperactivity Disorder. (2020). General Prevalence of ADHD. Retrieved from https://chadd.org/about-adhd/general-prevalence/ on 4th Oct 2020.

Chu, K. C., Lu, H. K., Huang, M. C., Lin, S. J., Liu, W. I., Huang, Y. S., & Wang, C. H. (2020). Using mobile electroencephalography and actigraphy to diagnose attention-deficit/hyperactivity disorder: Case-control comparison study. *JMIR Mental Health, 7*(6), e12158.

CPG, Clinical Practice Guidelines. (2008). Ministry of Health, Malaysia. Retrieved on 6th June from https://translate.google.com/translate?hl=en&sl=ms&u=https://www.moh.gov.my/index.php/pages/view/948&prev=search

Dane, A. V., Schachar, R. J., & Tannock, R. (2000). Does actigraphy differentiate ADHD subtypes in a clinical research setting? *Journal of the American Academy of Child and Adolescent Psychiatry, 39*, 752–760.

Das, W., & Khanna, S. (2021). A robust machine learning based framework for the automated detection of ADHD using pupillometric biomarkers and time series analysis. *Scientific Reports, 11*(1), 16370. https://doi.org/10.1038/s41598-021-95673-5

De Crescenzo, F., Armando, M., Mazzone, L., Ciliberto, M., Sciannamea, M., Figueroa, C., & Vicari, S. (2014). The use of actigraphy in the monitoring of methylphenidate versus placebo in ADHD: A meta-analysis. *ADHD Attention Deficit and Hyperactivity Disorders, 6*(1), 49–58.

De Crescenzo, F., Licchelli, S., Ciabattini, M., Menghini, D., Armando, M., Alfieri, P., & Quested, D. (2016). The use of actigraphy in the monitoring of sleep and activity in ADHD: A meta-analysis. *Sleep Medicine Reviews, 26*, 9–20.

Donnelly, M., Rapoport, J. L., Potter, W. Z., Oliver, J., Keysor, C. S., & Murphy, D. L. (1989). Fenfluramine and dextroamphetamine treatment of childhood hyperactivity: Clinical and biochemical findings. *Archives of General Psychiatry, 46*, 205–212.

DSM-5; American Psychiatric Association. (2013). Diagnostic and Statistical Manual of Mental Disorders, Fifth Edition, DSM-5. Washington, DC: American Psychiatric Association.

Duda, M., Haber, N., Daniels, J., & Wall, D. P. (2017). Crowdsourced validation of a machine-learning classification system for autism and ADHD. *Translational Psychiatry, 7*(5), e1133. https://doi.org/10.1038/tp.2017.86

Faedda, G. L., Ohashi, K., Hernandez, M., McGreenery, C. E., Grant, M. C., Baroni, A., & Teicher, M. H. (2016). Actigraph measures discriminate pediatric bipolar disorder from attention-deficit/hyperactivity disorder and typically developing controls. *Journal of Child Psychology and Psychiatry, 57*(6), 706–716.

Find-A-Code. (2023). 6A05 Attention deficit hyperactivity disorder. *International Classification of Diseases for Mortality and Morbidity Statistics, 11th Revision, v2023-01.* Retrieved online on 27th Apr 2023 from https://www.findacode.com/icd-11/code-821852937.html#:~:text=6A05%20Attention%20deficit%20hyperactivity%20 disorder%20%2D%20ICD%2D11%20MMS

Gapin, J. I. (2009). *Associations among physical activity, ADHD symptoms, and executive function in children with ADHD.* The University of North Carolina at Greensboro.

Ghiassian, S., Greiner, R., Jin, P., & Brown, M. R. (2016). Using functional or structural magnetic resonance images and personal characteristic data to identify ADHD and autism. *PloS One, 11*(12), e0166934.

Gilbert, H., Qin, L., Li, D., Zhang, X., & Johnstone, S. J. (2016). Aiding the diagnosis of AD/HD in childhood: Using actigraphy and a continuous performance test to objectively quantify symptoms. *Research in Developmental Disabilities, 59*, 35–42.

Ginsberg, Y., Quintero, J., Anand, E., Casillas, M., & Upadhyaya, H. P. (2014). Underdiagnosis of attention-deficit/hyperactivity disorder in adult patients: A review of the literature. *The Primary Care Companion for CNS Disorders, 16*(3), 23591.

Griffiths, K. R., Quintana, D. S., Hermens, D. F., Spooner, C., Tsang, T. W., Clarke, S., & Kohn, M. R. (2017). Sustained attention and heart rate variability in children and adolescents with ADHD. *Biological Psychology, 124*, 11–20.

Gunther, T., Kahraman-Lanzerath, B., Knospe, E. L., HerpertzDahlmann, B., & Konrad, K. (2012). Modulation of attention-deficit/hyperactivity disorder symptoms by short- and long-acting methylphenidate over the course of a day. *Journal of Child and Adolescent Psychopharmacology, 22*, 131–138.

Güven, A., Altınkaynak, M., Dolu, N. et al. (2020). Combining functional near-infrared spectroscopy and EEG measurements for the diagnosis of attention-deficit hyperactivity disorder. *Neural Comput & Applic, 32*, 8367–8380. https://doi.org/10.1007/s00521-019-04294-7

Hall, S., Halperin, J., Schwartz, S., & Newcorn, J. (1997). Behavioral and executive functions in children with attention-deficit hyperactivity disorder and reading disability. *Journal of Attention Disorders, 1*, 235–243.

Hall, C. L., Valentine, A. Z., Groom, M. J., Walker, G. M., Sayal, K., Daley, D., & Hollis, C. (2016). The clinical utility of the continuous performance test and objective measures of activity for diagnosing and monitoring ADHD in children: A systematic review. *European Child & Adolescent Psychiatry, 25*(7), 677–699.

Halperin, J. M., Matier, K., Bedi, G., Sharma, V., & Newcorn, J. H. (1992). Specificity of inat-
    tention, impulsivity, and hyperactivity to the diagnosis of attention-deficit hyperactivity
    disorder. *Journal of the American Academy of Child and Adolescent Psychiatry, 31*,
    190–196.
Hamrakova, A., Ondrejka, I., Sekaninova, N., Peregrim, L., & Tonhajzerova, I. (2019).
    Pupillary light reflex in children with ADHD. *Acta Medica Martiniana, 19*(1), 30–37.
Heller, M. D., Roots, K., Srivastava, S., Schumann, J., Srivastava, J., & Hale, T. S. (2013). A
    machine learning-based analysis of game data for attention deficit hyperactivity dis-
    order assessment. *Games for Health Journal, 2*(5), 291–298. https://doi.org/10.1089/
    g4h.2013.0058
ICD-11, International Classification of Diseases, 11th revision. (2019). World Health
    Organization, Geneva.
IMH.org [Institute of Mental Health]. (2020). A Randomised Controlled Trial of a Brain-
    Computer Interface Based Intervention for the Treatment of Attention Deficit
    Hyperactivity Disorder (ADHD). Retrieved from https://www.imh.com.sg/research/
    page on 4th Oct 2020.
Inoue, K., Nadaoka, T., Oiji, A., Morioka, Y., Totsuka, S., Kanbayashi, Y., & Hukui, T. (1998).
    Clinical evaluation of attention-deficit hyperactivity disorder by objective quantitative
    measures. *Child Psychiatry and Human Development, 28*(3), 179–188
James, M. E., King-Dowling, S., & Graham, J. D. et al. (2022). Effects of comorbid devel-
    opmental coordination disorder and symptoms of attention deficit hyperactivity dis-
    order on physical activity in children aged 4–5 years. *Child Psychiatry & Human
    Development, 53*, 786–796. https://doi.org/10.1007/s10578-021-01155-0
Jensen, P. S. (2001). AD/HD: What's up, what's next? *Attention! 7*, 24–27.
Jiang, X., Chen, Y., Huang, W., Zhang, T., Gao, C., Xing, Y., & Zheng, Y. (2020). WeDA:
    Designing and Evaluating a Scale-driven Wearable Diagnostic Assessment System for
    Children with ADHD. *CHI '20: Proceedings of the 2020 CHI Conference on Human
    Factors in Computing Systems, 1*–12. https://doi.org/10.1145/3313831.3376374
Kaufmann, F., Kalbfleisch, M. L., & Castellanos, F. X. (2000). Attention Deficit Disorders
    and Gifted Students: What Do We Really Know? *The National Research Center on the
    Gifted and Talented, Senior School Series.* Connecticut, U.S.
Kofler, M. J., Spiegel, J. A., Austin, K. E., Irwin, L. N., Soto, E. F., & Sarver, D. E. (2017).
    Are episodic buffer processes intact in ADHD? Experimental evidence and linkage
    with hyperactive behavior. *Journal of Abnormal Child Psychology, 46*(6), 1171–1185.
Konrad, K., Gunther, T., Heinzel-Gutenbrunner, M., & Herpertz-Dahlmann, B. (2005).
    Clinical evaluation of subjective and objective changes in motor activity and attention
    in children with attention-deficit/hyperactivity disorder in a double-blind methylpheni-
    date trial. *Journal of Child and Adolescent Psychopharmacology, 15*, 180–190.
Lerner, L., & Lerner, B. W. (Eds.). (2008). *The gale encyclopedia of science* (4th ed.).
    Thomson Gale, Detroit.
Lewin, A. B. (2003). Laboratory Measures of ADHD. PowerPoint PPT Presentation. Retrieved
    on 20th Oct 2019 from https://www.slideserve.com/omer/laboratory-measures-of-adhd-
    powerpoint-ppt-presentation
Loh, H. W., Ooi, C. P., Barua, P. D., Palmer, E. E., Molinari, F., & Acharya, U. (2022).
    Automated detection of ADHD: Current trends and future perspective. *Computers in
    Biology and Medicine*, 105525.
Marcano, J. L. L., Bell, M. A., & Beex, A. L. (2017, February). Classification of ADHD and
    Non-ADHD using theta/beta power ratio features. In *2017 IEEE EMBS International
    Conference on Biomedical & Health Informatics (BHI)* (pp. 345–348). IEEE.
Marks, D. J., Himelstein, J., Newcorn, J. H., & Halperin, J. M. (1999). Identification of AD/
    HD subtypes using laboratory-based measures: A cluster analysis. *Journal of Abnormal
    Child Psychology, 27*, 167–175.

Muñoz-Organero, M., Powell, L., Heller, B., Harpin, V., & Parker, J. (2018). Automatic extraction and detection of characteristic movement patterns in children with ADHD based on a convolutional neural network (CNN) and acceleration images. *Sensors, 18*(11), 3924.

Myhealth.gov.my. (2020). Attention Deficit Hyperactivity Disorder. Retrieved from http://www.myhealth.gov.my/en/attention-deficit-hyperactivity-disorder/ on 4th Oct 2020.

NIMH, National Institute of Mental Health. (2006). Attention deficit hyperactivity disorder (NIH) Publication No. 3572. Bethesda, MD: U.S. Department of Health and Human Services.

O'Mahony, N., Florentino-Liano, B., Carballo, J. J., Baca-García, E., & Rodríguez, A. A. (2014). Objective diagnosis of ADHD using IMUs. *Medical Engineering and Physics, 36*, 922–926.

Oztekin, I., Finlayson, M. A., Graziano, P. A., & Dick, A. S. (2021). Is there any incremental benefit to conducting neuroimaging and neurocognitive assessments in the diagnosis of ADHD in young children? A machine learning investigation. *Developmental Cognitive Neuroscience, 49*, 100966. https://doi.org/10.1016/j.dcn.2021.100966

Paloyelis, Y., Mehta, M. A., Kuntsi, J., & Asherson, P. (2007). Functional MRI in ADHD: A systematic literature review. *Expert Review of Neurotherapeutics, 7*(10), 1337–1356.

Pierangelo, R., & Giuliani, G. (2007). *Classroom management techniques for students with ADHD: A step-by-step guide for educators.* Corwin Press, Thousand Oaks, CA.

Porrino, L. J., Rapoport, J. L., Behar, D., Sceery, W., Ismond, D. R., & Bunney, W. E. Jr. (1983). A naturalistic assessment of the motor activity of hyperactive boys. I. Comparison with normal controls. *Archives of General Psychiatry, 40*, 681–687.

Rajendran, K., O'Neill, S., Marks, D. J., & Halperin, J. M. (2015). Latent profile analysis of neuropsychological measures to determine preschoolers' risk for ADHD. *Journal of Child Psychology and Psychiatry, 56*(9), 958–965.

Rapoport, J. L., Tepsic, P. N., Grice, J., Johnson, C., & Langer, D. (1980). Decreased motor activity of hyperactive children on dextroamphetamine during active gym program. *Psychiatry Research, 2*, 225–229.

SAMHSA: Substance Abuse and Mental Health Services Administration. (2016). DSM-5 Changes: Implications for Child Serious Emotional Disturbance [Internet]. *Substance Abuse and Mental Health Services Administration* Table 7, DSM-IV to DSM-5 Attention-Deficit/Hyperactivity Disorder Comparison. Rockville, Maryland, U.S.

Serrano-Barroso, A., Siugzdaite, R., Guerrero-Cubero, J., Molina-Cantero, A. J., Gomez-Gonzalez, I. M., Lopez, J. C., Vargas, J. P. (2021). Detecting Attention Levels in ADHD Children with a Video Game and the Measurement of Brain Activity with a Single-Channel BCI Headset. *Sensors (Basel), 21*(9), 3221. doi: 10.3390/s21093221. PMID: 34066492; PMCID: PMC8124980.

Soref, S. (2019). What is the role of lab testing in the diagnosis of attention deficit hyperactivity disorder (ADHD)? Retrieved from MedScape website on 10th September from https://www.medscape.com/answers/289350-4478/what-is-the-role-of-lab-testing-in-the-diagnosis-of-attention-deficit-hyperactivity-disorderadhd#:~:text=The%20 diagnosis%20of%20attention%20deficit%20hyperactivity%20disorder%20 (ADHD)%20is%20based,Serum%20CBC%20count%20with%20differential

Tanko, D., Barua, P. D., Dogan, S., Tuncer, T., Palmer, E., Ciaccio, E. J., & Acharya, U. R. (2022). EPSPatNet86: Eight-pointed star pattern learning network for detection ADHD disorder using EEG signals. *Physiol Meas, 43*(3). doi: 10.1088/1361-6579/ac59dc. PMID: 35377344.

Teicher, M. H. (1995). Actigraphy and motion analysis: New tools for psychiatry. *Harvard Review of Psychiatry, 3*, 18–35.

Varela, Casal P., et al. (2019). Clinical validation of eye vergence as an objective marker for diagnosis of ADHD in children. *Journal of Attention Disorders, 23*(6), 599–614. https://doi.org/10.1177/1087054717749931

Wang, Z. (2017). Neurofeedback training intervention for enhancing working memory function in attention deficit and hyperactivity disorder (ADHD) Chinese students. *NeuroQuantology, 15*(2), 277–183.

WHO: World Health Organization. (2023). ICD-11 2022 release. Retrieved online on 26th Apr 2023 from https://www.who.int/news/item/11-02-2022-icd-11-2022-release

Wiguna, T., Wigantara, N. A., Ismail, R. I., Kaligis, F., Minayati, K., Bahana, R., & Dirgantoro, B. (2020). A four-step method for the development of an ADHD-VR digital game diagnostic tool prototype for children using a DL model. *Frontiers in Psychiatry, 11*, 829.

Wood, A. C., Asherson, P., Rijsdijk, F., & Kuntsi, J. (2009). Is overactivity a core feature in ADHD? Familial and receiver operating characteristic curve analysis of mechanically assessed activity level. *Journal of the American Academy of Child & Adolescent Psychiatry, 48*(10), 1023–1030.

Ye, H., Bhatt, S., Zhong, W., Watson, J., Sargent, A., Topoglu, Y., & Suri, R. (2019). The Effects of Advertising on Cognitive Performance. In *International conference on applied human factors and ergonomics* (pp. 78–83). Springer.

Yeh, S. C., Lin, S. Y., Wu, E. H. K., Zhang, K. F., Xiu, X., Rizzo, A., & Chung, C. R. (2020). A virtual-reality system integrated with neuro-behavior sensing for attention-deficit/hyperactivity disorder intelligent assessment. *IEEE Transactions on Neural Systems and Rehabilitation Engineering, 28*(9), 1899–1907.

Yim, D., Lee, W. H., Kim, J. I., Kim, K., Ahn, D. H., Lim, Y. H., & Cho, S. H. (2019). Quantified activity measurement for medical use in movement disorders through IR-UWB radar sensor. *Sensors, 19*(3), 688.

Yu, C. L., Chueh, T. Y., Hsieh, S. S., Tsai, Y. J., Hung, C. L., Huang, C. J., & Hung, T. M. (2019). Motor competence moderates relationship between moderate to vigorous physical activity and resting EEG in children with ADHD. *Mental Health and Physical Activity, 17*, 100302.

Zentall, S. S. (2006). *ADHD and education: Foundations, characteristics, methods, and collaboration.* PEARSON, US.

20 Security of Medical Image Information by Cryptography and Watermarking Using Python

Pallavi R. Waghmare[1], Jayshree M. Waghmare[2], and Deepak D. Kshirsagar[1]
[1]Department of Computer Engineering & IT,
COEP Technological University (COEP Tech), Pune, India
[2]Department of Computer Science & Engineering,
SGGS IE & T, Nanded, India

CONTENTS

20.1 INTRODUCTION

Medical imaging such as ultrasound, X-rays, computerized tomography (CT) scans, and magnetic resonance imaging (MRI). It has a crucial function in identifying various disorders (Magdy et al., 2022). With the recent advancements in the Internet, massive volumes of information can now be shared and transferred online from diagnostic centers to physicians (Venkatasubramanian et al., 2012). We can download medical data or images without any approval from the owner, and this may cause all kinds of

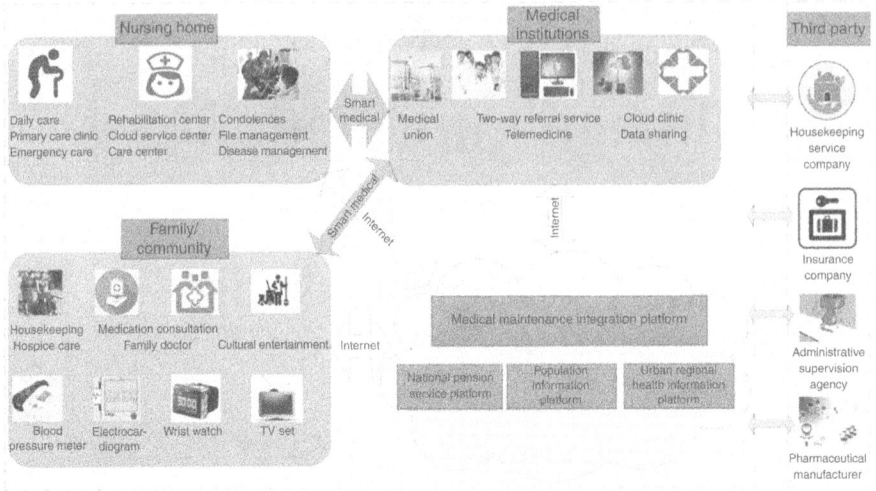

FIGURE 20.1 Medical health information data flow given by Jiang et al. (2019).

problems, such as proof of ownership, security, copyright protection, etc. (Cheddad et al., 2010). Especially in this computer technology era, the growth of telemedicine services like telesurgery and teleconsultation has increased a lot. The development in healthcare and medical information data flow is given by Jiang et al. (2019), seen in Figure 20.1, which also mentions the information demand for medical image exchange between patients, doctors, scan facilities, and insurance data sources.

Medical images contain essential and sensitive information compared to other digital images. Each and every pixel in the image is necessary for diagnosis, and small malpractice can be a cause of faulty diagnosis. Medical imaging seeks to locate and treat disease and reveal internal organs and bone and skin structures. Figure 20.1 shows how healthcare information begins from a nursing home, family, or community centers, and that information is shared with medical institutes either using the cloud or a local server by Internet. Hence, to safeguard patients' sensitive information during the transmission of medical pictures, this medical data should be communicated using a secure communication channel. So, false diagnoses may result if the attacker intercepts and modifies the transmitted healthcare information. Thus, maintaining confidentiality and integrity in transmitting healthcare data has become a major challenge. Therefore, greater care must be taken to protect healthcare information transfers over public networks. The three common methods for medical picture security are watermarking, steganography, and cryptography.

20.1.1 RECENT TRENDS

Researchers have reported various methods to secure information in digital images to address medical information security, such as digital signing, etc. Kuang et al. (2009) and Begum and Uddin (2020) have discussed digital watermarking and described image watermarking to solve various types of cybersecurity issues using copyright protection techniques. For example, Maurya et al. (2020) shows an extended visual cryptography technique for medical data protection. Kaur and Sharma (2013) introduces the novel cryptosystem TJ-ACA in the CBC mode algorithm for encrypting color images. Haidekker (2013), Magdy et al. (2022), Mitra (2016), and Santos et al. (2021) discussed the systematic review of security techniques and the improvement of image security in healthcare systems. Jasra and Moon (2020) described and analyze multimedia data security across public networks. Hasavari and Song (2019) and Venkateswarlu (2020) proposed both watermarking security with encryption. Katzenbeisser and Petitcolas (2000) suggested the techniques of information security in medical data. This is necessary for confidentiality between patients' diagnosis data and their medical history, e.g., physician, name of the patient, address, diseases, and other particulars. Jain and Kumar (2016a, 2016b) present the segmentation of liver ultrasound (US) images to extract patient health information. Further, Usman and Usman (2018) have presented a novel way to picture steganography. For securing medical data, Swapped Huffman tree coding is used to apply compression algorithm and manifold encoding to the payload before integrating it into the cover image. Tambe et al. (2018) and Wayner (2009) suggested that the framework adds an extra degree of protection by combining cryptography and steganography. The encrypted data are then incorporated into the default image of a system using the LSB algorithm. Using the uniform split and merge technique, the steganography default picture is partitioned into uniform portions and merged in reverse order. Rani and Kumar (2019) used the pixel values variance between a genuine image and its JPEG version to detect the image forgery techniques. Chen et al. (2012) listed a popular probabilistic model using the Markov random field (MRF) for representing the interplay of several events. To resolve these security requirements (Jasra and Moon, 2020), a variety of solutions have been proposed, including picture scrambling, digital watermarking, image steganography (Cheddad et al., 2010), and image cryptography (Zain and Fauzi, 2006). The visual cryptography technique by Saturwar and Chaudhari (2017) is a secret sharing system in which an original image is broken down into image shares and piled on top of one another to disclose a concealed secret image (Pape, 2014).

20.1.2 Motivation

However, all these methods are used by most individuals. Thus, in this chapter, we propose a hybrid approach for robust security in healthcare applications. The proposed hybrid method uses cryptography and watermarking techniques. Watermarking has the unique virtue of visually decoding the secret image by superimposing patient information for copyright or validation. Along with the password key for encryption, the approach is also used to make the visual cryptography image sharing safer and more robust in nature. The proposed methodology is implemented using a GUI in open-source Python programming. Further details are given in the subsequent sections. Section 20.2 explains the types of healthcare information standards and provides an overview of cyberattacks and existing security methods. Section 20.3 discusses the proposed hybrid methodology using cryptography and watermarking methods, with GUI steps described. Afterward, in Section 20.4, results and discussions of proposed and existing techniques are elucidated. In addition to this, in Section 20.4.2 quantitative analysis is carried out for PSNR, MSE, AD, MD, NAE, and NCC performance measures for original and decrypted medical images. The conclusion is presented in Section 20.5.

20.1.3 CONTRIBUTION

Overall, this chapter contributes as follows:

- We explain the necessity and types of cyberattacks on medical healthcare sensitive data.
- The chapter introduces existing technologies for image safety.
- We propose a hybrid approach for healthcare image security.
- Five different types of medical images data sets are taken into consideration.
- We develop an open-source Python-based GUI to demonstrate the proposed hybrid approach.
- The analysis by qualitative and quantitative performance measures such as PSNR, MSE, AD, MD, NAE, and NCC is computed.
- Original medical images with watermarked, encrypted, and watermarked + encrypted along with passkey images are compared.

20.2 TYPES OF CYBERCRIME ATTACKS IN HEALTHCARE AND THE STANDARD MEDICAL IMAGES DATA SET

In Southwick (2022), many cyberattacks in the health sector have been reported and documented in the USA. Florida's Broward Health Department announced earlier that such attacks may have affected more than 1.3 million customers. The US Department of Health and Human Services monitors hacks and security lapses at healthcare organizations (Zhang et al., 2020); the attacks are listed in Table 20.1. According to the agency, 618 breaches and assaults in 2021 affected at least 500 persons. According to a survey by IBM, the average cost of a healthcare breach increased to $9.4 million, up from $2 million the previous year. Healthcare ransomware attacks typically cost $4.6 million per (Southwick, 2022). The scope of this chapter is restricted to the following medical imaging types: ultrasound, X-rays, CT scans, MRI, and nuclear images. Figure 20.2 shows these imaging

---

TABLE 20.1

Types of Medical Image Cyber Attacks

Medical Cyber Attack	Category	Illustration
Median filter	Denoising	Algorithm of non-linear filter for removal of noise
Compression of image	JPEG compression	A digital compression of pixels
Scaling of image	JPEG compression	A linear transformation to modify the size of image large (scale up) and small (scale down)
Rotation	Geometric	Circulate the orientation of image around a point
Cropping	Geometric	Cutout the portion of image
Shearing	Geometric	Pushing part of the image from one location to other in the image through transformation
Salt and pepper	Noise attack	Deliberately add white and black pixels into the image
Gaussian	Noise attack	Statistical noise with a probability density function known as a Gaussian distribution
Histogram equalization	Image processing	Changes the contrast, intensity of the image

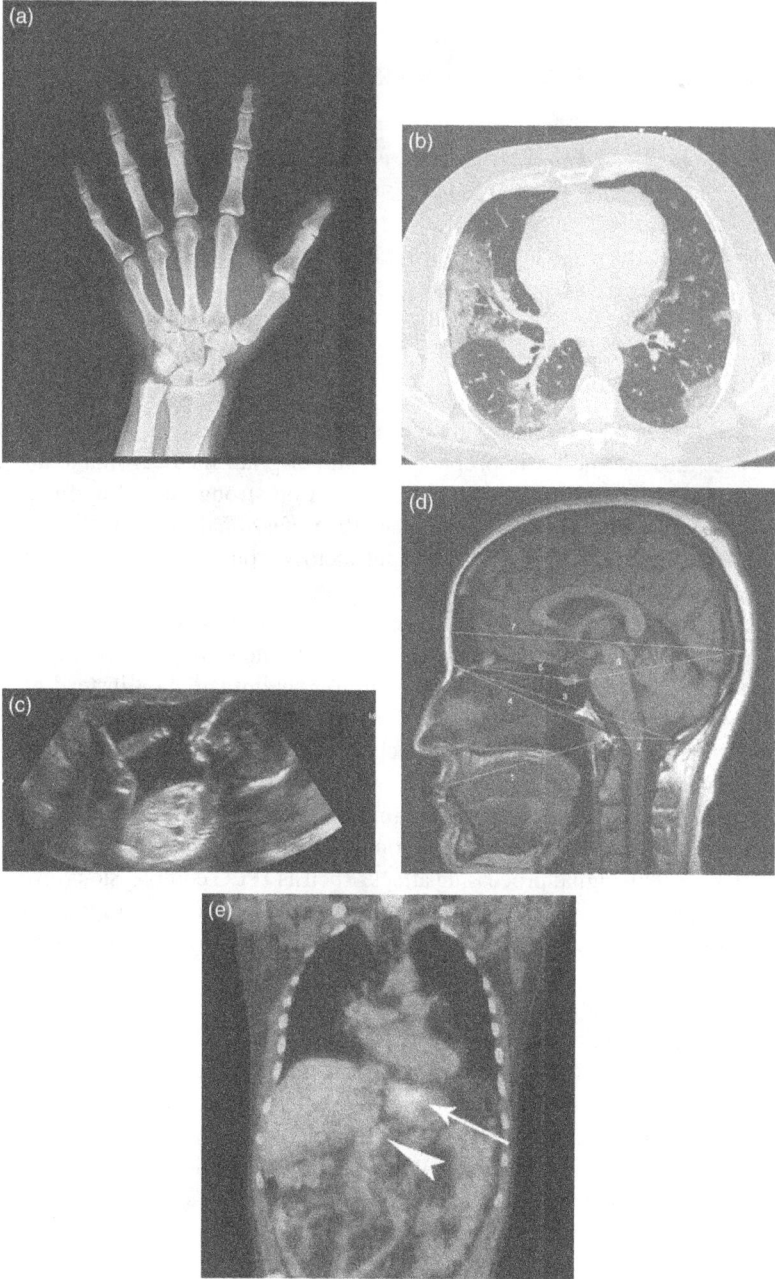

FIGURE 20.2 Medical original images of (a) Patient 1: X-ray (b) Patient 2: ultrasonic (c) Patient 3: CT scan (d) Patient 4: MRI (e) Patient 5: nuclear image.

TABLE 20.2

Properties of Original Medical Image Referred

Sr. No. of Image	Type of Image	File Format	File Size	Resolution	DPI	Bit Depth	Entropy
Patient 1	X-ray	JPG	1.73 MB	5967 × 7175	72 dpi	24	5.371382065
Patient 2	Ultrasound	JPG	62.2 KB	1600 × 761	72 dpi	24	6.568867939
Patient 3	CT scan	PNG	6.56 MB	2825 × 2500	600 dpi	32	7.018814499Ss
Patient 4	MRI	JPG	51.4 KB	542 × 546	300 dpi	24	6.450015398
Patient 5	Nuclear image	JPG	472 KB	500 × 500	72 dpi	24	7.109913478

types, which help physicians to find the functionality of patient medical disorders (PhysioNet, 2022). The basic properties of the original medical image are given in Table 20.2. Medical image security is based on strong ethical and regulatory norms that offer patients' rights and health professionals responsibilities. This necessitates the following three important factors: confidentiality, dependability, and availability (Santos et al., 2021).

During transmission over e-health networks, medical pictures may be impacted by a variety of threats. Tampering with a protected medical image is a cyberattack on the healthcare sector. These attacks aim to contaminate data instead of cracking cyphers and damaging protected information are listed in Table 20.1. Scaling, rotation, translation, cropping, and stretching are examples of geometric assaults. Signal processing cyberattack techniques include adaptive histogram, gamma correction, contrast adjustment, and histogram equalization. On the other hand, denoising attacks include image filtering techniques like median, average, and Sobel filters. In addition, various signal processing attacks such as JPEG compressions are used in picture compression strategies. These attacks distort the medical original information of patients, and due to these attacks, a wrong diagnosis may happen, and patients be harmed.

To prevent a cyberattack, for the last several years, researchers have been finding new methodologies to communicate and transmit information secretly. An example is the cryptography method, which is concerned with the method of encrypted communication. Further subdivisions are visual cryptography and digital signing. The visual cryptography scheme is a safe way to encrypt a secret document or image by splitting it down into image shares (Wayner, 2009). Visual cryptography has subtypes such as symmetric key, asymmetric key, and hash functions (Liu and Yan, 2014). Digital signing is another cryptography technique mostly used in the digital transmission of signals such as online payments, secure gateway, and a few public social sharing applications, etc. (Batten, 2013). The most efficient authentication mechanism in financial applications is symmetric key sharing, preferred by Maurya et al. (2020). Further, in digital watermarking, like steganography (Tambe et al., 2018), the information is embedded into the image. Two types of steganography are linguistic and technical. Technical steganography is classified into digital images, video, audio, and text content. The steps are given in Figure 20.3. Thus, it is seen

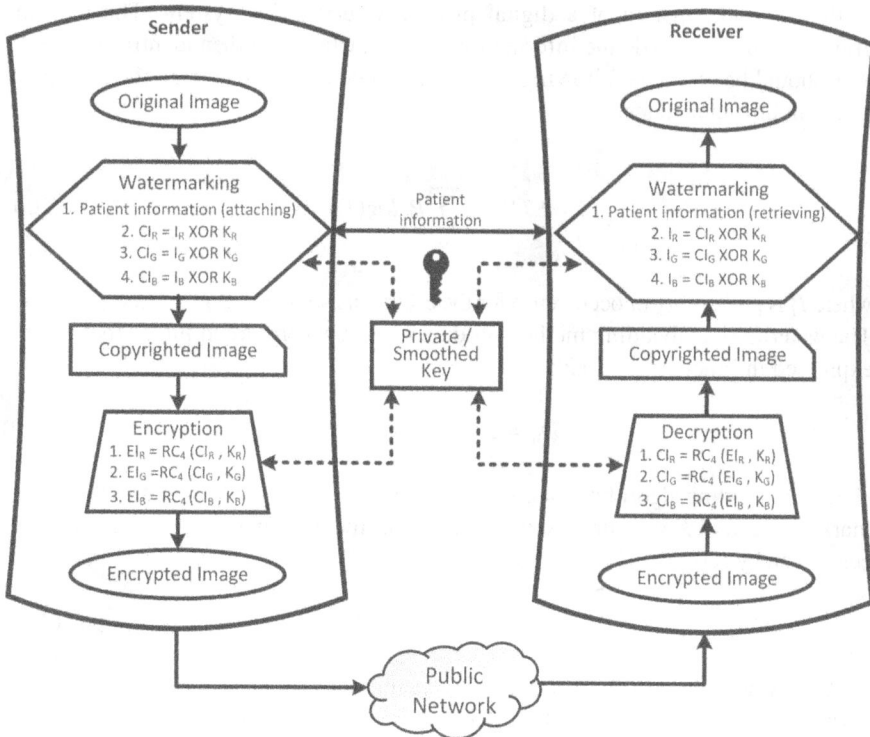

FIGURE 20.3 Steps of watermarking. Steps by Venkateswarlu (2020, 8).

that few requirements exist for characteristics and performance of watermarking, cryptography, and steganography techniques. Must have flaws such as robustness, security, capacity, computational cost, false positive, watermark keys, and tamper resistance.

20.3 PROPOSED HYBRID METHOD OF WATERMARKING AND CRYPTOGRAPHY TECHNIQUE

In the past, various researchers (Cheddad et al., 2010; Magdy et al., 2022) have developed and applied information hiding techniques that are discussed and enlisted in Waghmare and Waghmare (2022). Therefore, the proposed hybrid approach uses digital watermarking, cryptography, and a security key. The digital watermarking added a watermark into multimedia data to ensure the authenticity and copyright holder. Digital watermarking was founded in 1988 enabling secrecy, integrity, and availability (Cheddad et al., 2010). A symbol of owner authenticity (a watermark) is implanted in the host signal using watermarking methods, and the watermark data may then be retrieved. Information entropy is used in the digital picture watermarking strategy to mimic the human visual perception system. A just noticeable difference (JND) model may be used to create an ideal balance among imperceptibility, resilience, and capacity of a digital picture watermarking system. The masking effect may be used to define information entropy, which can then identify where the data should be put. The following equations can be used to calculate the entropy of a system having n states.

$$ETP = -\sum_{i=1}^{n} P_i \ log(P_i) \tag{20.1}$$

where P_i is probability of occurrence for the event i; its value is $0 \le P_i \le 1$ and $\sum_{i=1}^{n} P_i = 1$. The watermark embedding method produces D_W, a watermarked image that may be expressed in function as (20.2):

$$D_W = E(I, \ ETP, \ W, \ K) \tag{20.2}$$

Here E = encoding algorithm, I = cover image, ETP = entropy information, W = watermark image, and K = security key. Similarly, for the watermark extraction (W') process given by (20.3):

$$W' = e(D_W, \ K, \ ETP, \ I) \tag{20.3}$$

After watermarking the watermarked medical image, the next step is to go for cryptography with a security key. The public key encryption technology secures picture sharing to the point where it's difficult for a third party to decipher the secret image information without the appropriate data, without the security key. The picture encrypting approach M. Kaur et al. (2021), is based on one of two principles: permutation or diffusion, or a mix of both. The location of pixel values is modified in permutation alone approaches without affecting the pixel values themselves. Figure 20.4 depict the steps of image encryption from sender to receiver and then decrypting it at the receiver side.

The secret information embedding process is similar to Figure 20.4, and the difference can be seen in equations (20.4) and (20.5):

$$Emb: C \oplus K \oplus \rightarrow CEmb: g_k = (C, M) \tag{20.4}$$

Here C = cover image, M = file to hide, g_k = algorithm, and K = passkey (used for the encrypting message):

$$Ext\left[Emb(c, \ k, \ m)\right] \approx m, \ \forall \ c \in C, \ k \in K, \ m \in M \tag{20.5}$$

Hence, to implement the proposed methodology, a GUI for healthcare applications was developed using Python programming. The GUI is shown in Figure 20.5, where all the input and menu panels can be seen. To create a watermarked image, the suggested method begins by embedding a smoothened key photo (K) and patient information over the original image $(I) \times (W)$. Then, using the same

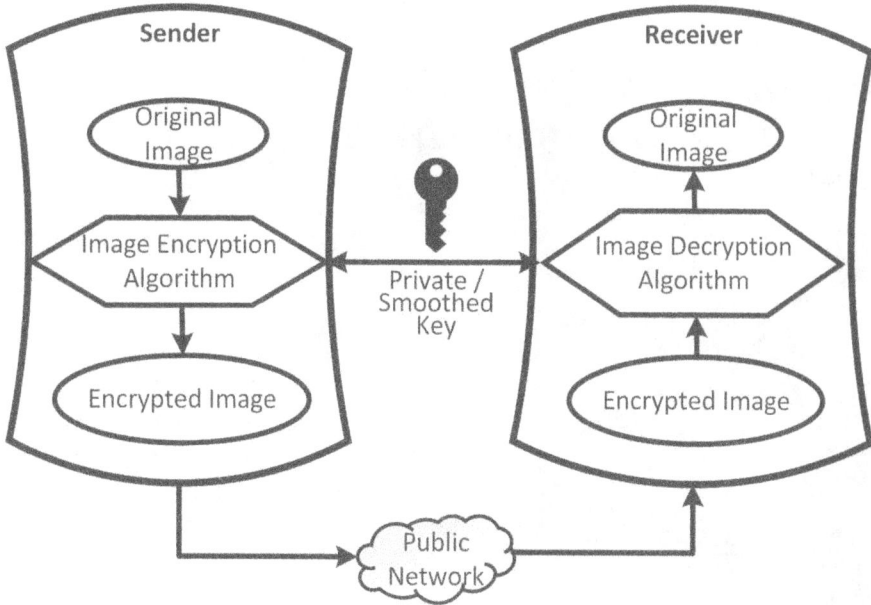

FIGURE 20.4 Image encryption steps.

smoothened key picture, each color channel of the watermarked picture (W) is encrypted individually to produce an encrypted picture $(E) \times (K)$. This image can be transmitted over an untrusted network, and the (I) can be recovered using a decryption technique, followed by de-watermarking at the recipient using the same key image (K). There are several languages that are employed in various contexts. However, there are certain languages that are widely applicable and universal. For example, Python is one language that is utilized and favored for development on a global scale. It is a widely used, general-purpose, high-level object-oriented programming (OOP)-based interpreted language for dynamic applications. Python is exceptionally well liked for its adaptability and range of uses. Here it is used the Tkinter library to develop GUI.

After encryption, the output file can't be read by the other software. Figure 20.6 shows an error message popup by other image software from the computer.

20.4   RESULTS AND DISCUSSION

It's also important to make sure that the picture file's header matches the image data. For image encryption, the basic requirements are as follows: The encryption of any type of data produces cypher text or data that must be distinct from the original picture, with no remnants or hints of the original data preferred. There are challenges for the image watermarking method, such as watermark attacks (harmful detection or impairment). These attacks can be intentional or unintentional and may cause distortion in the watermarked images. They fall into various categories, including active, passive,

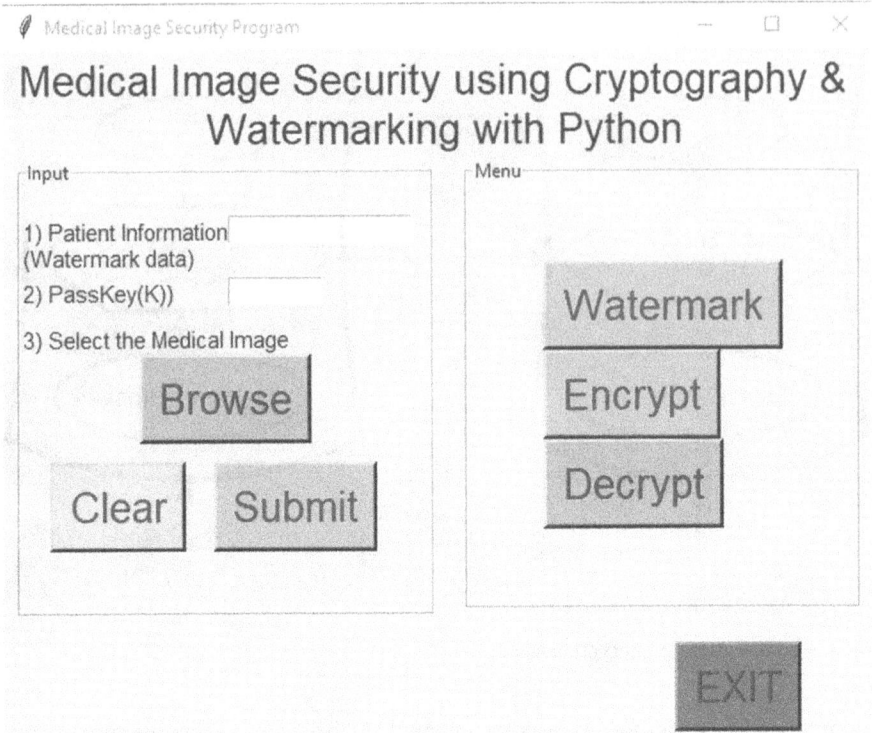

FIGURE 20.5   Medical image security program graphical user interface front panel.

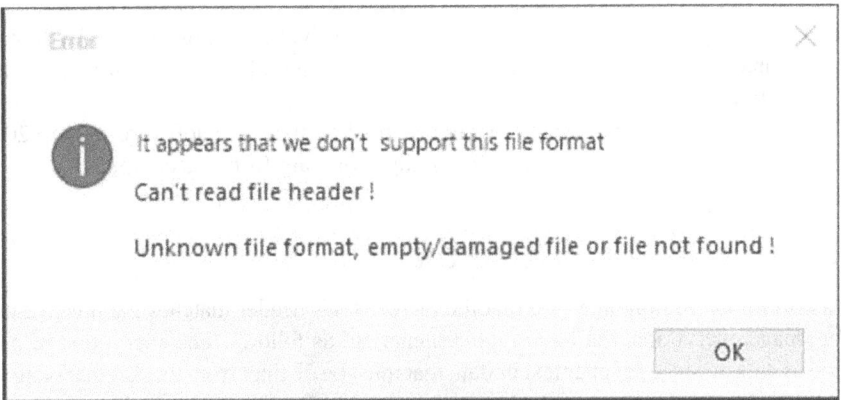

FIGURE 20.6   Encryption image popup message.

geometric, removal, protocol, blind, tampering, and destruction types. Additionally, it is important to fulfill security constraints and ensure compatibility with compression and decompression techniques. Moreover, the impact on compression efficiency must be considered. The image can be encrypted and compressed in three ways: (1) compression after encryption, (2) compression before encryption, and (3) compression and encryption together.

20.4.1 RESULTS OF HISTOGRAM AND PROPOSED METHOD STEPS

The number of pixels in a picture at each distinct intensity value may be seen graphically by finding a histogram. The term *histogram* in image processing often refers to gray pixel intensity values. Figures 20.7–20.11 show a histogram of original and watermarked images of patients one to five respectively.

Figure 20.12 shows medical image security at each stage and results of using watermarking and cryptography (encryption and decryption) of (a) patient 1 X-ray (Figure 20.12k), (b) patient 2 ultrasonic (Figure 20.12l), (c) patient 3 CT scan (Figure 20.12m), (d) patient 4 MRI (Figure 20.12n), and (e) patient 5 nuclear image (Figure 20.12n).

20.4.2 QUALITATIVE AND QUANTITATIVE RESULTS ANALYSIS

Modern communication systems, which include a variety of networks such as local and wide area networks, are used to share these medical records. Medical photographs make up more than 90% of all medical data stored in electronic health records

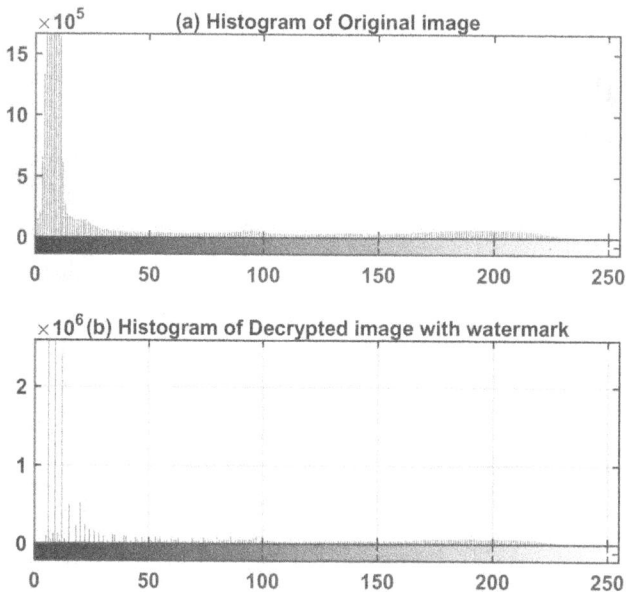

FIGURE 20.7   Histogram of patient 1 image shows (a) Original image (b) Decrypted image with watermark.

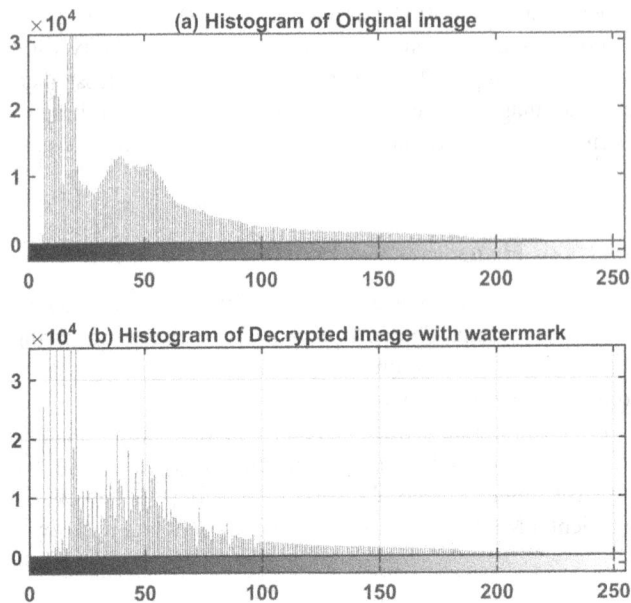

FIGURE 20.8   Histogram of patient 2 image shows (a) Original image (b) Decrypted image with watermark.

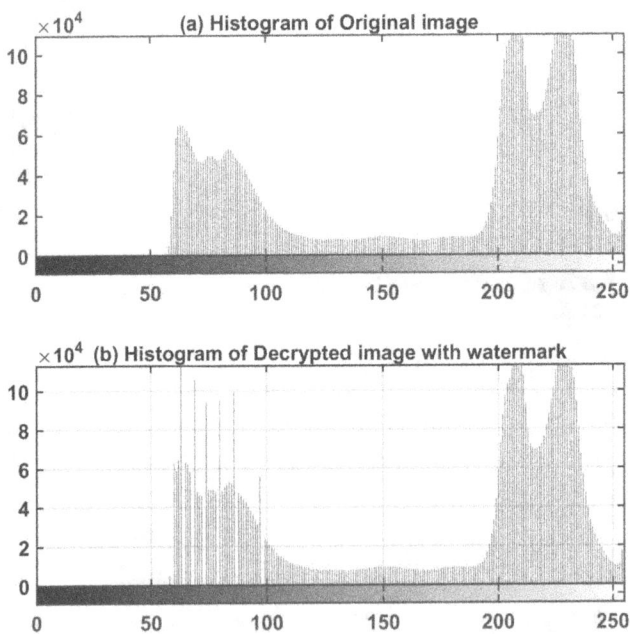

FIGURE 20.9   Histogram of patient 3 image shows (a) Original image (b) Decrypted image with watermark.

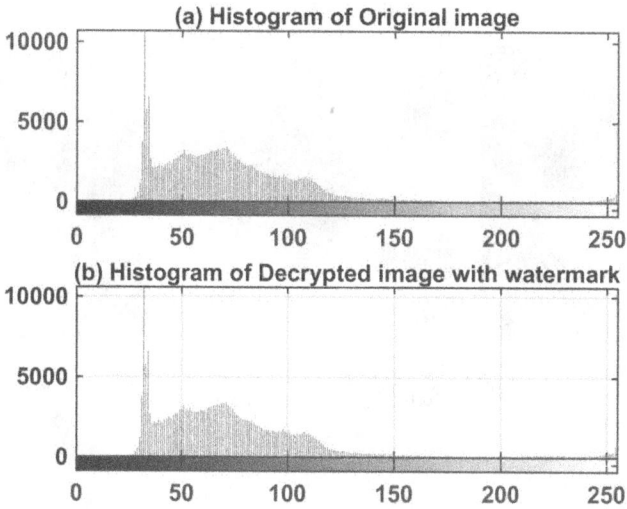

FIGURE 20.10 Histogram of patient 4 image shows (a) Original image (b) Decrypted image with watermark.

(Usman and Usman, 2018; Zain and Fauzi, 2006). In order to maintain confidence between patients and healthcare facilities, medical records must maintain their confidentiality. Electronic health records (EHR) are maintained in vast databases used by medical organizations to keep track of patients' medical details (Santos et al., 2021; Venkateswarlu, 2020). The Digital Imaging and Communications in Medicine (DICOM) standard is used to store, process, and transmit medical pictures such as

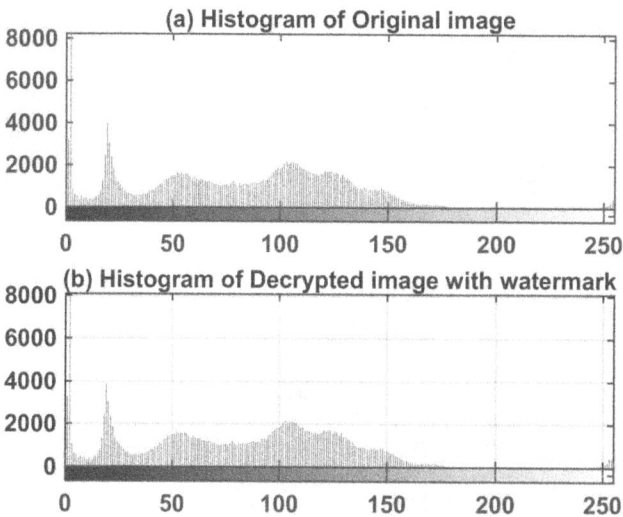

FIGURE 20.11 Histogram of patient 5 image shows (a) Original image (b) Decrypted image with watermark.

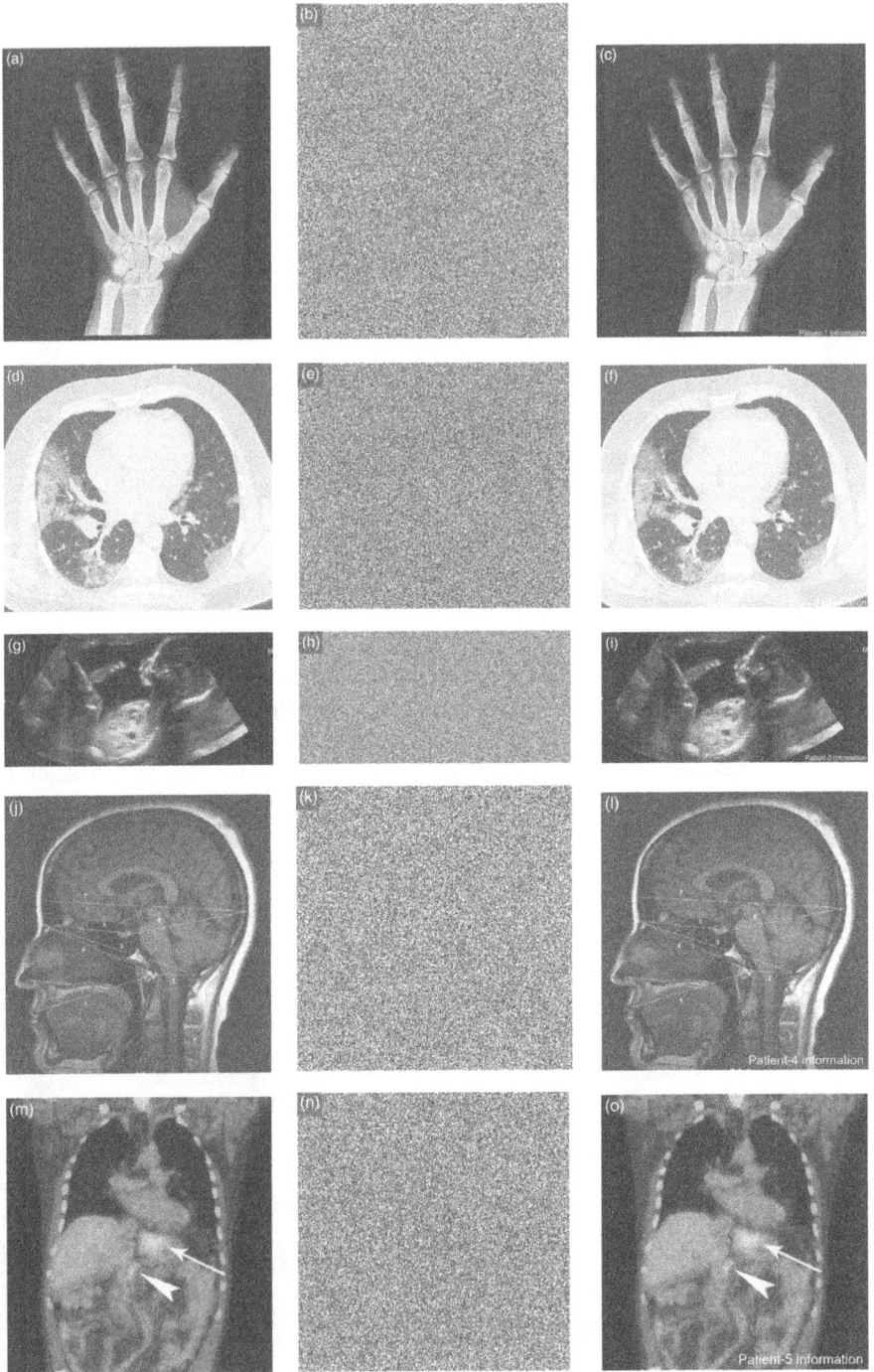

FIGURE 20.12 Medical image security stages and results using watermarking and Cryptography (Encryption and Decryption).

TABLE 20.3
Properties and Performance Measure of Watermarked and Original Medical Image

Sr. No. of Image	File Format	File Size	Resolution	DPI	Bit Depth	MSE	PSNR	NCC	AD	MD	NAE
Patient 1	PNG	5.84 MB	5967 × 7175	96 dpi	24	73.7365	48.7425	1.0001	−0.2978	7	0.0247
Patient 2	JPG	274 KB	1600 × 761	96 dpi	24	131.1553	52.3650	1.0034	−0.7243	5	0.022
Patient 3	PNG	3.51 MB	2825 × 2500	400 dpi	24	21.662	49.5591	1.0007	−0.1858	1	0.0013
Patient 4	JPG	73.7 KB	542 × 546	96 dpi	24	144.5189	47.4341	1.0061	−0.8156	1	0.0124
Patient 5	JPG	121 KB	500 × 500	96 dpi	24	169.7312	46.8129	1.0058	1.0058	2	0.015

X-rays, endoscopic images and movies, MR (magnetic resonance) images, and so on. To avoid tampering with patient data, prevent unauthorized copying, and ensure copyright protection, it is imperative to keep patient information in DICOM files secret. Quantitative analysis using the formula from Magdy et al. (2022) is carried out for PSNR, MSE, AD, MD, NAE, and NCC performance measures for original and decrypted medical images. Table 20.3 shows the properties and performance measures of watermarked and original medical images, and Table 20.4 shows the decrypted watermarked image and original image performance indices.

20.5 CONCLUSION

This chapter explored the importance of medical image security, the existing methodology, and how it will help humankind to minimize medical-related cybercrime. The chapter proposes a hybrid technique of cryptography, watermarking, and a passkey to protect from cyberattacks. This is implemented and demonstrated by

TABLE 20.4
Performance Measure of a Decrypted Image with Watermarked and Original Medical Image

Sr. No. of Image	Watermarked Text	Pass Key	Entropy	MSE	PSNR	NCC	AD	MD	NAE
Patient 1	Patient-1 information	35	4.343903383	73.7365	48.7425	1.0001	−0.2978	7	0.0247
Patient 2	Patient-2 information	35	6.257934989	131.1553	52.3650	1.0034	−0.7243	5	0.022
Patient 3	Patient-3 information	35	6.927448356	21.662	49.5591	1.0007	−0.1858	1	0.0013
Patient 4	Patient-4 information	35	6.470275013	144.5189	47.4342	1.0061	−0.8156	1	0.0124
Patient 5	Patient-5 information	35	7.139422485	169.7312	46.8129	1.0058	−0.9429	2	0.015

developing a GUI using open-source Python programming for healthcare information security. Further, qualitative and quantitative analysis is carried out by obtaining PSNR, MSE, AD, MD, NAE, and NCC performance measures for original and decrypted medical images, which shows the proposed method outperforming individually used techniques.

20.6 FUTURE SCOPE

Even the proposed hybrid approach shows better performance and robustness as compared to other individual techniques. However, in future work, this methodology can be enhanced using nested watermarks in colored images with encryption invertible techniques or Region of Interest (ROI) approaches to enhance the robustness.

REFERENCES

Batten, L. M. (2013). *Public key cryptography applications and attacks*. Wiley-IEEE Press.

Begum, M., & Uddin, M. S. (2020). Digital image watermarking techniques: A review. *Information, 11* (2), 110.

Cheddad, A., Condell, J., Curran, K., & Kevitt, P. M. (2010). Digital image steganography: Survey and analysis of current methods. *Signal Processing, 90,* 727–752.

Chen, S. Y., Tong, H., & Cattani, C. (2012). Markov models for image labelling. *Mathematical Problems in Engineering, 2012.* https://doi.org/10.1155/2012/814356

Haidekker, M. A. (2013). *Medical imaging technology* (1st ed.). Springer, New York, NY.

Hasavari, S., & Song, Y. T. (2019, 5). A secure and scalable data source for emergency medical care using blockchain technology. Proceedings - *2019 IEEE/ACIS 17th International Conference on Software Engineering Research, Management and Application, SERA 2019,* 71–75.

Jain, N., & Kumar, V. (2016a). IFCM based segmentation method for liver ultrasound images. *Journal of Medical Systems, 40* (11), 1–12.

Jain, N., & Kumar, V. (2016b). Liver ultrasound image segmentation using region-difference filters. *Journal of Digital Imaging, 30* (3), 376–390.

Jasra, B., & Moon, A. H. (2020, 1). Image encryption techniques: A review. *Proceedings of the Confluence 2020 - 10th International Conference on Cloud Computing, Data Science and Engineering,* 221–226.

Jiang, R., Shi, M., & Zhou, W. (2019). A privacy security risk analysis method for medical big data in urban computing. *IEEE Access, 7,* 143841–143854.

Katzenbeisser, S., & Petitcolas, F. A. (2000). *Information hiding techniques for steganography and digital watermarking* (1st ed.). Artech House, Inc, USA.

Kaur, T., & Sharma, R. (2013). Newly framed cryptosystem for color images: TJ-ACA, TJ-SCA and TJ-ACA in CBC mode image encrypting algorithms are discussed and security decisive tests are compared. *2013 IEEE 2nd International Conference on Image Information Processing, IEEE ICIIP 2013,* 666–671.

Kaur, M., Singh, S., & Kaur, M. (2021). Computational image encryption techniques: A comprehensive review. *Mathematical Problems in Engineering, 2021* (6). https://doi.org/10.1155/2021/5012496

Kuang, L. Q., Zhang, Y., & Han, X. (2009). Watermarking image authentication in hospital information system. Proceedings – *2009 International Conference on Information Engineering and Computer Science, ICIECS 2009.*

Liu, F., & Yan, W. Q. (2014). *Visual cryptography for image processing and security: Theory, methods, and applications* (1st ed.). Springer International Publishing.

Magdy, M., Hosny, K. M., Ghali, N. I., & Ghoniemy, S. (2022). Security of medical images for telemedicine: A systematic review. *Multimedia Tools and Applications, 81*, 25101–25145.

Maurya, R., Kannojiya, A. K., & Rajitha, B. (2020, 3). An extended visual cryptography technique for medical image security. *2nd International Conference on Innovative Mechanisms for Industry Applications, ICIMIA 2020 – Conference Proceedings*, 415–421.

Mitra, A. (2016, 1). Investigating scopes for automata based designs targeting image security in health system. *2015 E-Health and Bioengineering Conference, EHB 2015*.

Pape, S. (2014). *Authentication in insecure environments: Using visual cryptography and non-transferable credentials in practise* (1st ed.). Springer Vieweg+Teubner Verlag.

PhysioNet. (2022). *Medical image dataset.* Retrieved 2021-12-29, from https://physionet.org

Rani, P. B. S., & Kumar, A. (2019, 6). Digital image forgery detection techniques: A comprehensive review. *Proceedings of the 3rd International Conference on Electronics and Communication and Aerospace Technology, ICECA 2019*, 959–963.

Santos, N., Younis, W., Ghita, B., & Masala, G. (2021, 7). Enhancing medical data security on public cloud. *Proceedings of the 2021 IEEE International Conference on Cyber Security and Resilience, CSR 2021*, 103–108.

Saturwar, J., & Chaudhari, D. N. (2017, 11). Secure visual secret sharing scheme for color images using visual cryptography and digital watermarking. *Proceedings of the 2017 2nd IEEE International Conference on Electrical, Computer and Communication Technologies, ICECCT 2017*.

Southwick, R. (2022). *Cyberattacks in healthcare surged last year, and 2022 could be even worse.* Retrieved 2022-08-24, from https://www.chiefhealthcareexecutive.com

Tambe, S., Naik, D., Parab, V., & Doiphode, S. (2018, 1). Image steganography using uniform split and merge technique. *Proceedings of 2017 International Conference on Innovations in Information, Embedded and Communication Systems, ICIIECS 2017, 2018-January*, 1–6.

Usman, M. A., & Usman, M. R. (2018, 3). Using image steganography for providing enhanced medical data security. *CCNC 2018 - 2018 15th IEEE Annual Consumer Communications and Networking Conference, 2018-January*, 1–4.

Venkatasubramanian, K. K., Vasserman, E. Y., Sokolsky, O., & Lee, I. (2012). Security and interoperable-medical-device systems, part 1. *IEEE Security and Privacy, 10*, 61–63.

Venkateswarlu, I. B. (2020, 8). Fast medical image security using colour channel encryption. *Brazilian Archives of Biology and Technology, 63*, e20180473.

Waghmare, P. R., & Waghmare, J. M. (2022). A Methods of Medical Image Security Using Visual-Cryptography Techniques. In *IEEE 6th international conference on computing, communication, control and automation (ICCUBEA)* (pp. 1–6). Pune: IEEE Explorer.

Wayner, P. (2009). *Disappearing cryptography: Information hiding—steganography & watermarking.* Morgan Kaufmann Publishers.

Zain, J. M., & Fauzi, A. R. (2006). Medical image watermarking with tamper detection and recovery. *Annual International Conference of the IEEE Engineering in Medicine and Biology - Proceedings*, 3270–3273.

Zhang, B., Rahmatullah, B., Wang, S. L., Zaidan, A. A., Zaidan, B. B., & Liu, P. (2020). A review of research on medical image confidentiality related technology coherent taxonomy, motivations, open challenges and recommendations. *Multimedia Tools and Applications, 82* (1). https://doi.org/10.1007/s11042-020-09629-4

21 Integration of Biosensors and Drug Delivery Systems for Biomedical Applications

Jithu Jerin James and Sandhya K. V.
Department of Pharmaceutics, Faculty of Pharmacy,
M.S. Ramaiah University of Applied Sciences,
Bengaluru, Karnataka, India

CONTENTS

21.1 Introduction 354
21.2 Biosensors 354
    21.2.1 Structure of a Biosensor 355
    21.2.2 Properties of a Biosensor 355
    21.2.3 Biosensors Based on Nanotechnology 356
    21.2.4 Biosensing Drug Delivery Applications 356
21.3 MEMS (Microelectromechanical Systems) or Microtechnology 357
    21.3.1 MEMS Drug Delivery Devices 357
    21.3.2 Fabrication of Microneedles 359
    21.3.3 Stimuli-Responsive Microneedles 360
    21.3.4 Therapeutic Delivery to the Brain Using MEMS 361
21.4 Robotics in Drug Delivery 361
    21.4.1 Power-Driven Micro/Nanorobots 361
    21.4.2 Exogenous Power-Driven Micro/Nanorobots 363
    21.4.3 Endogenous Power-Driven Micro/Nanorobots 363
    21.4.4 DNA Origami 364
21.5 Biomechanics 364
    21.5.1 Electroporation Technique 364
    21.5.2 Microbubbles 365
    21.5.3 Biomechanics-Based Suprachoroidal Drug Delivery 366
    21.5.4 Biomechanics-Based Transdermal Drug Delivery System (TDDS) 366
21.6 Transplants 367
    21.6.1 Hydrogel-Mediated Drug Release 367
    21.6.2 Normothermic Machine Perfusion (NMP) 368
21.7 Conclusion 369
Reference 369

DOI: 10.1201/9781003324430-26

21.1   INTRODUCTION

A drug delivery system needs autonomous and controlled propulsion, cell perme-ation, payload transportation, and release to deliver therapeutic payloads precisely. Drug delivery technologies that detect biological signals and then release therapeu-tic payloads might change the delicate control and treatment of chronic illnesses. Platforms that integrate sensing and medication delivery might open the way for more effective biomedical therapy options. Because of significant advances in nano-technology, scientists and engineers have been able to build much smaller devices that can be implanted or delivered like drugs. The ability to analyze various physical and chemical signals is one of the most important aspects that indicate bodily states and sickness status. Hence, sensing platforms are a fascinating component of such devices. Furthermore, delivery carriers for various therapeutic drugs may be incor-porated into such platforms for regulated release.

Drug delivery approaches integrating biosensors include microneedles (MNs), magnetic nanoparticles (NPs), tetrahedral DNA nanostructures, responsive hydro-gels, etc. The sensing fractions can be glucose responsive linkers for diabetes [Fu et al., 2022] and pH-sensitive lipids for cancer drug delivery [Yan et al., 2020]. Stimuli-responsive microneedles, implantable devices and hydrogels categorized as MEMS are designed to respond to physiological cues. Treatment of chronic infected wounds [Mir et al., 2020] with carvacrol and bacterial lipase-sensitive poly(caprolactone) (PCL) nanoparticles incorporated into dissolving MN was another approach.

Biohybrid micro- and nanorobots that combine biological substances with inor-ganic or polymer matrix offer a promising drug delivery strategy. Andhari et al. [2020] developed a magnetic nanobot by chemically fusing antiepithelial cell adhe-sion molecule antibodies, magnetic Fe_3O_4 nanoparticles, and multiwalled carbon nanotubes with the anticancer medication doxorubicin hydrochloride (DOX).

Techniques like electroporation, microbubbles, and MNs powered by biome-chanical energy can be effectively used in illness prediction, diagnosis, and therapy. Liu et al. [2019] designed a triboelectric nanogenerator (TENG)-driven electropora-tion device powered by biomechanical energy for intracellular delivery of drugs. Formulations like NPs, microspheres, and hydrogels can be employed as delivery approach in transplantation medicine for immunosuppressive therapy. Deng et al. [2021] proposed that subcutaneous administration of FK506-loaded poly(lactide-co-glycolide) nanoparticles could treat acute rejection after heart transplantation.

This chapter focuses on the biosensors used in various drug delivery strategies, the role of MEMS, robotics, biomechanical devices, and transplants for various bio-medical applications. In addition, case studies of these devices' biomedical applica-tions to treat chronic diseases are explained on the basis of drug delivery approaches, sensing fraction, characterization, and *in vitro* and *in vivo* evaluation.

21.2   BIOSENSORS

Biosensors can identify and monitor a variety of physical and chemical stimuli in the body, as well as release therapeutic substances in a regulated manner. They are either surgically implanted or given orally. The objective of a biosensing drug delivery system is to more effectively treat chronic illnesses by combining diagnosis and therapy [Akolpoglu et al., 2019; Yazdi et al., 2020].

21.2.1 STRUCTURE OF A BIOSENSOR

A biosensor consists of a bioreceptor, a physicochemical detector, and an electrical system, as shown in Figure 21.1. Synthetic compounds, cells, enzymes, nucleotides, and antibodies are examples of bioreceptors. Different processes, including electrochemical, optical, thermal, and piezoelectric, might be used for transduction. The electrical system is for signal amplification and processing and also contains read out devices [Yazdi et al., 2020].

21.2.2 PROPERTIES OF A BIOSENSOR

The ideal biosensor for use in a drug delivery system should be immune to biofouling, sensitive, noncytotoxic, biocompatible, less intrusive, scalable, affordable, and able to respond quickly over long periods of time. Materials having high surface area and physical, chemical, electrical, mechanical, thermal, magnetic, and optical characteristics are favored for designing and producing biosensors with improved sensitivity and specificity. Polymers such as polyethylene glycol, chitosan, dextran, hyaluronan, collagen, and alginate are indicated to increase biocompatibility. Biosensors have been made using gold nanostructures, noble metal nanoparticles, carbon nanotubes, and conjugated polymers such as polyaniline, polypyrrole, and poly(3,4-ethylenedioxythiophene) (PEDOT). Analyte recognition components such as enzymes (e.g., oxidases), polymeric membranes, or size exclusion membranes may be employed to build selective biosensors [Akolpoglu et al. 2019; Ngoepe et al. 2013; Yazdi et al. 2020].

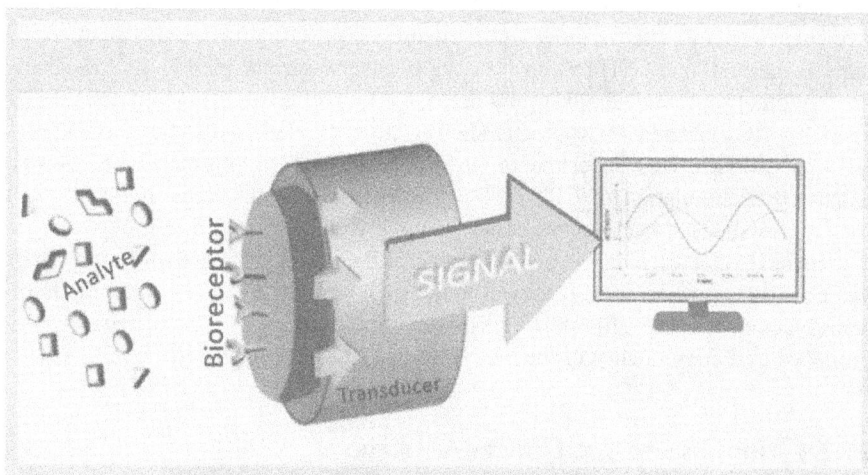

FIGURE 21.1 Structure of a biosensor.

21.2.3 BIOSENSORS BASED ON NANOTECHNOLOGY

Nanotechnology-based biosensors such as the DNA (tetrahedron, walker, G-quadruplex, dendrimer, chain, and origami) have been employed to determine cancer biomarkers. In the field of biomedicals such as tissue engineering, medical imaging, biosensing, and drug administration, nanocarriers with sensing and actuation mechanisms that respond to cues like temperature, pH, and glucose concentration in the microenvironment have been employed. Nanogels, bioresponsive polymers, and mesoporous silica are examples of nanocarriers [Yazdi et al., 2020].

Acyclovir-loaded magnetic nanoparticles (NPs) coated with 3-(triethoxysilyl)-propylamine was analyzed by scanning electron microscopy (SEM), transmission electron microscopy (TEM), vibrating sample magnetometer (VSM), dynamic light scattering (DLS), and zeta potential. The results proved that acyclovir reduced the saturation magnetization and zeta potential of NPs. The effects of pH, loading time, and temperature were also investigated. The best loading was accomplished at pH 9 at 39°C after five hours. Density functional theory (DFT) was used to analyze acyclovir's adsorption on untreated and modified magnetic nanoparticles. The study found that modified and metal-doped magnetic nanoparticles could be used as nanobiosensors for acyclovir detection and distribution [Xie et al., 2020].

Camptothecin-loaded DNA tetrahedral nanostructure (CPT-TET) with stimuli-responsive feature, i.e., glutathione (GSH) responsive disulfide linkage was formulated. The prodrug, i.e., a chemodrug was modified using disulfide linker containing the carbonethyl bromide group. Successful formation was analyzed using nuclear magnetic resonance (NMR) and verified its purity using liquid chromatography–mass spectrometry (LCMS). The drug grafting on nanostructure was confirmed using ultraviolet visible spectroscopy (UV-Vis) and PAGE. PAGE also revealed nanostructures' stability in physiological conditions. The particle size of nanostructures was analyzed using DLS and atomic force microscopy (AFM). Using DLS, the average hydrodynamic size was found to be 24 nm. AFM showed that the 18 nm-sized nanostructures had a rather homogeneous shape. Drug release was analyzed by dialysis method, and GSH responsive drug release was confirmed by LCMS. Using flow cytometry, it was demonstrated that CPT-TET effectively entered cells. MTT assay on HCT116 and MCF-7 cells showed higher cytotoxicity of nanostructures to tumor cells. *In vivo* experiments on HCT116 tumor-bearing nude mice showed enhanced accumulation of CPT-TET at the tumor site and better suppression of tumor growth. Histopathology studies using hematoxylin and eosin, hematoxylin and eosin (H&E) staining showed apoptosis of the tumor cells in the treated group, and no adverse effects were observed in the major organs. A drug-containing tetrahedral framework with stimuli responsiveness and improved anticancer activity was produced as a consequence of the investigation [Zhang et al., 2019].

21.2.4 BIOSENSING DRUG DELIVERY APPLICATIONS

Electrochemical sensors, bioMEMS, and responsive hydrogels are used in biosensing drug delivery applications. The chemical signal is converted into an electrical signal by electrodes in electrochemical biosensors. Electrochemical sensors can detect DNA, hemoglobin, blood ketones, glucose, lactate, cholesterol, uric acid, and other biomolecules in the human body. Electrochemical biosensors based on enzymes and proteins have been extensively investigated for detecting particular analytes. These biosensors immobilize proteins on the detector and detect analytes using electroactive by-products. Responsive hydrogels detect specific biomolecules, and drugs are released as a consequence of the interaction between these molecules and the polymer matrix. These hydrogels are also responsive to cues like temperature, pH, and light. The disadvantage of hydrogel is the delayed diffusion of therapeutics after stimulation; nevertheless, research is under way to address this problem [Akolpoglu et al., 2019; Ngoepe et al., 2013]. Biosensor applications in drug delivery systems are included in Table 21.1.

21.3 MEMS (MICROELECTROMECHANICAL SYSTEMS) OR MICROTECHNOLOGY

Biomedical or biological microelectromechanical systems (bioMEMS) are MEMS built for biomedical applications and are utilized for biomolecular analysis and sensing. In an ideal bioMEMS, physiochemical or biological cues are transformed into electrical impulses, which activate medication release. BioMEMS have a number of advantages in biosensing applications, including a faster reaction time, high scalability, repeatable manufacturing, and high sensitivity [Akolpoglu et al., 2019].

Integrated circuits (ICs) for MEMS and other sensors have been made using microfabrication methods. When the biologicals are used in combination with MEMS, it has been possible to design innovative systems that are ideal for disease detection and treatment. Implantable and wearable MEMS drug delivery systems have advanced significantly. Blood pressure sensors, biosensors, and microvalves are examples of current MEMS, and MEMS applications have shown biotechnological breakthroughs in DNA sequencing and drug discovery [Yazdi et al., 2020].

21.3.1 MEMS Drug Delivery Devices

Implantable devices for drug delivery consist of reservoirs that are stocked with drugs that are distributed. Polydimethylsiloxane, medical grade silicone rubber, polyacrylamide, and pyrex are most often used as reservoir materials due to their ideal physicochemical qualities, biocompatibility, bonding, and optical visibility. Drugs are commonly placed into single or multiple reservoirs in MEMS drug delivery systems. Pumps use several actuation techniques such as piezoelectric, phase-change, magnetic, electrochemical, and transdermal to deliver the reservoir-loaded drug in single reservoir-based devices to achieve a precise and controlled drug release. Multiple reservoir-based devices employ actuation techniques such as near infrared radiation (NIR), passive release, electrothermal, and electrochemical methods to release medication in a regulated way [Villarruel Mendoza et al., 2020].

TABLE 21.1

Biosensors and Drug Delivery Systems

Sl. No	Author and Year	Drug	Delivery Approach	Sensing Fraction	Application
1	Fu et al., 2022	Insulin	Microneedle patch	Phenylboronic acid-based fluorescent probes (glucose responsive linkers)	Controlled insulin delivery system for type 1 diabetes
2	Xie et al., 2020	Acyclovir	Magnetic nanoparticles	3-(triethoxysilyl)-propylamine	Delivery of acyclovir for cancer therapy
3	Zhang et al., 2019	Camptothecin (CPT)	Tetrahedral DNA nanostructures (TDN)	Carbonethyl bromide-modified CPT in phosphorothioate modified DNAs, with a GSH-responsive disulfide linkage	Chemotherapy
4	Yan et al., 2020	Doxorubicin	D-(KLAKLAK)2 (KLA) conjugated tetrahedral DNA nanostructures (TDN)	KLA modified with 2,3-dimethylmaleic anhydride and coupled to 1,2-disteroyl-sn-glycero-3-phosphoethanolamine resulted in a pH sensitive lipid	Mitochondrial delivery of the cancer drug
5	Lee et al., 2016	Metformin	Wearable polymeric microneedle patch with heater, temperature, humidity, glucose and pH sensors	Gold mesh with graphene doped with gold Sensors used in patch includes PEDOT, Prussian Blue, polyaniline, and graphene	Diabetes monitoring and therapy
6	Wu et al., 2010	Insulin	Hybrid nanogels	Copolymer gel shell of poly (4-vinylphenylboronic acid-co-2-(dimethylamino)ethyl acrylate)	Glucose detection, self-regulated drug delivery for diabetes

The MEMS micropump technology continuously provides pharmaceuticals via a reservoir while allowing active control over drug release. The dynamic interaction between a microtechnology component and electrical components boosts the innovative medication delivery systems' efficiency and functionality. Wireless transmission enables smart medication release and correct dosing over several occasions. Advances in microtechnology and biocompatible materials have extended drug delivery systems' target locations, routes of administration, patient compliance, drug spectrum, and dosing techniques [Lee et al., 2018].

A pulsatile distribution of human growth hormone (HGH) [Lee et al., 2019] was achieved by using an implantable device with several drug reservoirs topped with an NIR stimulus-responsive membrane (SRM). SRMs are composed of thermosensitive polymer POSS(MEO2MA-co-OEGMA) and varying concentrations of reduced graphene oxide (RGO) nanoparticles. The SRMs were characterized using field emission-SEM (FE-SEM), Fourier-transform infrared spectroscopy (FTIR), and differential scanning calorimetry (DSC). FE-SEM images showed that all SRMs exhibited a similar surface morphology. There were no peak shifts in the FTIR spectra of RGO NPs and SRMs. According to DSC data, RGO addition had no significant effects on the properties of the polymer, and the melting temperature of SRMs remained constant. After NIR irradiation, optical images demonstrated that only SRM3 could be sufficiently ruptured to completely access the drug reservoir. *In vitro* drug release of the device was measured using reverse-phase high-performance liquid chromatography (RP-HPLC), and after irradiation complete release of drug was seen within one hour in SRM3. *In vivo* experiments were performed on male hypophysectomized rats, followed by pharmacokinetic, pharmacodynamic analysis and histopathological evaluation using H&E staining. The implanted device could release HGH when NIR was delivered from outside the body, according to the findings of *in vivo* trials. Due to the quick dissolution of HGH from the exposed drug reservoir, the pharmacokinetic and pharmacodynamic parameters of the HGH were equivalent to those of the conventional subcutaneously injected HGH. Therefore, it was determined that the present device could be a suitable, less invasive method for pulsatile, on-demand medication administration.

The release of pharmaceutical was according to sensor feedback on implanting BioMEMS into the human body. As a result, BioMEMS offer a lot of potential for precisely monitoring and directing the release of medications. The key challenge is the immunological response of the host when sensing devices are implanted [Akolpoglu et al., 2019].

21.3.2 FABRICATION OF MICRONEEDLES

Microneedles (solid or hollow) and their molds are made using MEMS. The manufacturing process comprises depositing, patterning, etching, and photoresist removal. Different materials' etchant selectivities generate complex 3-D structures. First, a chemical or physical vapor deposition forms a thin coating on a substrate. The second phase, patterning, transfers a two-dimensional master pattern of the desired material from the original photomask to the photosensitive-coated substrate. The transferring method uses a radiation source with one of the lithography processes (photolithography, ion beam lithography, or X-ray lithography). Using a strong acid or caustic chemical, the exposed sections of the substrate are etched to produce a pattern. Last, the photoresist layer is removed to get the molds for microneedles.

21.3.3 STIMULI-RESPONSIVE MICRONEEDLES

Recently, stimuli-responsive microneedles based on polymeric matrices have been used to regulate payload release. Stimuli-responsive materials respond to changes in their surroundings. These systems release payloads in response to physiological cues like pH, glucose, enzymes, redox potential, or physical signals like temperature, electric current, light, and mechanical force. External and internal stimuli responsive payload release by transdermal microneedle patch is shown in Figure 21.2.

A single removable transdermal patch with insulin and nondegradable polymeric matrix-loaded microneedle with glucose-responsive moiety, i.e., phenylboronic acid (PBA), was designed by Yu et al. [2020]. The glucose-responsive MNs (GR-MN) vfluorescence image showed that each needle's matrix had insulin in a consistent amount. The mechanical strength of microneedles using a tensile compression machine was found to be $0.90 \pm 0.35N$ per needle, which is sufficient for skin penetration without breaking. The amount of released monomers was estimated by high-performance liquid chromatography (HPLC). The insulin molecule was intact during the polymerization procedure, according to mass spectrometry (MS). Additionally, a high loading capacity of 20 weight percent was achieved with a 100% encapsulation efficiency of insulin. *In vitro* glucose binding and drug release by microplate protein assay was carried out. The findings supported that the insulin release rate from the polymeric matrix was controlled in a glucose-dependent way. *In vivo* efficacy was studied on streptozotocin (STZ) induced adult diabetic mice/minipigs and plasma insulin concentration was recorded by enzyme-linked immunosorbent assay (ELISA). GR-MNs regulate glucose levels for a long period of time with a decreased risk of hypoglycemia.

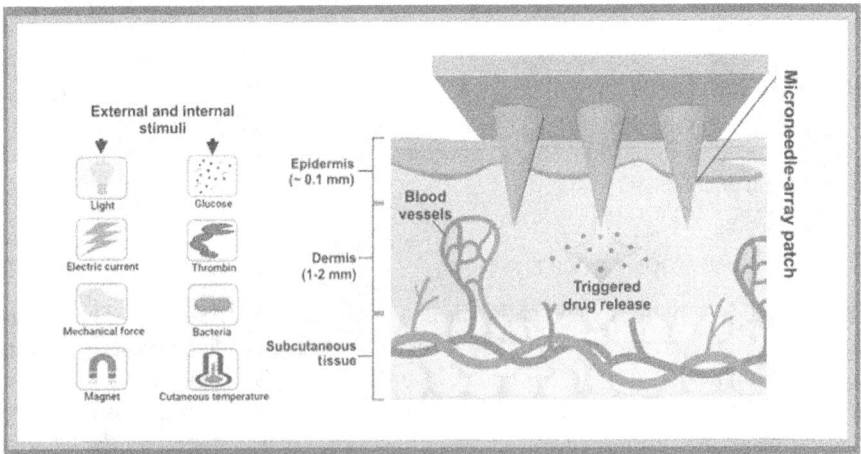

FIGURE 21.2   External and internal stimuli responsive transdermal microneedle patch.

21.3.4 Therapeutic Delivery to the Brain Using MEMS

Transcranial direct brain infusion and targeted ultrasonic blood brain barrier (BBB) disruption benefit from microtechnology. Convection-enhanced diffusion (CED) is utilized for human transcranial brain medication delivery. CED employs external pressure to deliver medicines into the brain using a hollow cannula or needle. MEMS-based microneedles or neural probes with an integrated microfluidic channel are proposed for *in vivo* brain infusion. By overcoming BBB, drugs can be delivered to the brain via the bloodstream. On application of focused ultrasound (FUS) to a small region in the brain can temporarily damage or destroy the BBB. When a medicine containing an ultrasound contrast agent like microbubbles is given intravenously, the drug only enters the brain where the BBB has been disrupted.

DNAs, genes, small molecules, hydrophilic substances, drug-loaded microbeads, and macromolecules can all benefit from this noninvasive approach. There will be no damage to the surrounding tissue. Drugs have been administered transdermally, transcorneally, and orally using FUS technology. The development of such tiny MEMS ultrasonic transducer arrays for sonication is under progress [Lee et al., 2018].

MEMS technology is ideal for spatiotemporal and dosage-controlled drug administration because of its miniaturization, integration of many functionalities, and electromechanical actuation. MEMS for controlled medication release are used as therapeutic agent delivery devices. High-potency medicines that elicit a reaction at low concentrations may be released via various devices [Lee et al., 2018]. Table 21.2 lists applications of MEMS in drug delivery systems.

21.4 ROBOTICS IN DRUG DELIVERY

Medical robotics builds and deploys programmable, reconfigurable micro/nanomachines with physical, chemical, or biological propulsion to perform a variety of medical tasks, such as delivering drugs, targeting diseased cells, and conducting microsurgery within a complex body condition. Biohybrid micro- and nanorobots combine biological substances like DNA, enzymes, cytomembranes, blood cells, sperms, and bacteria with artificial components like inorganic or polymer particles. Biological features, onboard actuation, and sensory capacities may be inherited [Li et al., 2022].

Unlike conventional medication delivery, which depends on blood circulation, micro/nanorobots may move autonomously, delivering pharmaceuticals to hard-to-reach locations, as shown in Figure 21.3. Micro/nanorobot systems have an internal payload and an exterior shell to reach a target [Hu et al., 2020]. Electroless plating, template-assisted electrodeposition, physical vapor deposition, strain engineering, 3-D printing, capillary micromolding, material assembly, bioinspired design, and biohybridizing are conventional micro/nanorobot production processes [Li et al., 2022].

21.4.1 Power-Driven Micro/Nanorobots

Micro/nanorobots uses exogenous power from magnetic fields, light energy, acoustic fields, electric fields, etc., to overcome Brownian motion or endogenous power from

TABLE 21.2
MEMS and Drug Delivery System

Sl. No	Author and Year	Drug	Device	Stimuli	Application
1	Yu et al. [2020]	Insulin	MN patch with PBA	Glucose	Diabetes
2	Mir et al. [2020]	Carvacrol	Dissolving MNs loaded with PCL NPs	Bacterial lipases	Wound healing
3	Lee et al. [2019]	Growth hormone (human)	Implantable device with a membrane that responds to stimuli made of POSS (MEO2MA-co-OEGMA) and reduced graphene oxide	NIR irradiation	For deficiency treatment
4	Liu et al. [2018]	Metformin	Polymer-nanodots, i.e., bismuth nanodots stabilized by poly(vinylpyrrolidone) composite dissolvable MNs coated with lauric acid	NIR irradiation	Transdermal drug delivery for diabetes treatment
5	Dong et al. [2018]	Doxorubicin (DOX)	Gold nanocage and drug-loaded hyaluronic acid dissolving MN	NIR	Transdermal therapy for superficial skin tumors
6	Zhang et al. [2018]	Metformin	Separable microneedles arrowheads made of PCL	Electrothermal	Diabetes
7	Yu et al. [2017]	Nepafenac	Hydrogel composed of carboxymethyl chitosan and poloxamer cross-linked by glutaraldehyde	pH and temperature	Ophthalmic drug delivery system
8	Hardy et al. [2016]	Ibuprofen	Hydrogel-forming microneedle arrays loaded with 3,5-dimethoxybenzoin conjugate	UV light	On-demand transdermal drug delivery for pain relief
9	Goldwirt et al. [2016]	Carboplatin	Implantable ultrasound device	Ultrasound in combination with systemic injection of microbubbles	Treatment of brain tumors by opening BBB

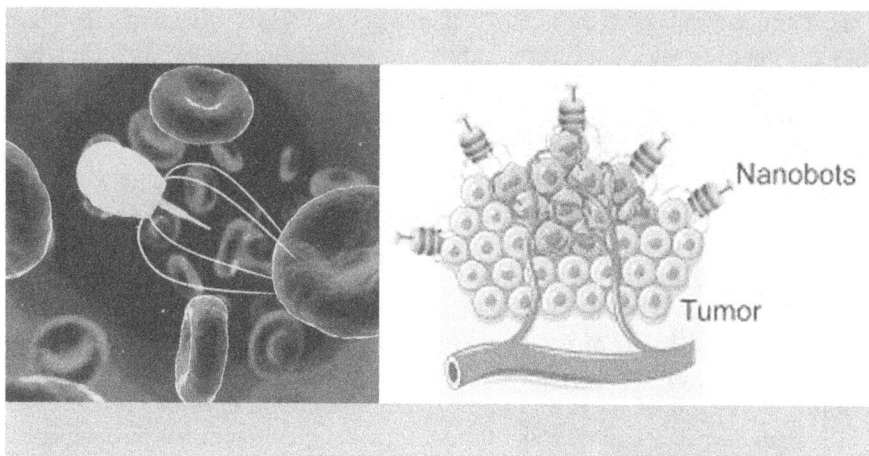

FIGURE 21.3   Nanobots leave blood vessels and deliver payloads to tumor cells.

biological reactions like enzyme catalysis/microorganisms motility or energy from chemical reactions [Hu et al., 2020].

21.4.2   EXOGENOUS POWER-DRIVEN MICRO/NANOROBOTS

The magnetic energy-driven micro/nanorobot has precise positioning, changeable direction, and a broad motion range. Micro/nanorobots operate under a moderate, safe magnetic field. Adding metal to the base material or surface coating may elicit immunological or inflammatory responses in the body, necessitating the development of safer, nontoxic alternatives. Although freely accessible, electric energy has a lower penetration than a magnetic field, and hence its intensity increases in practical use. The applications of micro/nanorobots driven by electric field, excessive current on the body, and the use of metals should be addressed. Light-powered therapeutic micro/nanorobots are rare. Light energy combines with other sources to move micro/nanorobots or trigger drug release. Compared to other propelled technologies, ultrasound provides adequate penetration and propulsion for nanorobots to overcome human body boundaries. Ultrasound may cause oxidative stress in cells, harming both targeted and normal cells.

21.4.3   ENDOGENOUS POWER-DRIVEN MICRO/NANOROBOTS

The use of a redox reaction to convert chemical energy into a motor force for a nanorobot is a popular method. The chemical energy drive simply needs to direct the target site by using magnetic field attraction, not continual control of the micro/nanorobots. The robot's movement is reversed by the gas produced by the chemical reaction, which is suited for the gastrointestinal environment. However, the chemical energy-driven self-propelled nanorobot has some flaws, such as difficulty controlling movement direction and movement being readily disrupted by the ionic medium.

One of its disadvantages is the lack of continuity of movement; the micro/nanorobots may run out of power as the chemical reaction progresses. Another significant barrier to its use is the safety of the reaction products generated.

Microrobots were prepared by coloading citric acid–coated superparamagnetic NPs (CA-MNPs) and DOX containing thermosensitive nanoliposomes (DOX-TSLPs) into the macrophages [Nguyen et al., 2021]. Temperature of CA-MNP solution rapidly increased when exposed to NIR, confirming its NIR laser responsive characteristics, which in turn induced drug release from TSLPs. VSM studies indicated that CA-MNPs are superparamagnetic, with a magnetic value of 50.22 emu/g. Techniques such as controlled low-strength material (CLSM), fluorescence spectroscopy, and bio-TEM were used for characterization of microrobots. CLSM showed macrophage nanoparticle uptake. Fluorescence spectroscopy and bio-TEM confirmed NPs and DOX-TSLPs loading into macrophages. *In vitro* cytotoxicity by MTT assay revealed that NPs and drug-loaded nanoliposomes are biocompatible with macrophages. In 2-D and 3-D tumor spheroids *in vitro* studies, microrobots penetrated tumors and caused cell death. *In vivo* investigations on tumor-bearing BALB/c mice showed that microrobots inhibited tumor development with a subtherapeutic dosage of DOX and a single injection. The research outlines a strategy for successful anticancer therapy utilizing microrobots.

21.4.4   DNA ORIGAMI

DNA origami is a technique for making DNA nanorobots that has a lot of potential in the realm of medication delivery. Complementary base pairing is used to fold single-stranded DNA and bind it to multiple short oligonucleotides resulting in DNA nanostructures. Functional ligands, biomolecules, and nanoscale objects may be accurately constructed on DNA origami's surface, improving nanorobot targeting. Most DNA origami robots can't move autonomously but can deliver medications precisely to targets [Hu et al., 2020]. Nano/microrobot applications in drug delivery systems are listed in Table 21.3.

21.5   BIOMECHANICS

Biomechanics involves application of methods derived from mechanics to study biological systems, particularly their structure and function. Hence it could effectively be used in illness prediction, diagnosis, and therapy. Some popular approaches include microbubble, microneedle, electroporation techniques, etc.

Liu et al. [2019] designed a TENG-driven electroporation device powered by biomechanical energy for intracellular delivery of drugs, and the system proved its efficiency and low cell damage in *in vitro* and *in vivo* studies.

21.5.1   ELECTROPORATION TECHNIQUE

In electroporation, the applied electric field significantly depolarizes and hyperpolarizes the cell's transmembrane potentials. This is followed by the breakdown of the cell's electric membrane. When the membrane potential exceeds a critical

TABLE 21.3
Robotics and Drug Delivery System

Sl. No	Author and Year	Drug	Micro/Nano Robots	Application
1	Nguyen et al. [2021]	Doxorubicin	Macrophage-based microrobots	Tumor therapy
2	Liu et al. [2021]	Antigen (OVA peptide) and two adjuvants (dsRNA and CpG loop oligonucleotides)	DNA nanodevice vaccine	DNA nanodevice-based vaccine for cancer immunotherapy
3	Andhari et al. [2020]	Doxorubicin hydrochloride	Magnetic nanorobots	Targeted cancer therapy
4	Xu et al. [2018]	Doxorubicin hydrochloride	Sperm-hybrid micromotor	Gynecological care, diagnosis and treatment of cancers and other disorders of the female reproductive system.
5	Li et al. [2018]	Thrombin	DNA nanorobot	Drug delivery in cancer therapy

value, it results in pores. Solutes that cannot pass through the cell membrane enter during "pore open time." If the electric field is weak, membrane breakdown is reversed after the pulse. High electric fields leave holes following the pulse, triggering membrane damage and cell death. Pulse voltage, duration of pulse, pH, waveform, and ionic strength of suspending media influence pore number and size [Matsuki, 2018].

Propidium iodide (a membrane-impermeable chemical) was given to MCF-7 human breast cancer cells via electroporation, and the molecule was effectively delivered with an 85% efficiency. Dextran-fluorescein isothiocyanate (FITC) (10 and 70 kDa) was given with propidium iodide as a dead cell indicator (staining was performed 24 hours after electroporation). Ten kDa and 70 kDa dextran-FITC delivery effectiveness was 86% and 49% respectively. TENG-enabled electroporation delivered 82% siRNA to MCF-7 cells with 94% viability. HeLa and rat bone mesenchymal stem cells (rBMSCs) proved the system's flexibility. HeLa and rBMSCs absorbed 63% and 51% of dextran-FITC (70 kDa), respectively. After electroporation, all cell lines had viabilities over 94%. TENG has been extensively employed in self-powered and wearable devices as a new age energy technology [Liu et al., 2019].

21.5.2 MICROBUBBLES

Microbubbles are employed in ultrasound-based pharmaceutical or gene delivery systems. Microbubbles are oxygen or air bubbles in liquids with a size of 50 μm or less in diameter. They stay steady in water or rise slowly, shrivel, and collapse. In addition, their high inner pressure enhances gas solubility in liquid. They can also generate free radicals and have a negatively charged surface. This prevents them from forming bigger bubbles.

Mechanical agitation, sonication, and pressured gas–liquid mixing produces microbubble suspensions. Mechanical agitation produces big, wide, inhomogeneous microbubbles. Sonication produces finer, homogeneous microbubbles of diameter less than 1.5 μm. Gas–liquid mixing systems produce enormous volumes of micro-bubble suspensions with small bubble diameters. These microbubbles, which have a diameter less than 1.5 μm, are regarded as clinically safe [Matsuki, 2018].

21.5.3 BIOMECHANICS-BASED SUPRACHOROIDAL DRUG DELIVERY

As research on suprachoroidal drug delivery develops and therapeutic potential of small molecule suspensions to gene therapy has advanced via clinical trials, it is crucial to understand suprachoroidal space (SCS) biomechanics. To provide treatments to the back of the eye, the SCS can be accessed via a catheter, hypodermic needle, or microneedle. Biomechanics of suprachoroidal injection includes injection pressures, force measurements, as well as the effects of fluid mechanics features such as viscosity, suspension particle size, volume, and osmotic properties on fluid distribution in SCS.

Hancock et al. [2021] suggested in his review that suprachoroidal injection with the SCS microinjector required no extra mechanical aid beyond a physician's manual pressures. Increasing injection volume was found to increase SCS circumferential coverage. Based on viscosity, the amount of injectates dispersed in the SCS can be modified and altered. Particle size and molecular weight could be modified to increase design flexibility of the formulation. Fluid spread in the SCS has also been shown to be influenced by the formulation's osmotic properties, such as its capacity to absorb fluid and swell. Ionic charge of medication formulation affected iontophoresis drug distribution.

Peripheral choroidal disorders required widespread coverage of drug delivery. Low-viscosity, high-volume formulations were recommended. For macula-focused disorders, low-viscosity, high-volume formulations were preferred. Hydrogel pushing or iontophoresis could guarantee the drug candidate reached the back of the eye. For glaucoma medications, a low-degrading, high-viscosity polymer was required. It is possible to adapt biomechanics-based medication delivery in SCS to a variety of biological applications [Hancock et al., 2021].

21.5.4 BIOMECHANICS-BASED TRANSDERMAL DRUG DELIVERY SYSTEM (TDDS)

TDDS was sought to increase the dosage quantity of transdermal drugs. By physically stimulating the skin with heat, noncavitational/cavitational ultrasound, thermal ablation, etc., the mechanical advances of TDD have improved the physical penetration of drugs through the skin surface.

By penetrating the stratum corneum, microneedles improve transdermal delivery of small and large therapeutics. Using microfabrication techniques, solid, coated, dissolving, and hollow microneedles for TDD were prepared. Solid microneedles were designed in different sizes and shapes to promote skin permeability. After inserting and withdrawing microneedles, skin pores were found to enhance drug permeability. Drug-coated microneedles dissolve in the skin to release drugs directly. Mechanical transdermal delivery improvements are a fast-growing technology [Kikuchi, 2018].

21.6 TRANSPLANTS

Transplantation entails transplanting an organ or group of cells from a donor to a recipient or to various sites inside the same individual to save lives or enhance quality of life [Anggelia et al., 2022]. The recipient's immune reaction to the donor graft and the graft's alloimmune response after transplantation contribute to rejection.

Nanoparticles can serve as pharmaceutical or biological delivery techniques in transplantation medicine to increase the donor organ supply by sustaining graft viability, preventing or treating ischemia reperfusion damage, and preventing graft rejection, thereby promoting tolerance. Nanoparticles have minimal toxicity and low effective dose requirement and can be used for graft and recipient therapy [Yao and Martins, 2020].

For *ex situ* grafts, before transplantation as well as for transplant patients, researchers are looking at integrating nanoparticles into diagnostic or therapeutic procedures. With *ex vivo* machine perfusion preservation, graft therapy seems to be more appealing, and nanoparticles have significant promise.

21.6.1 HYDROGEL-MEDIATED DRUG RELEASE

Researchers collaborated to give immunosuppressants locally to prevent transplant rejection. This was done with a biomaterial that forms a hydrogel. This mechanism targets and controls drug release. Researchers developed a hydrogel–tacrolimus combination. After transplantation, this mixture was injected. The hydrogel remained inactive until it detected inflammation or an immunological reaction at the transplant site. Then it released the immunosuppressive medication in the graft tissue. This activity could extend for several months. Local administration of immunosuppressant medication to grafted tissue reduces toxicity and improves therapeutic results and may lead to a paradigm change in clinical immunosuppressive therapy in transplant surgery.

Methoxy-poly(ethylene glycol)-co-poly(lactic acid)-poly(e-caprolactone) hydrogel was developed by Wu et al. [2021] and used as a drug depot. FTIR, gel permeation chromatography, and 1H-NMR were used to characterize the hydrogel. The vial inverted method used to explore the behavior of the sol–gel transition, examined the rheological characteristics of the gel, quantified drug concentration, and measured the effectiveness of drug encapsulation and release using HPLC. Using the MTT assay, the biocompatibility of formulation was evaluated. A Lewis rat's dorsal thorax received a tail-skin graft from a male Brown-Norway rat. Blood samples were collected from Lewis rats, and drug concentrations were found. H&E staining was used for histopathological analyses. The results showed that sustained drug release could be maintained within 30 days. The formulated hydrogel underwent significant degradation during that time. Improved allograft survival was also attained.

21.6.2 Normothermic Machine Perfusion (NMP)

Targeted nanoparticles enhance pharmaceutical delivery to organs. *Ex vivo* NMP might enhance transplantable organs. It delivers medications to vascular endothelial cells (ECs), the initial site of interaction with a transplant recipient's immune system. NMP eliminates many of the constraints of systemic medication delivery. The study used slowly hydrolyzable polymeric nanoparticles as a delivery vehicle to target the vascular endothelium of the organ. This study implies renal vascular ECs might be a target for transplant therapy.

Tietjen et al. [2017] studied on a protein, CD31, that might be utilized by examining EC surface indicators in human kidneys. They used a polymeric nanoparticle linked to anti-CD31 to target transplant ECs. CD31-targeting increased the accumulation of drug-filled nanoparticles by fivefold.

Antigen-presenting cells that are involved in the systemic immune response have their receptors targeted by nanoparticle therapy. Targeting by nanoparticles offers sustained and controlled drug delivery. Mycophenolic acid in PLGA NPs bound to dendritic cells and macrophages in murine skin grafts increased graft survival to 100% at 20 days posttransplantation. Polymer NPs encapsulating donor antigens improved graft protection and were cheaper than standard cell delivery methods. Prior to being placed to clinical use, nanoparticles must first have their toxicity fully evaluated, particularly with regard to how they interact with other biological molecules found in the human body [Yao and Martins, 2020]. Table 21.4 comprises transplants in drug delivery systems.

TABLE 21.4
Transplants and Drug Delivery System

Sl. No	Author and Year	Drug	Delivery Approach	Application
1	Deng et al. [2021]	FK506	PLGA – nanoparticles	Immunosuppressive treatments
2	Wu et al. [2021]	Tacrolimus	Thermosensitive polyester hydrogel	Immunosuppressive treatments
3	Wang et al. [2020]	Tacrolimus (FK506), mycophenolate mofetil (MMF), and prednisolone	PLGA – microspheres	In vascularized composite allotransplantation, long-term immunological rejection prevention
4	Lin et al. [2019]	Tacrolimus	Polypeptide thermosensitive hydrogel	Immunosuppressive therapy
5	Dzhonova et al. [2018]	Tacrolimus	Inflammation responsive hydrogel	Impact on immunology, toxicology, and long-term graft survival

21.7 CONCLUSION

Technological advancement in the design and sensing efficiency in combination with research in drug delivery systems will go a long way toward better diagnosis and treatment, thereby ensuring good patient compliance. Various approaches like bioMEMS and biomechanics offer superior therapeutic activity and are a proficient approach. However, proper selection of biomarkers remains a vital key for designing any responsive drug delivery systems.

REFERENCE

Akolpoglu, M. B., Bozuyuk, U., Erkoc, P., & Kizilel, S. (2019). Biosensing–Drug Delivery Systems for In Vivo Applications. In *Advanced biosensors for health care applications.* Elsevier Inc. https://doi.org/10.1016/b978-0-12-815743-5.00009-3

Andhari, S. S., Wavhale, R. D., Dhobale, K. D., Tawade, B. V., Chate, G. P., Patil, Y. N., Khandare, J. J., & Banerjee, S. S. (2020). Self-propelling targeted magneto-nanobots for deep tumor penetration and pH-responsive intracellular drug delivery. *Scientific Reports, 10* (1), 1–16. https://doi.org/10.1038/s41598-020-61586-y

Anggelia, M. R., Huang, R. W., Cheng, H. Y., Lin, C. H., & Lin, C. H. (2022). Implantable immunosuppressant delivery to prevent rejection in transplantation. *International Journal of Molecular Sciences, 23* (3). https://doi.org/10.3390/ijms23031592

Deng, C., Jin, Q., Wu, Y., Li, H., Yi, L., Chen, Y., Gao, T., Wang, W., Wang, J., Lv, Q., Yang, Y., Xu, J., Fu, W., Zhang, L., & Xie, M. (2021). Immunosuppressive effect of PLGA-FK506-NPs in treatment of acute cardiac rejection via topical subcutaneous injection. *Drug Delivery, 28* (1), 1759–1768. https://doi.org/10.1080/10717544.2021.1968978

Dong, L., Li, Y., Li, Z., Xu, N., Liu, P., Du, H., Zhang, Y., Huang, Y., Zhu, J., Ren, G., Xie, J., Wang, K., Zhou, Y., Shen, C., Zhu, J., & Tao, J. (2018). Au nanocage-strengthened dissolving microneedles for chemo-photothermal combined therapy of superficial skin tumors. *ACS Applied Materials and Interfaces, 10* (11), 9247–9256. https://doi.org/10.1021/acsami.7b18293

Dzhonova, D. V., Olariu, R., Leckenby, J., Banz, Y., Prost, J. C., Dhayani, A., Vemula, P. K., Voegelin, E., Taddeo, A., & Rieben, R. (2018). Local injections of tacrolimus-loaded hydrogel reduce systemic immunosuppression-related toxicity in vascularized composite allotransplantation. *Transplantation, 102* (10), 1684–1694. https://doi.org/10.1097/TP.0000000000002283

Fu, Y., Liu, P., Chen, M., Jin, T., Wu, H., Hei, M., Wang, C., Xu, Y., Qian, X., & Zhu, W. (2022). On-demand transdermal insulin delivery system for type 1 diabetes therapy with no hypoglycemia risks. *Journal of Colloid and Interface Science, 605,* 582–591. https://doi.org/10.1016/j.jcis.2021.07.126

Goldwirt, L., Canney, M., Horodyckid, C., Poupon, J., Mourah, S., Vignot, A., Chapelon, J. Y., & Carpentier, A. (2016). Enhanced brain distribution of carboplatin in a primate model after blood-brain barrier disruption using an implantable ultrasound device. *Cancer Chemotherapy and Pharmacology, 77* (1), 211–216. https://doi.org/10.1007/s00280-015-2930-5

Hancock, S. E., Wan, C. R., Fisher, N. E., Andino, R. V., & Ciulla, T. A. (2021). Biomechanics of suprachoroidal drug delivery: From benchtop to clinical investigation in ocular therapies. *Expert Opinion on Drug Delivery, 18* (6), 777–788. https://doi.org/10.1080/17425247.2021.1867532

Hardy, J. G., Larrañeta, E., Donnelly, R. F., McGoldrick, N., Migalska, K., McCrudden, M. T. C., Irwin, N. J., Donnelly, L., & McCoy, C. P. (2016). Hydrogel-forming microneedle arrays made from light-responsive materials for on-demand transdermal drug delivery. *Molecular Pharmaceutics*, *13* (3), 907–914. https://doi.org/10.1021/acs.molpharmaceut.5b00807

Hu, M., Ge, X., Chen, X., Mao, W., Qian, X., & Yuan, W. E. (2020). Micro/nanorobot: A promising targeted drug delivery system. *Pharmaceutics*, *12* (7), 1–18. https://doi.org/10.3390/pharmaceutics12070665

Kikuchi, K., Matsuki, N., & Shimogonya, Y. (2018). Biomechanics for Pathology and Treatment. In Yamaguchi, T., Ishikawa, T., and Imai, Y., editors. *Integrated nanobiomechanics*. Boston: Elsevier; 101–146. https://doi.org/10.1016/b978-0-323-38944-0.00004-8

Lee, H., Choi, T. K., Lee, Y. B., Cho, H. R., Ghaffari, R., Wang, L., Choi, H. J., Chung, T. D., Lu, N., Hyeon, T., Choi, S. H., & Kim, D. H. (2016). A graphene-based electrochemical device with thermoresponsive microneedles for diabetes monitoring and therapy. *Nature Nanotechnology*, *11* (6), 566–572. https://doi.org/10.1038/nnano.2016.38

Lee, H. J., Choi, N., Yoon, E. S., & Cho, I. J. (2018). MEMS devices for drug delivery. *Advanced Drug Delivery Reviews*, *128*, 132–147. https://doi.org/10.1016/j.addr.2017.11.003

Lee, S. H., Piao, H., Cho, Y. C., Kim, S. N., Choi, G., Kim, C. R., Ji, H. B., Park, C. G., Lee, C., Shin, C. I., Koh, W. G., Choy, Y. B., & Choy, J. H. (2019). Implantable multireservoir device with stimulus-responsive membrane for on-demand and pulsatile delivery of growth hormone. *Proceedings of the National Academy of Sciences of the United States of America*, *116* (24), 11664–11672. https://doi.org/10.1073/pnas.1906931116

Li, J., Dekanovsky, L., Khezri, B., Wu, B., Zhou, H., & Sofer, Z. (2022). Biohybrid micro- and nanorobots for intelligent drug delivery. *Cyborg and Bionic Systems*, *2022*, 1–13. https://doi.org/10.34133/2022/9824057

Li, S., Jiang, Q., Liu, S., Zhang, Y., Tian, Y., Song, C., Wang, J., Zou, Y., Anderson, G. J., Han, J. Y., Chang, Y., Liu, Y., Zhang, C., Chen, L., Zhou, G., Nie, G., Yan, H., Ding, B., & Zhao, Y. (2018). A DNA nanorobot functions as a cancer therapeutic in response to a molecular trigger in vivo. *Nature Biotechnology*, *36* (3), 258–264. https://doi.org/10.1038/nbt.4071

Lin, C. H., Anggelia, M. R., Cheng, H. Y., Wen, C. J., & Wang, A. Y. L. (2019). A mixed thermosensitive hydrogel system for sustained delivery of tacrolimus for immunosuppressive therapy. *Pharmaceutics*, *11* (8). https://doi.org/10.3390/pharmaceutics11080413

Liu, S., Jiang, Q., Zhao, X., Zhao, R., Wang, Y., Wang, Y., Liu, J., Shang, Y., Zhao, S., Wu, T., Zhang, Y., Nie, G., & Ding, B. (2021). A DNA nanodevice-based vaccine for cancer immunotherapy. *Nature Materials*, *20* (3), 421–430. https://doi.org/10.1038/s41563-020-0793-6

Liu, Z., Nie, J., Miao, B., Li, J., Cui, Y., Wang, S., Zhang, X., Zhao, G., Deng, Y., Wu, Y., Li, Z., Li, L., & Wang, Z. L. (2019). Self-powered intracellular drug delivery by a biomechanical energy-driven triboelectric nanogenerator. *Advanced Materials*, *31* (12), 1–8. https://doi.org/10.1002/adma.201807795

Liu, D., Zhang, Y., Jiang, G., Yu, W., Xu, B., & Zhu, J. (2018). Fabrication of dissolving microneedles with thermal-responsive coating for NIR-triggered transdermal delivery of metformin on diabetic rats. *ACS Biomaterials Science and Engineering*, *4* (5), 1687–1695. https://doi.org/10.1021/acsbiomaterials.8b00159

Mir, M., Permana, A. D., Ahmed, N., Khan, G. M., Rehman, A. ur, & Donnelly, R. F. (2020). Enhancement in site-specific delivery of carvacrol for potential treatment of infected wounds using infection responsive nanoparticles loaded into dissolving microneedles: A proof of concept study. *European Journal of Pharmaceutics and Biopharmaceutics*, *147*, 57–68. https://doi.org/10.1016/j.ejpb.2019.12.008

Ngoepe, M., Choonara, Y. E., Tyagi, C., Tomar, L. K., du Toit, L. C., Kumar, P., Ndesendo, V. M. K., & Pillay, V. (2013). Integration of biosensors and drug delivery technologies for early detection and chronic management of illness. *Sensors (Switzerland), 13* (6), 7680–7713. https://doi.org/10.3390/s130607680

Nguyen, V. D., Min, H. K., Kim, H. Y., Han, J., Choi, Y. H., Kim, C. S., Park, J. O., & Choi, E. (2021). Primary macrophage-based microrobots: An effective tumor therapy in vivo by dual-targeting function and near-infrared-triggered drug release. *ACS Nano, 15* (5), 8492–8506. https://doi.org/10.1021/acsnano.1c00114

Tietjen, G. T., Hosgood, S. A., DiRito, J., Cui, J., Deep, D., Song, E., Kraehling, J. R., Piotrowski-Daspit, A. S., Kirkiles-Smith, N. C., Al-Lamki, R., Thiru, S., Bradley, J. A., Saeb-Parsy, K., Bradley, J. R., Nicholson, M. L., Saltzman, W. M., & Pober, J. S. (2017). Nanoparticle targeting to the endothelium during normothermic machine perfusion of human kidneys. *Science Translational Medicine, 9* (418). https://doi.org/10.1126/scitranslmed.aam6764

Villarruel Mendoza, L. A., Scilletta, N. A., Bellino, M. G., Desimone, M. F., & Catalano, P. N. (2020). Recent advances in micro-electro-mechanical devices for controlled drug release applications. *Frontiers in Bioengineering and Biotechnology, 8* (July 29), 1–28. https://doi.org/10.3389/fbioe.2020.00827

Wang, S., Xiong, Y., Wang, Y., Chen, J., Yang, J., & Sun, B. (2020). Evaluation of PLGA microspheres with triple regimen on long-term survival of vascularized composite allograft–an experimental study. *Transplant International, 33* (4), 450–461. https://doi.org/10.1111/tri.13574

Wu, I. E., Anggelia, M. R., Lin, S. Y., Chen, C. Y., Chu, I. M., & Lin, C. H. (2021). Thermosensitive polyester hydrogel for application of immunosuppressive drug delivery system in skin allograft. *Gels, 7* (4). https://doi.org/10.3390/gels7040229

Wu, W., Mitra, N., Yan, E. C. Y., & Zhou, S. (2010). Multifunctional hybrid nanogel for integration of optical glucose sensing and self-regulated insulin release at physiological pH. *ACS Nano, 4* (8), 4831–4839. https://doi.org/10.1021/nn1008319

Xie, X., Zhang, L., Zhang, W., Tayebee, R., Hoseininasr, A., Vatanpour, H. H., Behjati, Z., Li, S., Nasrabadi, M., & Liu, L. (2020). Fabrication of temperature and pH sensitive decorated magnetic nanoparticles as effective biosensors for targeted delivery of acyclovir anti-cancer drug. *Journal of Molecular Liquids, 309*, 113024. https://doi.org/10.1016/j.molliq.2020.113024

Xu, H., Medina-Sánchez, M., Magdanz, V., Schwarz, L., Hebenstreit, F., & Schmidt, O. G. (2018). Sperm-hybrid micromotor for targeted drug delivery. *ACS Nano, 12* (1), 327–337. https://doi.org/10.1021/acsnano.7b06398

Yan, J., Chen, J., Zhang, N., Yang, Y., Zhu, W., Li, L., & He, B. (2020). Mitochondria-targeted tetrahedral DNA nanostructures for doxorubicin delivery and enhancement of apoptosis. *Journal of Materials Chemistry B, 8* (3), 492–503. https://doi.org/10.1039/c9tb02266j

Yao, C. G., & Martins, P. N. (2020). Nanotechnology applications in transplantation medicine. *Transplantation, 104* (4). https://doi.org/10.1097/TP.0000000000003032

Yazdi, M. K., Zarrintaj, P., Bagheri, B., Kim, Y. C., Ganjali, M. R., & Saeb, M. R. (2020). Nanotechnology-based biosensors in drug delivery. In *Nanoengineered biomaterials for advanced drug delivery*. Elsevier Ltd. https://doi.org/10.1016/B978-0-08-102985-5.00032-2

Yu, J., Wang, J., Zhang, Y., Chen, G., Mao, W., Ye, Y., Kahkoska, A. R., Buse, J. B., Langer, R., & Gu, Z. (2020). Glucose-responsive insulin patch for the regulation of blood glucose in mice and minipigs. *Nature Biomedical Engineering, 4* (5), 499–506. https://doi.org/10.1038/s41551-019-0508-y

Yu, S., Zhang, X., Tan, G., Tian, L., Liu, D., Liu, Y., Yang, X., & Pan, W. (2017). A novel pH-induced thermosensitive hydrogel composed of carboxymethyl chitosan and poloxamer cross-linked by glutaraldehyde for ophthalmic drug delivery. *Carbohydrate Polymers, 155*, 208–217. https://doi.org/10.1016/j.carbpol.2016.08.073

Zhang, Y., Chai, D., Gao, M., Xu, B., & Jiang, G. (2018). Thermal ablation of separable microneedles for transdermal delivery of metformin on diabetic rats. *International Journal of Polymeric Materials and Polymeric Biomaterials*, *68* (14), 850–858. https://doi.org/10.1080/00914037.2018.1517347

Zhang, J., Guo, Y., Ding, F., Pan, G., Zhu, X., & Zhang, C. (2019). A camptothecin-grafted DNA tetrahedron as a precise nanomedicine to inhibit tumor growth. *Angewandte Chemie – International Edition*, *58* (39), 13794–13798. https://doi.org/10.1002/anie.201907380

22 Automatic Liver and Lesion Segmentation in CT Using 3-D Context Convolutional Neural Network: 3-D Context U-Net

Lida Daryani Ghazani and M. A. Balafar
Department of Software Engineering, Faculty of Electrical and Computer Engineering, University of Tabriz, Tabriz, Iran

CONTENTS

22.1 INTRODUCTION

Because of the liver tissue, it is difficult and important to diagnose liver diseases. Liver and liver lesions segmentation in medical images with precise automated methods are prerequisites for computer-aided diagnostic systems (CADx). In the liver tissue, benign and malignant tumors are difficult to distinguish because of low contrast. Hence, researchers are trying to provide methods for a more accurate diagnosis. Therefore, challenges to increase the accuracy of liver segmentation have been conducted since 2007 [1, 2]. In the case of segmentation, many image processing methods have been used. Meanwhile, thresholding is a simple but effective tool used for liver segmentation and liver lesions [3, 4]. In recent research, the region-based method has also been used [5, 6]. Yan et al. segmented liver metastases in contrast-enhanced computed tomography (CECT) images based on the watering method [7]. The active cantour method was used in a similar study for lung segmentation [8]. Recent work on medical image segmentation also employs graph-based techniques [9, 10].

However, these methods have low speed and low robustness, so they are not suitable for 3-D and large images. In addition, automatic methods rather than inter-active methods are more suitable for use in clinics. Other methods such as K-means clustering and random subspace method are used in this field of study [11–13].

In this field, deep neural networks provide automated models with more reliable results at higher speeds. The convolutional neural network (CNN) is one of the deep neural networks used in image segmentation, which is used in [14, 15]. The fully convolutional network (FCN) also has attracted the attention of researchers for their abilities [16, 17].

In 2015, Ronneberger et al. [18] introduced an architecture of convolutional neural networks that called U-Net. This network provides a satisfactory end-to-end result with a low train set, so it is very useful in medical images segmentation, as medical images labeling is cost intensive and time consuming. This architecture is made of a contracting path to catch context and a symmetric expanding path to achieve accurate localization.

Using the UNet architecture, an accurate pixel prediction algorithm has been designed by combining spatial and contextual information. It consists of the frequent use of two 3 × 3 convolutions (unpadded convolutions), each performed by a modified linear unit (ReLU), and a 2 × 2 max merge operation with a second step for downsampling. In the expansive path, each step consists of an upsampling of the feature map that is followed by a 2 × 2 convolution ("up-convolution") that reduces the number of feature channels by half, a concatenation with a feature map cut from the contraction path, and two 3 × 3 convolutions, each followed by a ReLU.

In the field of liver segmentation, new methods are mostly based on deep neural networks, and the architecture of the U-Net has been most used. There are several advantages of using U-Net with a cascaded framework for segmentation of hierarchical structures [19]. In another research study, Liu et al. [20] used U-Net for liver segmentation and then improved the network output by the graph cutting method.

The difference between lesions and non-lesions in the liver is difficult. In this case, 3D context information can be useful and extract more local features. Convulsion neural networks are often made for two-dimensional input images, but with a slight change in the CNN network, 3D context information given as input, and network extraction capabilities increase. Yan et al. [21] proposed a context-based 3D region-based CNN (3DCE) to efficiently combine 3D context information by collecting feature maps from 2D images.

Han et al. [22] propose 2.5-D perpendicular UNet to combine the segmentation results of three perpendicular 2.5-D Res-UNets for the task of liver and hepatic tumor segmentation.

In [23], Yang and Wu present an efficient 3-D U-Net equipped with ResNet architecture and a two-way deep monitoring method to increase the capacity of the network to learn a richer representation of lung tumors from global and local points of view. In [24], Chi and Zhang propose a multi-input-directional UNet (MID-UNet) for segmentation of COVID-19 putridity in lung CT images.

In this chapter, we provide an automatic segmentation of the liver and liver lesions in high-contrast CT abdominal images using deep learning and image processing. The deep learning network presented in this study is based on the well-known U-Net convolutional neural network powered by the 3-D context information.

22.2   THE PROPOSED METHOD

For liver segmentation, a neural network based on U-Net architecture is proposed in this chapter. In addition, images are preprocessed in a variety of ways before they start learning by model. To improve the quality of the learning process, we used the data augmentation. Finally, the threshold is applied to improve the output image. This chapter presents the following three main steps:

- At this point, preprocessing and data augmentation are performed on images in the dataset.
- The learning model is performed using deep convolutional neural network architecture to identify and segment the liver and its lesions.
- To measure the output with defined criteria, a threshold method is applied to the output of the second step.

22.2.1   DATASET

In this research, the 3D-IRCADb-01 [25] dataset was used. The dataset consists of three-dimensional high-contrast CT abdominal images of the venous phase. In the dataset, the liver, liver lesions, heart, lung, kidneys, skin, esophagus, spinal column, spleen, pancreas, and bone have been segmented and labeled, but we have only used the ground truth of liver and liver lesions.

We have defined three labels 0, 1, and 2. The value of 0 as the foreground, the value of 1 as the healthy tissue of the liver, and the value of 2 as liver lesions (tumors, cysts, and metastases) are considered.

22.2.2   DATA PREPROCESSING AND DATA AUGMENTATION

In this step, existing data are adapted for usability in the model. Also, to reduce computational costs, the collected data should be checked to eliminate inappropriate, irrelevant, and ineffective data but not to reduce the generality of the data. And there must be different data in different test conditions since in this case, the model will have more generalizability. Therefore, we use data augmentation. For this case, we used normalization, adjusting the brightness and contrast of the image, adding

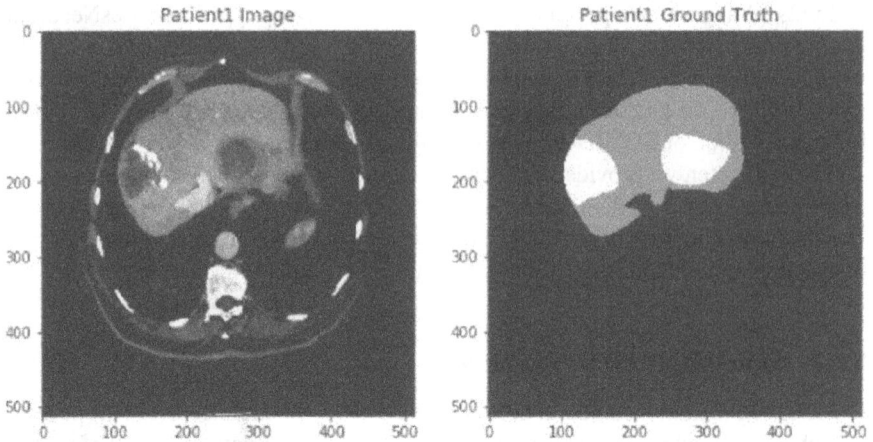

FIGURE 22.1 The first step is for data augmentation of overlapping areas. The image on the left is the image of the CT scan of the first patient, and the image on the right is the label of the liver and its liver tumors.

noise and elastic deformation, adding data overlapping regions, and including liver segmentation using image processing [26–29].

The described methods are almost common, but it is best to review the overlapping area data addition method used in this research. Two slices are taken from two patients, and a part of their liver tissue or liver lesion is replaced together. If the liver lesion area of the first image overlaps the liver lesion area of the second image, the overlapped part of the first image is replaced by the pixels of the second image in the overlapped part.

This method has also been used for healthy liver tissue in the slices where there is no lesion, which means that the liver tissue of the first patient has been replaced with the tissue of the second patient. It should be noted that the liver tissue of the first patient should completely overlap with the liver of the second patient. In this case, the entire tissue of the patient's liver will be replaced. This method can be used in slices where the size of the liver in the first patient is small. In this research, we have used this method to increase data. The result of this type of data addition can be seen in Figures 22.1–22.3.

22.2.3 CREATING 3-D CONTEXT INFORMATION

The 3-D context information includes a slice of CT images that are concatenated with two neighboring slices. As a result, a three-channel image is formed, each channel containing a 2-D slice of the CT image. If the input slice is S, the image created will be $[S_{i-1}, S_i, S_{i+1}]$. This is a prerequisite for the proposed deep neural network. The ground truth will not change. Considering the purpose of the proposed deep neural network, if the ground truth of the slice S is G, for 3-D context information with the input $[S_{i-1}, S_i, S_{i+1}]$, we will have G_i.

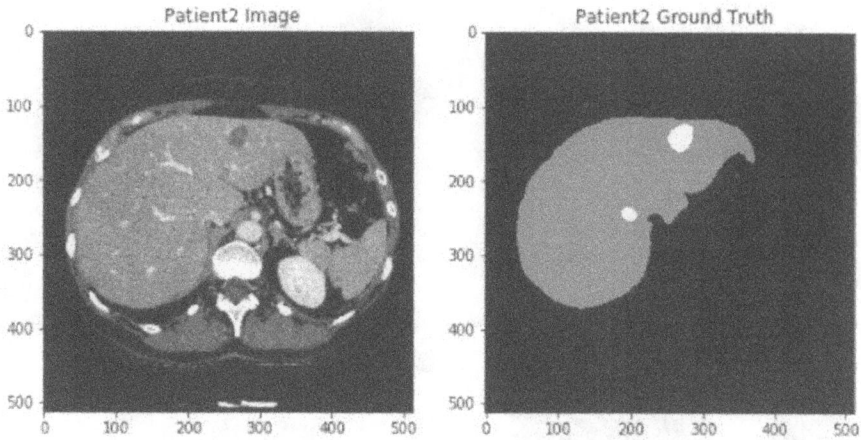

FIGURE 22.2 The second step is for data augmentation of overlapping areas. The image on the left is the image of the CT scan of the second patient, and the image on the right is the label of the liver and its liver tumors.

22.2.4 THE PROPOSED NETWORK (3-D CONTEXT U-NET)

As stated in the introduction, the basis of the proposed network is the use of U-Net architecture, and given the kind of problem that targets medical images, and given that the CT scan image is stored as a set of slices, then new features can be extracted from slices as new local features, because each pixel is associated with the pixels in the same position in neighboring slices.

In this proposed approach, the network is fed with 3-D context information. There are three subnets in the proposed network, each subset of which is a U-Net, called sub U-Net. Each sub U-Net takes a slice from the 3-D context input and gives a feature map as output, each of the three feature maps combines, and then a convolution layer is applied on them to create the final output. The proposed network is shown in Figure 22.4.

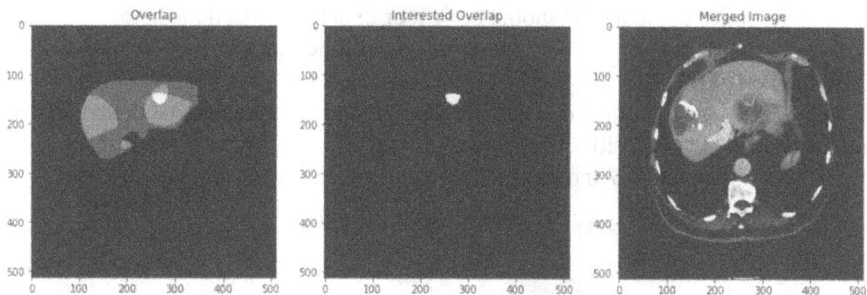

FIGURE 22.3 The third step is for data augmentation of overlapping areas. The image on the left side shows the overlap of the tumor of the second patient on the liver and the tumors of the first patient. The middle image is the sharing of the tumor of the first patient.

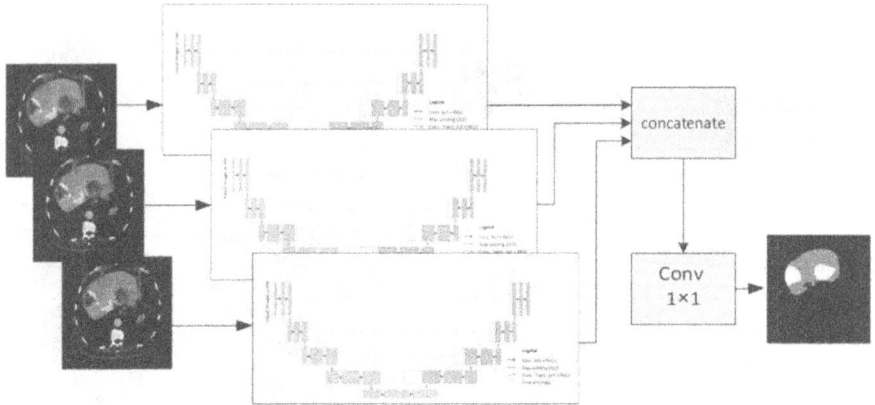

FIGURE 22.4 Proposed network structure (3-D context U-Net).

It is noteworthy that sub U-Nets used in this architecture do not have the final
1×1 convolutional layer. Also, after each convolution layer, the batch normalization method is used. An advantage of this method is that it can increase the speed of the network [30] because the proposed network is three times larger than the basic method and its use is beneficial in this step.

The network input is a tensor of [1, 3, 512, 512], which is 3-D context information, each dimension of which is a slice of the gray level of the CT scan image. Each dimension of the entry matrix enters a subnet, each subnet creates a features map.

By combining these three maps, new features will be created that will make the final output more accurate. After combining the three feature maps, a 1×1 convolutional layer is applied, and the final output is a matrix equal to [1, 3, 512, 512]. The three values in the output matrix means having three categories. In each dimension of this output, there is an existing segmental image that belongs to one of the categories. Dimensions of the matrix belong to the foreground, liver, and liver lesions, respectively.

The output of the U-Net network and as a result the output of the proposed networks are transferable with a uniform distribution. For the output with a correct map, the segmentation sections with the defined criteria must be the same. It means that the output image of the model should be 0, 1, or 2. In the works done before, methods have been done for this purpose, and the sigmoid function is one of the most widely used methods.

Sigmoid is a real, bounded, and differentiable function that can be defined for all real values and has a positive derivative. Graphically, this function has a shape similar to the English letter S and has the following general relationship Equation (22.1):

$$S_{(t)} = \frac{1}{1 + e^{-t}} \tag{22.1}$$

This function receives input values in the range of real numbers and produces an output value between 1 and 0 based on the preceding formula. But using this method reduces the accuracy of the output to some extent. At this stage, the use of a threshold-setting method is suggested to find the best threshold to improve the accuracy of the output.

In this research, instead of using the sigmoid function, we have used a thresholding method that we call the dynamic thresholding method, because this method searches for the best threshold in the range of network output image values, and the result is the selection of the thresholding value with the best value for the Dice criterion. This search is performed by a loop, and the lower limit and upper limit for the search are the range of network output image values. In each step of the loop iteration, one step is added to the current threshold, and the best result of the previous steps is benchmarked with the new threshold. In each iteration, it is checked whether the Dice value is better than the previous values. At the end of the loop, the best threshold is introduced. The output of the network is approached by the obtained threshold.

22.2.5 Dice Coefficient

To measure the effectiveness of the proposed model to improve the segmentation accuracy of liver tumors, the Dice score coefficient error criterion from Equation (22.2) has been used:

$$DSC = 2 * \frac{|A \cap B|}{|A| + |B|} \tag{22.2}$$

A and B in Equation (22.2) are two sets. This measure determines the overlap of the segmented region with the correct segmentation map. This method has been used a lot in natural sciences. The range of this evaluation criterion is between 0 and 1, and the best result is determined by a value of 1.

22.2.6 Specifications of the Proposed Model

Table 22.1 presents the specification of the U-Net subnet, which is derived from the U-Net architecture, from which the last convolutional layer has been removed. The specifications and details of the proposed model (3-D-Context U-Net) are also listed in Table 22.2. It should be noted that the layers introduced in Tables 22.1 and 22.2 are executed from top to bottom respectively.

22.2.7 Select the Optimizer Function

To choose a suitable optimizer function, 3-D-Context U-Net network with several different optimizer functions, including the following.

We have tested SGD, RMSProp, AraGrad, AraDelta, and Momentum in 100 training iterations. The results of this test show that the RMSProp function has a fast convergence compared to other functions to have a suitable Dice criterion.

In Figure 22.5, it can be seen how to train with different optimizer functions, whose vertical axis shows the average Dice evaluation criterion in each repetition of the training. In addition to the fast convergence in training, the results show that the RMSProp cost function performs better even in slices with very small liver size,

TABLE 22.1
Specifications of the U-Net Subnetwork

Layer	Output	Layer Type	Output Size
2D Slice	Input	Input	$1 \times 1 \times 512 \times 512$
inConv	X1	(conv 3×3, ReLU / conv 3×3, ReLU)	$1 \times 64 \times 512 \times 512$
Encoder1	X2	Max pool 2×2/ (conv 3×3, batchNorm, ReLU / conv 3×3, batchNorm, ReLU)	$1 \times 128 \times 256 \times 256$
Encoder2	X3	Max pool 2×2/ (conv 3×3, batchNorm, ReLU / conv 3×3, batchNorm, ReLU)	$1 \times 256 \times 128 \times 128$
Encoder3	X4	Max pool 2×2/ (conv 3×3, batchNorm, ReLU / conv 3×3, batchNorm, ReLU)	$1 \times 512 \times 64 \times 64$
Encoder4	X5	Max pool 2×2/ (conv 3×3, batchNorm, ReLU / conv 3×3, batchNorm, ReLU)	$1 \times 512 \times 32 \times 32$
Decoder1	X6	Cat ($\times4$, $\times5$)/ (conv 3×3, batchNorm, ReLU / conv 3×3, batchNorm, ReLU)	$1 \times 256 \times 64 \times 64$
Decoder2	X7	Cat ($\times3$, $\times6$)/ (conv 3×3, batchNorm, ReLU / conv 3×3, batchNorm, ReLU)	$1 \times 128 \times 128 \times 128$
Decoder3	X8	Cat ($\times2$, $\times7$)/ (conv 3×3, batchNorm, ReLU / conv 3×3, batchNorm, ReLU)	$1 \times 64 \times 256 \times 256$
Decoder4	X9	Cat ($\times1$, $\times8$)/ (conv 3×3, batchNorm, ReLU / conv 3×3, batchNorm, ReLU)	$1 \times 64 \times 512 \times 512$

and the detection network gives more accurate results than other functions in this condition. For this reason, a very significant difference can be seen in Figure 22.5.

22.2.8 THE EFFECT OF DATA AUGMENTATION

During the training of the proposed network and U-Net, we noticed that the network sometimes fluctuates in the early stages of training and abandons the decreasing trend of the cost function and finds an upward jump state.

By studying the causes of fluctuation during education, we realized the effect of data augmentation in improving the quality of education. In Figure 22.6, the

TABLE 22.2
Specifications of the 3-D-Context U-Net

Layer	Output	Layer Type	Output Size
3-D-Context image	Input	Input	$1 \times 3 \times 512 \times 512$
U-Net1	X1	SubU-Net	$1 \times 64 \times 512 \times 512$
U-Net2	X2	SubU-Net	$1 \times 64 \times 512 \times 512$
U-Net3	X3	SubU-Net	$1 \times 64 \times 512 \times 512$
concatenate	X	Cat ($\times1$, $\times2$, $\times3$)	$1 \times 192 \times 512 \times 512$
convOut	X	Conv 1×1	$1 \times 3 \times 512 \times 512$

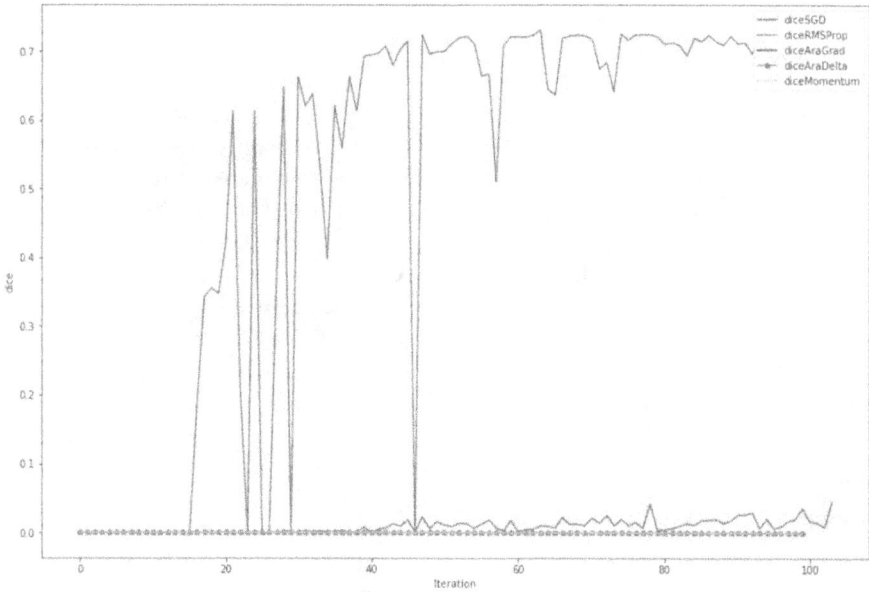

FIGURE 22.5   3-D-context U-Net network training with different optimizer functions.

comparison of two modes of training with data augmentation and without data augmentation can be seen in the number of 20 repetitions of training. In addition to the mentioned problem, in the learning of the proposed network, due to the repetition of three times the data in each repetition in the network, after performing an average of 50 repetitions, the training suffered from overfitting, which was partially resolved by increasing the data.

22.3   RESULTS AND DISCUSSION

To validate and evaluate the proposed network, we examine it with the U-Net network under the same conditions (the same parameters and hyperparameters). The number of training datasets is 17 CT scan images, equivalent to 2,405 2-D slices,

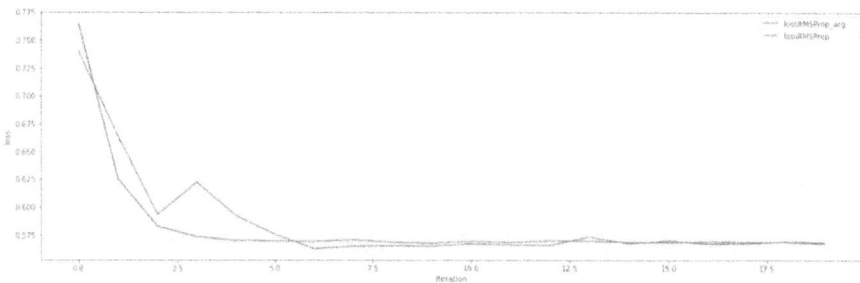

FIGURE 22.6   The effect of data augmentation in improving the quality of U-Net training. The red vector has data augmentation, and the green vector has no data augmentation.

and the number of validation datasets is three CT scan images, equivalent to 418 2-D slices. These values are independent of the number of images after data addition. The U-Net network outputs an image with a uniform distribution.

Normally, after training the proposed network, to evaluate the output with the defined criteria, the dynamic threshold method will be applied on the output of the network. Sigmoid function is used so that the image values are between 0 and 1. By using the dynamic threshold method, better results can be obtained than with the sigmoid function at this stage. The dynamic threshold method automatically searches for the threshold value, as described earlier.

The outputs of the U-Net network and the proposed network with the combination of the sigmoid function and dynamic thresholding with Dice, VOE, and RVD evaluation criteria are shown as an average in Tables 22.3–22.5. Also, in Figures 22.7–22.9, the output results with excellent, average, and bad standards are shown respectively.

TABLE 22.3
Comparison of the Results Obtained with the Dice Criterion

Method	Liver (Train)	Lesions (Train)	Liver (Test)	Lesions (Test)
U-Net + sigmoid	8293/0	4037/0	7413/0	0504/0
U-Net + thresholding	8369/0	4108/0	7818/0	0588/0
3-D-Context U-Net + sigmoid	9648/0	4263/0	8184/0	2403/0
3-D-Context U-Net + thresholding	9725/0	4341/0	8277/0	2480/0

TABLE 22.4
Comparison of the Results Obtained with the VOE Criterion

Method	Liver (Train)	Lesions (Train)	Liver (Test)	Lesions (Test)
U-Net + sigmoid	54/22	56/72	23/33	95/94
U-Net + thresholding	93/21	56/72	68/28	95/94
3-D-Context U-Net + sigmoid	96/5	85/65	65/23	96/75
3-D-Context U-Net + thresholding	78/5	41/63	06/20	96/75

TABLE 22.5
Comparison of the Results Obtained with the RVD Criterion

Method	Liver (Train)	Lesions (Train)	Liver (Test)	Lesions (Test)
U-Net + sigmoid	17/15	56/72	02/17	95/94
U-Net + thresholding	10/15	56/72	17/16	95/94
3-D-Context U-Net + sigmoid	81/1	85/65	54/11	96/75
3-D-Context U-Net + thresholding	78/1	41/63	15/11	96/75

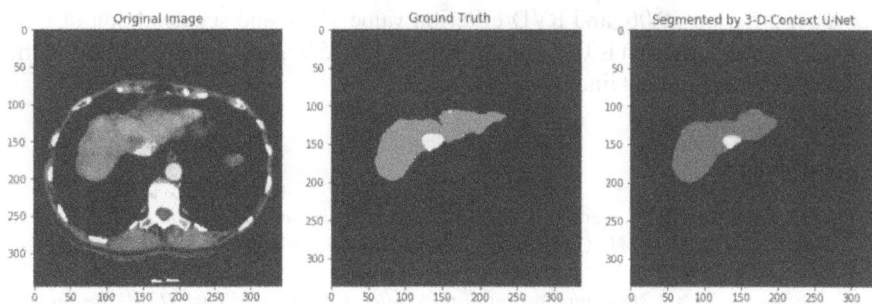

FIGURE 22.7   Excellent result.

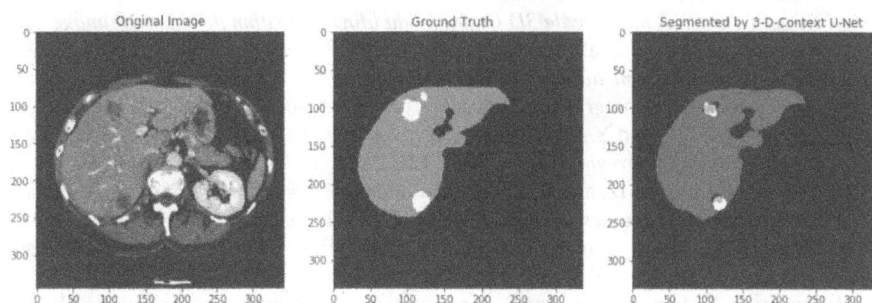

FIGURE 22.8   Average result.

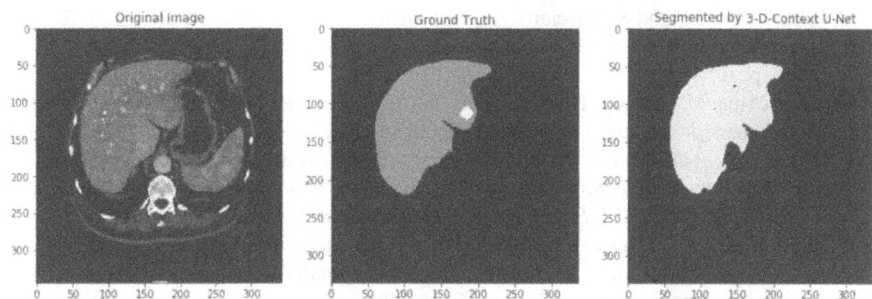

FIGURE 22.9   Bad result.

In the U-Net architecture, the input image is a two-dimensional slice of the CT scan image, and the output of gray-level images will be the number of problem categories. In this research, we present a convolutional neural network based on U-Net architecture using 3-D context information. The experimental results in this research show the effectiveness of the proposed method.

Three-dimensional context information improves final results by combining feature maps. Also, finding the best threshold to provide a two-state output (having values of 1 or 0) leads to better accuracy than using the sigmoid function. The average efficiency of the proposed method in liver segmentation for Dice criterion is 0.83, for VOE criterion 20.06, and RVD criterion value 11.15, and segmentation of liver lesions for Dice criterion is 0.25, for VOE criterion 75.96, and for RVD criterion the value 96/75 has been obtained.

REFERENCES

1. Van Ginneken, B., T. Heimann, and M. Styner, *3D segmentation in the clinic: A grand challenge*, 2007. In *MICCAI workshop on 3D segmentation in the clinic: A grand challenge* (Vol. 1, p. 7–15).
2. Styner, M., et al., *3D segmentation in the clinic: A grand challenge II–MS lesion segmentation*. MIDAS Journal, 2008. **2008**: p. 1–6.
3. Moltz, J.H., et al., *Segmentation of liver metastases in CT scans by adaptive thresholding and morphological processing*. In *MICCAI workshop*. 2008.
4. Feng, Y., et al., *A multi-scale 3D Otsu thresholding algorithm for medical image segmentation*. Digital Signal Processing, 2017. **60**: p. 186–199.
5. Zhou, Z., et al., *Semi-automatic liver segmentation in CT images through intensity separation and region growing*. Procedia Computer Science, 2018. **131**: p. 220–225.
6. Zhang, X., X. Li, and Y. Feng, *A medical image segmentation algorithm based on bi-directional region growing*. Optik, 2015. **126**(20): p. 2398–2404.
7. Yan, J., L.H. Schwartz, and B. Zhao, *Semiautomatic segmentation of liver metastases on volumetric CT images*. Medical Physics, 2015. **42**(11): p. 6283–6293.
8. Nithila, E.E., and S. Kumar, *Segmentation of lung from CT using various active contour models*. Biomedical Signal Processing and Control, 2019. **47**: p. 57–62.
9. Dogra, J., S. Jain, and M. Sood, *Segmentation of MR images using hybrid kMean-graph cut technique*. Procedia Computer Science, 2018. **132**: p. 775–784.
10. Huang, Q., et al., *Optimized graph-based segmentation for ultrasound images*. Neurocomputing, 2014. **129**: p. 216–224.
11. Massoptier, L., and S. Casciaro, *A new fully automatic and robust algorithm for fast segmentation of liver tissue and tumors from CT scans*. European Radiology, 2008. **18**(8): p. 1658.
12. Skurichina, M., and R.P. Duin, *Bagging, boosting and the random subspace method for linear classifiers*. Pattern Analysis & Applications, 2002. **5**(2): p. 121–135.
13. Huang, W., et al., *Random feature subspace ensemble based extreme learning machine for liver tumor detection and segmentation*. In *2014 36th Annual International Conference of the IEEE Engineering in Medicine and Biology Society*. 2014. IEEE.
14. Shin, H.-C., et al., *Deep convolutional neural networks for computer-aided detection: CNN architectures, dataset characteristics and transfer learning*. IEEE Transactions on Medical Imaging, 2016. **35**(5): p. 1285–1298.
15. Milletari, F., et al., *Hough-CNN: Deep learning for segmentation of deep brain regions in MRI and ultrasound*. Computer Vision and Image Understanding, 2017. **164**: p. 92–102.
16. Sun, C., et al., *Automatic segmentation of liver tumors from multiphase contrast-enhanced CT images based on FCNs*. Artificial Intelligence in Medicine, 2017. **83**: p. 58–66.
17. Krizhevsky, A., I. Sutskever, and G.E. Hinton, *Imagenet classification with deep convolutional neural networks*. Advances in Neural Information Processing Systems, 2012. **60**: p. 6.
18. Ronneberger, O., P. Fischer, and T. Brox, *U-Net: Convolutional networks for biomedical image segmentation*. In *International Conference on Medical Image Computing and Computer-Assisted Intervention*. 2015. Springer.
19. Christ, P.F., et al., *Automatic liver and lesion segmentation in CT using cascaded fully convolutional neural networks and 3D conditional random fields*. In *International Conference on Medical Image Computing and Computer-Assisted Intervention*. 2016. Springer.

20. Liu, Z., et al., *Liver CT sequence segmentation based with improved u-net and graph cut.* Expert Systems with Applications, 2019. **126**: p. 54–63.

21. Yan, K., M. Bagheri, and R.M. Summers, *3D context enhanced region-based convolutional neural network for end-to-end lesion detection.* In *International Conference on Medical Image Computing and Computer-Assisted Intervention.* 2018. Springer.

22. Han, L., et al., *Liver segmentation with 2.5D perpendicular UNets.* Computers and Electrical Engineering, 2021. **91**. https://doi.org/10.1016/j.compeleceng.2021.107118

23. Yang, J., and B. Wu, et al., *MSDS-UNet: A multi-scale deeply supervised 3D U-Net for automatic segmentation of lung tumor in CT.* Computerized Medical Imaging and Graphics, 2021. **92**: p. 101957.

24. Chi, J., and S. Zhang, et al., *MID-UNet: Multi-input directional UNet for COVID-19 lung infection segmentation from CT images.* Signal Processing: Image Communication, 2022. **108**: p. 116835.

25. Soler, L., et al., *3D Image reconstruction for comparison of algorithm database: A patient specific anatomical and medical image database.* IRCAD, Strasbourg, France, Tech. Rep, 2010.

26. Balafar, M.A., A.R. Ramli, and S. Mashohor, *Brain magnetic resonance image segmentation using novel improvement for expectation maximizing.* Neurosciences Journal, 2011. **16**(3): p. 242–247.

27. Balafar, M.A., *New spatial based MRI image de-noising algorithm.* Artificial Intelligence Review, 2013. **39**(3): p. 225–235.

28. Balafar, M.A., A.B.D. Rahman Ramli, M.I. Saripan, S. Mashohor, and R. Mahmud, *Medical image segmentation using fuzzy c-mean (FCM) and user specified data.* Journal of Circuits, Systems, and Computers, 2010. **19**(1): p. 1–14.

29. Balafar, M.A., A.B.D.R. Ramli, M.I. Saripan, and S. Mashohor, *Improved fast fuzzy C-mean and its application in medical image segmentation.* Journal of Circuits, Systems, and Computers, 2010. **19**(1): p. 203–214.

30. Ioffe, S., and C. Szegedy, *Batch normalization: Accelerating deep network training by reducing internal covariate shift.* arXiv preprint arXiv:1502.03167, 2015.

Index

For Product Safety Concerns and Information please contact our EU
representative GPSR@taylorandfrancis.com
Taylor & Francis Verlag GmbH, Kaufingerstraße 24, 80331 München, Germany

www.ingramcontent.com/pod-product-compliance
Lightning Source LLC
Chambersburg PA
CBHW060750220326
41598CB00022B/2390

* 9 7 8 1 0 3 2 3 4 9 1 5 2 *